PRAISE FOR
The Black Women's Health Book

"In a variety of ways the contributors redefine the notion of health . . . they affirm the need to heal the body and the spirit."
—*Women's Review of Books*

"This wonderful compendium of articles by black women is a must-buy reference for any library . . . Highly recommended."
—*Library Journal*

"Not only does it speak on health, it speaks to the heart; it is a fine piece of literature for the soul. The experiences it contains speak to all humanity."
—*Sojourner*

"*The Black Women's Health Book* breaks the silence, bursts the taboos, and mends many hearts along the way."
—*The San Francisco Chronicle*

"Through *The Black Women's Health Book,* women will begin to see they are not alone."
—*Emerge*

"This book makes a valuable contribution in an area where there are conspicuous gaps in our knowledge."
—*Women & Therapy*

"[The contributors] offer a compelling assortment of historical data, health statistics and information, gritty 'womanist' advice, and inventive strategies for turning the tide on the downward spiral of Black women's health."
—*Belles Lettres*

"Educators, administrators, health activists of all racial, ethnic groups and genders will find this essential reading."
—*New Directions for Women*

THE BLACK WOMEN'S HEALTH BOOK

SPEAKING FOR OURSELVES

EDITED BY EVELYN C. WHITE

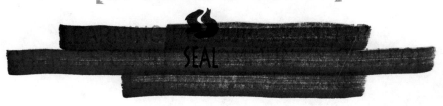

Publication and distribution of this book was made possible in part with support from The L.J. Skaggs and Mary C. Skaggs Foundation, The Open Meadows Foundation and The Henry J. Kaiser Family Foundation.

Cover design by Kris Morgan
Text design by Clare Conrad

Library of Congress Cataloging-in-Publication Data

The Black women's health book : speaking for ourselves / edited by
   Evelyn C. White
      p.   cm.
      Reissued with eleven new essays. Previously published: 1990.
      Includes bibliographical references.
      ISBN 1-878067-40-0
      1. Afro-American women—Health and hygiene. 2. Afro-American
   women—Medical care. 3. Afro-American women—Mental health.
   I. White, Evelyn C. 1954–
   RA778.B645   1994
   613'.0424'08996073—dc20   93-28901
                                                                    CIP

Printed in the United States of America

10 9 8 7 6 5 4 3 2

Distributed to the trade by Publishers Group West
Foreign Distribution:
In Canada: Publishers Group West Canada, Montreal West, Quebec
In the U.K. and Europe: Airlift Book Company, London, England

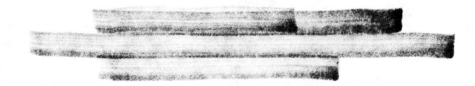

Editor's Acknowledgements

Many people helped me during the three years it took to compile and edit this collection. First of all, I give heartfelt thanks to the nearly forty contributors who all took time from their busy lives to bring words of solace and support to black women.

For their kind acts and encouraging comments that always lifted my spirits, I wish to thank: Judith Barrington, Laura Brown, Diane Bryant, Gwen Carmen, Leah Garchik, Roberta Goodman, Gladys Griffin, Ruth Gundle, Elaine Herscher, Lisa Keller, M.D., Elaine Lee, Fran Miller, Fran Staton, Ann Trauner, and Alice Walker.

I am exceedingly grateful to *San Francisco Chronicle* librarian Kathleen Rhodes, who provided invaluable research assistance. *Chronicle* city editor Daniel Rosenheim and special projects editor Judy Miller also supported this effort.

For their generous financial contributions, I wish to thank the Henry J. Kaiser Family Foundation, the Open Meadows Foundation, Inc. and the L. J. Skaggs and Mary C. Skaggs Foundation.

The women of Seal Press, especially publishers Faith Conlon and Barbara Wilson, again demonstrated their commitment to the ideals of the feminist movement by supporting this book every step of the way. As my editor, Faith provided honest and skilled direction that uplifted my soul and improved this book considerably.

Lastly, I thank Catherine A. S. Lyons for her love, patience and understanding as I worked on this project. She encouraged and enabled me to give my best to black women, which is, after all, exactly what we deserve.

To the memory of my parents
Amanda Cantrell White
and
Andrew Saja White

Contents

THREE: CLIMBING HIGHER MOUNTAINS

FOUR: ROCKA MY SOUL

FIVE: SOON AND VERY SOON

Introduction

The photograph that gave birth to this book hangs like a talisman on the wall of my study. It is a newspaper photo of an elderly black woman weeping over her dead daughter, who lies splayed like a Raggedy Ann doll on a grimy Chicago street.

At first glance, the photo does not seem any different than the thousands of others that have captured the demise of African-Americans in our cities. It is an image of blacks that makes most viewers ponder, usually with apathy: Drug overdose? Sex crime? Murder?

Under the photo, a terse caption reveals the truth about the twenty-six-year-old black woman's death. Afflicted with a serious coronary problem, the woman died of a heart attack after rescuing her mother and toddler children from the third story of a burning building.

For me, this photo has become a symbol for the scores of physically and emotionally scarred black women who have died before the severity of their wounds could be recognized or treated. In the tragic photo, I see the faces of singer Esther Phillips, vanquished by alcoholism at age forty-six; Chicago journalist Leanita McClain, a suicide victim at thirty-two; Olympic volleyball champion Flo Hyman, felled by Marfan's disease at thirty-one; playwright Lorraine Hansberry, silenced by cancer at thirty-four; actress Dorothy Dandridge, dead at forty-one of an overdose of Tofranil, a drug used to treat psychiatric depression.

The images of black women without such public personas are as compelling as the famous faces the photo evokes. For every well-known black woman whose death has been noted and marked, there are countless other black women who have died in the shadows. These are the black women in our neighborhoods and communities who suffer in silence from AIDS, hypertension, diabetes or domestic violence. They are the black women who die without anyone ever asking why death came to call so soon.

The Black Women's Health Book: Speaking For Ourselves is an effort to make the photo on my wall less haunting, less foreboding and less of a reality for black women. It is a book that has been propelled by words written in 1827 by the founders of America's first black newspaper, *Freedom's Journal:* "We wish to plead our own cause. Too long have others spoken for us."

This book is also a direct response to an alarming health crisis in the African-American community. Over the past few years, I have observed a growing number of vibrant black women being devastated by a multitude of physical and emotional ailments, ranging from drug addiction to cancer. Ironically, this downward trend has occurred at a time when this country has developed state-of-the-art medical technology that is envied around the world.

Without a sound body and mind, it is impossible for black women to attain personal goals or to provide the leadership our community needs as we approach the twenty-first century. For generations, we have taken care of everything and everyone but ourselves. Now is the time for us to put our well-being at the top of the program.

With the support of my publisher and the photo etched in my mind, I began compiling this collection in June 1987. In my search for authors I contacted a variety of sources throughout the country including black and feminist publications, black professional and community organizations, medical associations, leading health activists, colleagues and friends. Over time, the book began to take on what appeared to be a divinely inspired life of its own. While reading one author's piece, I'd notice a footnote that would lead me to another vital source on black women's health. While chatting with an author on the phone, she'd mention yet another topic that had to be included in the book. At times, it seemed as if the entire sisterhood was directing insight and energy to this collection. I welcomed all suggestions, both practical and psychic.

The most substantive influence and spiritual guide for this book has been the model set for me by Byllye Avery, founder and director of the National Black Women's Health Project (NBWHP) in Atlanta, Georgia. Organizing around wellness, Avery and her grassroots agency have created a black, *feminist* movement that is an inspiration to the black community.

As a participant in an NBWHP workshop held in the San Francisco Bay Area several years ago, I saw firsthand the inroads the NBWHP has made in helping black women address and overcome the numerous issues that have damaged our mental and physical health. Knowing that we were safe at the workshop and that our silence was killing us, we cried out about the racism, sexism, incest, domestic violence, homophobia, class and color issues that are crushing our spirits and breaking our hearts. For many of us, it was the first time since childhood that we permitted ourselves to be vulnerable and to reach out to other black women for solace. Every trembling shoulder was touched, every hand was held, no tear was shed alone.

Like the organizing principle of the NBWHP, this book is based on the belief that as black women, we can be our own best friends. Painful though it may be, we *must* look at what ails us and how we can get better. Without our health, we truly have nothing.

This book is also a heartfelt protest against the racism that cripples the medical establishment and consequently our lives. It says black women have had enough of the statistics that tell us that the life expectancy for whites is 75.3 years compared with 69.4 for blacks; that the infant mortality rate for blacks is 20 deaths per 1,000, about twice the rate suffered among whites; that 52 percent of the women with AIDS are black; that more than 50 percent of black women live in a state of emotional distress; and that black women stand a one in 104 chance of being murdered compared with a one in 369 chance for white women.

We have to address and *change* the dismal predictions about our lives because we've got glorious contributions to make to society. We've got songs to sing, pictures to paint, poems to recite, children to teach, books to write, pies to bake, hair to braid, flowers to grow, businesses to run and people to love. There's a whole lot of living left in us yet.

The contributions in this collection present a broad spectrum of black female experiences and insights about health matters. They range from scholarly evaluations of the politics of black women's health and teenage pregnancy to personal accounts of management of and recovery from a number of health problems, including diabetes, lupus, cancer, stress, obesity, alcoholism, sickle cell anemia and hypertension. The writings are an honest reflection of the health issues faced by many black women; however, they are not intended to provide a scientific study of disease. None of the information in this book should be used exclusively to diagnose or treat medical problems.

Within these pages, courageous black women write of the grief they've suffered in the face of family loss and the sexual abuse they've endured in their homes. Drawing not from impersonal data but rather from their own experiences, they offer advice and support for black women who are struggling to get and stay well. Black women poets, using their craft like a soothing tonic, share their enthusiasm for life in the book. In a poem published for the first time, the late poet Pat Parker writes poignantly of her struggle with breast cancer.

Many health care providers and activists also tell their stories in the collection. As nurses, physicians, dentists, therapists and midwives, these women serve as role models and invaluable links between the black community and an often uncaring medical establishment.

The writing styles and approaches to topics represent the diversity of black women who contributed to the anthology. The wide range of material—essays, historical pieces, political debates, poems, interviews and personal stories—mirrors our creative and multi-faceted existence. Black women have never been one-dimensional people.

In this gathering of voices, black women have come together to love and comfort each other. Within these pages are the dialogues and discussions, prayers and potions that many of us have shared privately. Like the photo on my wall, the stories in this book document our real pain and vulnerability as black women in a culture that devalues our very essence. They also testify to our energy, resilience and stalwart determination to lead peaceful, productive and healthy lives.

Please take this sisterly medicine and pass it on.

Evelyn C. White
January 1990
Oakland, California

Note to the Expanded Edition

In offering the expanded edition of *The Black Women's Health Book*, I'd like to share some thoughts about the vitality and vulnerability of black women.

These thoughts have been evoked by the multitudes of black women who have extended themselves to me since the initial publication of the book. These women—of all ages, incomes and backgrounds—have contacted me through letters and phone calls. They've looked up at me from classrooms, lecture halls, church pews, libraries and community centers across the nation. They have approached me in parking lots and as I stood in line at a restaurant trying to make, for a non-cook like myself, the major decision of the day: whether to order flautas or fajitas. They have politely introduced themselves to me at meetings and during intermission at dance concerts.

These black women have smiled warmly, wrapped their arms around me and told me how much better they felt after reading the book you hold in your hands. They have also revealed—through the sadness in their eyes, the tremor in their voices, the slump of their shoulders, the trembling of their hands and the bow of their heads— how much they still need to be comforted and loved.

In all of these women, I have seen the mirror reflection of myself. Through their visages, I've seen myself energized and elated, ready to "put my foot on the rock" and take on the world. At other times I've seen myself depleted and despairing, bearing the full weight of being the motherless and fatherless child that I am.

But through it all, whether they were extending themselves to me from wells of happiness or heartache, black women have shown me the multifaceted contours of our desire. They have shown me the desire with which we want to connect; the desire with which we want to belong; the desire with which we want to give; the desire with which we want to soothe and nurture those who look like us. Always reflected back to me, from black women, has been our fierce desire to have healthy bodies, minds and hearts. Read what you will about the misery and mayhem in our lives but here's what I know: *Sisters want and intend to be well.*

Sisters like the one struggling with lupus who told me that she fully intended to find a supportive group of black women with whom she could share her experiences, even though she lived in a predominately white community.

Sisters like the one who revealed to me that she'd suffered emotional problems after having an abortion, but that she'd started therapy and was feeling better about her decision to control her reproductive life.

Sisters like the one who sent me her vegetarian soul food cookbook (see Additional Reading in the back of the book) with a note that read: "We can change our eating habits and improve our health."

The expanded edition of *The Black Women's Health Book* is a response to our continuing desire to connect with each other and to heal. New additions to this collection include articles on fibroids, breastfeeding, non-Western medicine, love, menopause, the evolution of the African-American diet, the challenges black women face within medical settings and skin color issues. Because of its ongoing impact in our community, the volume features an update on HIV infection and black women. In an effort to reclaim and rectify our heritage as healers, there is an essay on Nurse Rivers, the black woman who played a pivotal role in the Tuskegee Syphilis Study. Unlike much of the other published works on the controversial experiment, the essay examines the episode from a *black feminist perspective*.

In addition to the women of Seal Press and the new contributors to the book, I extend my heartfelt gratitude to the following women whose support was both inspirational and invaluable to me: Joan Miura, Taigi Smith and Diane Hamer of the Schlesinger Library at Radcliffe College.

My work on this collection has been graced by the memory of poet Audre Lorde and of my journalist colleague Toni Y. Joseph, who died unexpectedly of a heart attack at age thirty-one. Both women taught me about purpose and passion.

Blessings to Toni Morrison for her generosity and to my beloved friend, Mona Vold.

Love Yourself. And again, pass it on.

Evelyn C. White
August 1993
Oakland, California

One: There Is a Balm in Gilead

In Answer to the Question:
Have You Ever Considered Suicide
Kate Rushin

Suicide?!?!
Gurl, is you crazy?
I'm scared I'm not gonna live long enough
As it is

I'm scared to death of high places
Fast cars
Rare diseases
Muggers
Drugs
Electricity
And folks who work roots

Now what would I look like
Jumpin offa somethin
I got everything to do
And I ain't got time for that

Let me tell you
If you ever hear me
Talkin bout killin my frail self
Come and get me
Sit with me until that spell passes
And if they ever
Find me layin up somewhere
Don't let them tell you it was suicide
Cause it wasn't

I'm scared of high places
Fast moving trucks
Electricity
Drugs
Folks who work roots
And home-canned string beans

Now with all I got
To worry about
What would I look like
Killin myself

3

In July 1989, Byllye Y. Avery, founder of the National Black Women's Health Project, was named one of twenty-nine people to receive a five-year grant from the MacArthur Foundation. Bestowed by an anonymous committee, the award can be used by recipients however they choose. It seems only fitting that Avery, a grassroots organizer who has never sought a personal spotlight, would receive such a prestigious award. Since 1981, she has worked tirelessly to help black women who are "sick and tired of being sick and tired" improve their mental and physical well-being through empowerment, healing and self-love.

Through its community-based self-help programs, the NBWHP has created a safe place for black women to talk about the multitude of hurts that have kept us from living full and healthy lives. NBWHP conferences, weekend retreats, educational films and publications are widely acclaimed for dealing with black women's health concerns within the context of black culture. Under Avery's determined leadership, the National Black Women's Health Project has created a vital wellspring of black feminist activism that will have a significant social impact in the 1990s and beyond.

The following piece is an edited version of a talk Avery gave in Cambridge, Massachusetts, in July 1988.

Breathing Life into Ourselves: The Evolution of the National Black Women's Health Project
Byllye Y. Avery

I got involved in women's health in the 1970s around the issue of abortion. There were three of us at the University of Florida, in Gainesville, who just seemed to get picked out by women who needed abortions. They came to us. I didn't know anything about abortions. In my life that word couldn't even be mentioned without having somebody look at you crazy. Then someone's talking to me about abortion. It seemed unreal. But as more women came (and at first they were mostly white women), we found out this New York number we could give them, and they could catch a plane and go there for their abortions. But then a black woman came and we gave

4

her the number, and she looked at us in awe: "I can't get to New York. . . . " We realized we needed a different plan of action, so in May 1974 we opened up the Gainesville Women's Health Center.

As we learned more about abortions and gynecological care, we immediately started to look at birth, and to realize that we are women with a total reproductive cycle. We might have to make different decisions about our lives, but whatever the decision, we deserved the best services available. So, in 1978, we opened up Birthplace, an alternative birthing center. It was exhilarating work; I assisted in probably around two hundred births. I understood life, and working in birth, I understood death, too. I certainly learned what's missing in prenatal care and why so many of our babies die.

Through my work at Birthplace, I learned the importance of being involved in our own health. We have to create environments that say "yes." Birthplace was a wonderful space. It was a big, old turn-of-the-century house that we decorated with antiques. We went to people's houses and, if we liked something, we begged for it—things off their walls, furniture, rugs. We fixed the place so that when women walked in, they would say, "Byllye, I was excited when I got up today because this was my day to come to Birthplace." That's how prenatal care needs to be given—so that people are excited when they come. It's about eight and a half or nine months that a woman comes on a continuous basis. That is the time to start affecting her life so that she can start making meaningful lifestyle changes. So you see, health provides us with all sorts of opportunities for empowerment.

Through Birthplace, I came to understand the importance of our attitudes about birthing. Many women don't get the exquisite care they deserve. They go to these large facilities, and they don't understand the importance of prenatal care. They ask, "Why is it so important for me to get in here and go through all this hassle?" We have to work around that.

Through the work of Birthplace, we have created a prenatal caring program that provides each woman who comes for care with a support group. She enters the group when she arrives, leaves the group to go for her physical checkup, and then returns to the group when she is finished. She doesn't sit in a waiting room for two hours. Most of these women have nobody to talk to. No one listens to them; no one helps them plan. They're asking: "Who's going to get me to the hospital if I go into labor in the middle of the night, or the middle of the day, for that matter? Who's going to help me get out of this abusive relationship? Who's going to make sure I have the food I need to eat?" Infant mortality is not a medical problem; it's a social problem.

One of the things that black women have started talking about regarding infant mortality is that many of us are like empty wells; we give a lot, but we don't get much back. We're asked to be strong. I have said, "If one more person says to me that black women are strong I'm going to scream in their face." I am so tired of that stuff. What are you going to do—just lay down and die? We have to do what's necessary to survive. It's just a part of living. But most of us are empty wells that never really get replenished. Most of us are dead inside. We are walking around dead. That's why we end up in relationships that reinforce that particular thought. So you're talking about a baby being alive inside of a dead person; it just won't work.

We need to stop letting doctors get away with piling up all this money, buying all these little machines. They can keep the tiniest little piece of protoplasm alive, and then it goes home and dies. All this foolishness with putting all this money back into their pockets on that end of the care and not on the other end has to stop. When are we going to wake up?

The National Black Women's Health Project

I left the birthing center around 1980 or '81, mostly because we needed more midwives and I wasn't willing to go to nursing school. But an important thing had happened for me in 1979. I began looking at myself as a black woman. Before that I had been looking at myself as a woman. When I left the birthing center, I went to work in a Comprehensive Employment Training Program (CETA) job at a community college and it brought me face-to-face with my sisters and face-to-face with myself. Just by the nature of the program and the population that I worked with, I had, for the first time in my life, a chance to ask a nineteen-year-old why—please give me the reason why—you have four babies and you're only nineteen years old. And I was able to listen, and bring these sisters together to talk about their lives. It was there that I started to understand the lives of black women and to realize that we live in a conspiracy of silence. It was hearing these women's stories that led me to start conceptualizing the National Black Women's Health Project.

First I wanted to do an hour-long presentation on black women's health issues, so I started doing research. I got all the books, and I was shocked at what I saw. I was angry—angry that the people who wrote these books didn't put it into a format that made sense to us, angry that nobody was saying anything to black women or to black men. I was so angry I threw one book across the room and it stayed there for three or four days, because I knew I had just seen the tip of the iceberg, but I also knew enough to know that I couldn't go back. I had opened my eyes, and I had to go on and look.

Instead of an hour-long presentation we had a conference. It didn't happen until 1983, but when it did, 2,000 women came. But I knew we couldn't just have a conference. From the health statistics I saw, I knew that there was a deeper problem. People needed to be able to work individually, and on a daily basis. So we got the idea of self-help groups. The first group we formed was in a rural area outside of Gainesville, with twenty-one women who were severely obese. I thought, "Oh this is a piece of cake. Obviously these sisters don't have any information. I'll go in there and talk to them about losing weight, talk to them about high blood pressure, talk to them about diabetes—it'll be easy."

Little did I know that when I got there, they would be able to tell me everything that went into a 1200-calorie-a-day diet. They all had been to Weight Watchers at least five or six times; they all had blood-pressure-reading machines in their homes as well as medications they were on. And when we sat down to talk, they said, "We know all that information, but what we also know is that living in the world that we are in, we feel like we are absolutely nothing." One woman said to me, "I work for General Electric making batteries, and, from the stuff they suit me up in, I know it's killing me." She said, "My home life is not working. My old man is an alcoholic. My kids got babies. Things are not well with me. And the one thing I know I can do when I come home is cook me a pot of food and sit down in front of the TV and eat it. And you can't take that away from me until you're ready to give me something in its place."

So that made me start to think that there was some other piece to this health puzzle that had been missing, that it's not just about giving information; people need something else. We just spent a lot of time talking. And while we were talking, we were planning the 1983 conference, so I took the information back to the planning committee. Lillie Allen (a trainer who works with NBWHP) was there. We worked with her to understand that we are dying inside. That unless we are able to go inside of ourselves and touch and breathe fire, breathe life into ourselves, that, of course, we couldn't be healthy. Lillie started working on a workshop that we named "Black and Female: What is the Reality?" This is a workshop that terrifies us all. And we are also terrified not to have it, because the conspiracy of silence is killing us.

Stopping Violence

As we started to talk, I looked at those health statistics in a new way. Now, I'm not saying that we are not suffering from the things we die from—that's what the statistics give us. But what causes all this sickness? Like cardiovascular disease—it's the number one killer. What causes all that heart pain? When sisters take their shoes off and start talking about what's happening, the first thing we cry about is violence. The violence in our lives. And if you look in statistics books, they mention violence in one paragraph. They don't even give numbers, because they can't count it: the violence is too pervasive.

The number one issue for most of our sisters is violence—battering, sexual abuse. Same thing for their daughters, whether they are twelve or four. We have to look at how violence is used, how violence and sexism go hand in hand, and how it affects the sexual response of females. We have to stop it, because violence is the training ground for us.

When you talk to young people about being pregnant, you find out a lot of things. Number one is that most of these girls did not get pregnant by teenage boys; most of them got pregnant by their mother's boyfriends or their brothers or their daddies. We've been sitting on that. We can't just tell our daughters, "just say no." What do they do about all those feelings running around their bodies? And we need to talk to our brothers. We need to tell them, the incest makes us crazy. It's something that stays on our minds all the time. We need the men to know that. And they need to know that when they hurt us, they hurt themselves. Because we are their mothers, their sisters, their wives; we are their allies on this planet. They can't just damage one part of it without damaging themselves. We need men to stop giving consent, by their silence, to rape, to sexual abuse, to violence. You need to talk to your boyfriends, your husbands, your sons, whatever males you have around you—talk to them about talking to other men. When they are sitting around womanizing, talking bad about women, make sure you have somebody stand up and be your ally and help stop this. For future generations, this has got to stop somewhere.

Mothers and Daughters

If violence is the number one thing women talk about, the next is being mothers too early and too long. We've developed a documentary called "On Becoming a Woman: Mothers and Daughters Talking Together." It's eight mothers and eight daughters—sixteen ordinary people talking about extraordinary things.

The idea of the film came out of my own experience with my daughter. When Sonja turned eleven, I started bemoaning that there were no rituals left; there was nothing to let a girl know that once you get your period your life can totally change, nothing to celebrate that something wonderful is happening. So I got a cake that said, "Happy Birthday! Happy Menstruation!" It had white icing with red writing. I talked about the importance of becoming a woman, and, out of that, I developed a workshop for mothers and daughters for the public schools. I did the workshops in Gainesville, and, when we came to Atlanta, I started doing them there. The film took ten years, from the first glimmer of an idea to completion.

The film is in three parts. In the first part all the mothers talk about when we got our periods. Then the daughters who have their periods talk about getting theirs, and the ones who are still waiting talk about that. The second part of the film deals with contraception, birth control, anatomy and physiology. This part of the film is animated, so it keeps the kids' attention. It's funny. It shows all the anxiety: passing around condoms, hating it, saying, "Oh no, we don't want to do this."

The third part of the film is the hardest. We worked on communication with the mothers and daughters. We feel that the key to birth control and to controlling reproduction is the nature of the relationship between the parents and their young people. And what's happening is that everybody is willing to beat up on the young kids, asking, "Why did you get pregnant? Why did you do this?" No one is saying to the parents, "Do you need some help with learning how to talk to your young person? Do you want someone to sit with you? Do you want to see what it feels like?" We don't have all the answers. In this film, you see us struggling.

What we created, which was hard for the parents, is a safe space where everybody can say anything they need to say. And if you think about that, as parents, we have that relationship with our kids: we can ask them anything. But when we talk about sex, it's special to be in a space where the kids can ask *us*, "Mama, what do you do when you start feeling funny all in your body?" What the kids want to know is, what about lust? What do we do about it? And that's the very information that we don't want to give up. That's "our business." But they want to hear it from us, because they can trust us. And we have to struggle with how we do that: How do we share that information? How do we deal with our feelings?

Realizing the Dream

The National Black Women's Health Project has ninety-six self-help groups in twenty-two states, six groups in Kenya, and a group in Barbados and in Belize. In addition, we were just funded by the W.K. Kellogg Foundation to do some work in three housing projects in Atlanta. We received $1,032,000 for a three-year period to set up three community centers. Our plan is to do health screening and referral for adolescents and women, and in addition to hook them up with whatever social services they need—to help cut through the red tape. There will be computerized learning programs and individualized tutorial programs to help young women get their General Equivalency Degrees (GED), along with a panel from the community who will be working on job readiness skills. And we'll be doing our self-help groups—talking about who we are, examining, looking at ourselves.

We hope this will be a model program that can be duplicated anywhere. And we're excited about it. Folks in Atlanta thought it was a big deal for a group of black women to get a million dollars. We thought it was pretty good, too. Our time is coming.

Studies show that stress is linked to several physical and emotional problems that disproportionately affect black women, including heart disease, depression, ulcers, hypertension and drug and alcohol abuse. Learning to manage stress, black female style, is key to achieving a healthier and more productive life.

Rocking in the Sun Light: Stress and Black Women
Opal Palmer Adisa

Rocking in the sun light, rocking the blues away, rocking in the sun light, rocking the tears away. When African women were forcefully brought to the shores of America and were worked and treated worse than cattle, they gritted their teeth, determined to survive their lot, and gave birth to the blues. Since then, all African-American women have been seeking a rocking chair and the sun light to rock themselves well.

"Stress!"

"Girl, ain't that the truth."

"Needing to have a change of face to put on depending on the occasion wears on my body."

"Always having to think six steps ahead, then some, is what gets to me."

"What I need is a rocking chair... "

"And the sun light to rock under... "

Silence. The two women wrapped in thought, dreaming of the rocking chair under the sun light. Their stress is like the blues. It has feet and teeth, and as they rock, slowly, ever so slowly, in the gentle, even, backward and forward motion, stress steps on its bunion feet and leaves these sisters' bodies. They doze. Smiles play around the corners of their mouths and the furrows of their brows smooth as they dream of themselves: walking on the water; shooting arrows like their Dahomey warrior sisters. The rocking continues; the women dream on.

All African-American women may not have rocking chairs, but

we have each other. The best doctor, best medicine, best antidote for what ails us is the mirror reflection of ourselves: our friendships, our bonds, the comfort we seek and the support we receive from each other. If truth be told, black women would cease to exist if we didn't have each other.

For who but a sister can you call up at 2:00 a.m. in the middle of the week and ask, "Do you have time to talk?" Who but a sister can you go to on payday to borrow twenty dollars to tide you over? Who but a sister will understand when you drop your kids off without notice because you have won free tickets to a concert? Who but a sister can you depend on to be at your graduation with champagne and roses like she earned that doctorate herself? Who but a sister can you gossip and laugh with, tears rolling down your cheeks, asses sliding off the chairs, bodies rolling on the floor in spasms? Sisters simply depend on and nurture each other. We use each other's strength and tenacity to fight the stress that would put us in our graves before our time.

I don't know one black woman, regardless of educational status, economic condition or social position, who is not faced with stress. Some people think stress is like the blues, but it's not. Blues is medicine because it's not meant to depress or pull one down—it has the opposite effect. The blues heals. The more you listen to the moans, the more blues singers belt out their sorrows and hard times, our collective hard times, the more the blues leaves them, leaves us, giving us space to continue living. The blues helps us laugh at our misfortune, make light of our hazardous lives, and reaffirms that living is what life is about no matter how many hurdles we have to jump over. Stress doesn't do that. Stress does not heal; it infects; it's only satisfied when you're dead. It is the venom that gets into all black women's blood, causing our bodies to swell and explode, extinguishing our lives.

But we have learned to create balm-yards to mix potions and perform a laying on of hands, to share our magic so that we can vanquish the stress that slaps us in the face every day. So sisters, let us sing the blues, moan and rock in the sun light.

Rocking in the sun light might mean me sitting in a sister's kitchen, sipping mandarin orange tea, talking while dishes in the sink remain unwashed and groceries to be packed away sit on the counter. Our children are acting the fools in the living room, but we ignore them as much as we can, and they leave us alone as much as they are able. We rock while we talk about needing a new job that pays better and provides benefits, about being taken for granted, about all the homeless people, particularly women and children that we try not to walk by everyday. Just talking, hearing ourselves cry, learning to say we've had enough. We know that the image of the strong black woman is a mask we wear that helps bring us closer to madness. Rocking in the sun light is our release. It's us, black women, allowing ourselves our humanity, refusing to be the mules, refusing to be strong for everyone but ourselves.

Stress leads black women to madness, so much so that we have become experts at camouflaging our angst. It is the theme of much of my poetry:

> Sometimes I mutter
> as I walk
> people stare/pass by
> on the far side
>
> To be
> one of those desolate men
> lounging in
> stench alley ways
> forever talking
> to the wind
> their words
> bullets
> people shy from
>
> But I'm woman
> conditioned to nurse
> like a mute child
>
> I write

As a writer, my poetry is viewed as an "acceptable" outlet for my stress. But many black women don't have such an escape. Many cannot even identify the stress that gnaws on them. Even more believe it's tantamount to treason to admit they can't cope. We bite our tongues until blood bubbles and silence swells big in our mouths; we are unable to utter a syllable.

Did you ever wonder why so many sisters look so angry? Why we walk like we've got bricks in our bags and will slash and curse you at the drop of a hat? It's because stress is hemmed into our dresses, pressed into our hair, mixed into our perfume and painted on our fingers. Stress from the deferred dreams, the dreams not voiced; stress from the broken promises, the blatant lies; stress from always being at the bottom, from never being thought beautiful, from always being taken for granted, taken advantage of; stress from being a black woman in white America. How long do you think you can hold your breath without asphixiating? Yes, black women do commit suicide!

We kill ourselves when we cease to smile; when we take drugs to deaden the pain of being black; when we allow a partner to physically and mentally abuse us because we are desperate to have "somebody"; when we allow ourselves to be divided by class privilege, income, preoccupation with skin color, looks or sexual preference; when night after week after month we sit alone in our apartments and cry, or eat packaged death, or watch television because there is no one to call and say, "Hey girl, what's happenin'?" We are stressed out.

We who have invented the blues and sung songs that were warm towels to wrap ourselves in, must find rocking chairs and we must find them soon. Let that rocking chair be a kiss from a sister, a hug, a squeeze of the hand, a makeshift dinner, a cup of coffee, an attentive ear, a walk together, or unsolicited ("Girl, I told you that romance was gonna flow downhill like water") but loving advice. Sisters know sisters; we have to turn to each other and get the rocking going.

Sisters are so mobile these days that the phone is often the cheapest way to rock with a dear friend. I can't imagine what we'd do without it. Sometimes I just need to check in with my "good-good" friend Lorna in Jamaica or Wendy in New York or Pamela in Baltimore. I hear their voices, their laughter, imagine the looks on their faces, share news and feel safe because the distance cushions my fears. I'm rocking myself well, feeling the hot tropical sunshine on my body. Rocking, rocking the troubles away.

If we are to triumph and leave a better world for our children, black women must rock with a vengeance. Rock the way we ran for freedom, rock the way we marched for justice, rock and rock and never stop. Gently, slowly, in an even, backward and forward motion, we must rock until the sun is right in our hearts. With such rocking we'll heal and grow well like radiant sunflowers with our heads held high.

Yes, we are rocking, rocking in the sun light, rocking our tears away . . .

Zora Neale Hurston (1901–1960) was a life-loving folklorist, novelist, critic and playwright. As a student at Barnard College in the 1920s, she studied with the noted anthropologist Dr. Franz Boas. A Florida native, Hurston went on to travel widely and write on a variety of black customs and folkways. After a long eclipse of her literary reputation, Hurston's achievements were resurrected in the 1970s by writer Alice Walker.

In 1935 Hurston published Mules and Men, *a vibrant and magical collection of black folklore she had gathered in the South. The following excerpt from the book is an invaluable contribution to our heritage and our understanding of traditional black folk medicine.*

Prescriptions of Root Doctors
Zora Neale Hurston

Folk medicine is practiced by a great number of persons. On the "jobs," that is, in the sawmill camps, the turpentine stills, mining camps and among the lowly generally, doctors are not generally called to prescribe for illnesses, certainly, nor for the social diseases. Nearly all of the conjure doctors practice "roots," but some of the root doctors are not hoodoo doctors. One of these latter at Bogaloosa, Louisiana, and one at Bartow, Florida, enjoy a huge patronage. They make medicine only, and white and colored swarm about them claiming cures.

The following are some prescriptions gathered here and there in Florida, Alabama and Louisiana:

Bladder Trouble

One pint of boiling water, two tablespoons of flaxseed, two tablespoons of cream of tartar. Drink one-half glass in the morning and one-half at night.

Fistula

Sweet gum bark and mullen cooked down with lard. Make a salve.

Rheumatism

Take mullen leaves (five or six) and steep in one quart of water. Drink three to four wine glasses a day.

Swelling

Oil of white rose (fifteen cents), oil of lavender (fifteen cents), Jockey Club (fifteen cents), Japanese honeysuckle (fifteen cents). Rub.

Blindness

a. Slate dust and pulverized sugar. Blow in the eyes. (It must be finely pulverized to remove film.)

b. Get somebody to catch a catfish. Get the gall and put it in a bottle. Drop one drop in each eye. Cut the skin off. It gives the sight a free look.

Lockjaw

a. Draw out the nail. Beat the wound and squeeze out all the blood possible. Then take a piece of fat bacon, some tobacco and a penny and tie it on the wound.

b. Draw out the nail and drive it in a green tree on the sunrise side, and the place will heal.

*Flooding**

One grated nutmeg, pinch of alum in a quart of water (cooked). Take one-half glass three times daily.

Sick at Stomach

Make a tea of parched rice and bay leaves (six). Give a cup at a time. Drink no other water.

Live Things in Stomach (Fits)

Take a silver quarter with a woman's head on it. Stand her on her head and file it in one-half cup of sweet milk. Add nine parts of garlic. Boil and give to drink after straining.

Medicine to Purge

Jack of War tea, one tablespoon to a cup of water with a pinch of soda after it is ready to drink.

---

*Menstruation

Loss of Mind

Sheep weed leaves, bay leaf, sarsaparilla root. Take the bark and cut it all up fine. Make a tea. Take one tablespoon and put in two cups of water and strain and sweeten. You drink some and give some to patient.

Put a fig leaf and poison oak in shoe. (Get fig leaves off a tree that hasn't borne fruit. Stem them so that nobody will know.)

To Make a Tonic

One quart of wine, three pinches of raw rice, three dusts of cinnamon (about one heaping teaspoon), five small pieces of the hull of pomegranate about the size of a fingernail, five tablespoons of sugar. Let it come to a boil, set one-half hour and strain. Dose: one tablespoon.

(When the pomegranate is in season, gather all the hulls you can for use at other times in the year.)

For more than three decades, activist Angela Y. Davis has fought tire-lessly for social justice and equality. Her incisive political analysis of health issues and her indictment of insensitive and inadequate United States health care policies challenge us to renew our efforts to make government more accountable for the physical and mental well-being of black women.

This address was first given in August 1987 at Bennett College, Greensboro, North Carolina, before a conference organized by the North Carolina Black Women's Health Project. As Davis tells it, it is time for black women to fight back on every front and reclaim our health.

Sick and Tired of Being Sick and Tired: The Politics of Black Women's Health
Angela Y. Davis

Politics do not stand in polar opposition to our lives. Whether we desire it or not, they permeate our existence, insinuating themselves into the most private spaces of our lives. As a starting point for this discussion of the politics of Black women's health, I propose we consider the lived experience of one courageous individual who, as she poignantly documents her own personal health battles, harvests lessons that elucidate our collective quest for wellness. "How do I provide myself," Audre Lorde asks,

> . . . with the best physical and psychic nourishment to repair past, and minimize future damage to my body? How do I give voice to my quests so that other women can take what they need from my experiences? How do my experiences with cancer fit into the larger tapestry of my work as a Black woman, into the history of all women? And most of all, how do I fight the despair born of fear and anger and powerlessness which is my greatest internal enemy?
>
> I have found that battling despair does not mean closing my eyes to the enormity of the tasks of effecting change, nor ignoring the strength and the barbarity of the forces aligned against

us. It means teaching, surviving and fighting with the most important resource I have, myself, and taking joy in that battle. It means, for me, recognizing the enemy outside and the enemy within, and knowing that my work is part of a continuum of women's work, of reclaiming this earth and our power, and knowing that this work did not begin with my birth nor will it end with my death. And it means knowing that within this continuum, my life and my love and my work has particular power and meaning relative to others.

It means trout fishing on the Missisquoi River at dawn and tasting the green silence, and knowing that this beauty too is mine forever.[1]

On this continuum of women's work, upon which Audre Lorde situates herself and her precious offerings, the pursuit of health in body, mind and spirit weaves in and out of every major struggle women have ever waged in our quest for social, economic and political emancipation. During the past decade, we have been the fortunate beneficiaries of the valuable work of health activists like Byllye Avery and Lillie Allen of the National Black Women's Health Project, who have perceptively and passionately addressed Black women's health issues and have begun to chart out paths toward wellness in all its myriad forms. The Project has chosen as its motto Fannie Lou Hamer's well-known lament: We are sick and tired of being sick and tired.

We have become cognizant of the urgency of contexualizing Black women's health in relation to the prevailing political conditions. While our health is undeniably assaulted by natural forces frequently beyond our control, all too often the enemies of our physical and emotional well-being are social and political. That is why we must strive to understand the complex politics of Black women's health.

One would assume that the U.S. Constitution, which guarantees all individuals "life, liberty and the pursuit of happiness," by implication assures that all citizens of this country are entitled to be healthy. However, it is not really necessary to derive this right from the Constitution, for health ought to be universally recognized as a basic human right. Yet in this society, dominated as it is by the profit-seeking ventures of monopoly corporations, health has been callously transformed into a commodity—a commodity that those with means are able to afford, but that is too often entirely beyond the reach of others. Pregnant Black women, uninsured and without the means to pay hospital entrance fees, have been known to give birth in parking lots outside the hospitals that have refused them entrance. In other instances, poor Black women who are subscribers to health plans have been denied treatment because hospital officials have presumptuously argued that they were lying about their insurance coverage.

Sharon Ford, a young Black woman on welfare in the San Francisco Bay Area, gave birth to a stillborn child because two hospitals declined to treat her, even though she was covered by a health plan. Aware of a serious problem with her pregnancy, Ms. Ford sought treatment at the hospital nearest her home. When she informed officials there that she was covered by a certain medical plan, she was sent by them to the hospital associated with that plan, despite the fact that her critical condition obviously warranted emergency intervention. Officials at the second hospital, who claimed that their computerized list of subscribers to that plan did not include her name, instructed her to go to yet another facility, known as the poor people's medical warehouse in that area. In the meantime, however, three hours had passed, and by the time she was treated by doctors at the third hospital, her unborn baby had died. Ironically, it was later discovered that the insurance company had been tardy in delivering the subscriber list that, indeed, contained Sharon Ford's name. While this is the tragic story of a single Black woman, it cannot be dismissed as an aberration. Rather, it is symptomatic of dangerous trends within the health-care industry.

Because so many programs designed to ameliorate the conditions of poor people—inadequate as they may have been—have been abolished or cut back in recent years, accessibility to health services has become an especially pressing problem. The major barrier to Black women's health is poverty—and during the Reagan years, our communities became increasingly impoverished. The number of poor people increased by more than six million, and according to the Physicians' Task Force on Hunger, as many as twenty million people in this country suffered from want of food. A dire consequence of poverty is malnutrition and a plethora of diseases emanating from the lack of adequate sustenance. Malnutrition, which can cause maternal anemia and toxemia, a potentially fatal condition for a pregnant woman, is also implicated in premature births and infant deaths.

Associated with higher rates of chronic illnesses such as heart disease, arthritis and diabetes, poverty causes its victims to be more susceptible to hypertension and lung, stomach and esophageal cancer. The National Black Women's Health Project has pointed out that while proportionately fewer Black women than white women suffer from breast cancer, more Black women are likely to die from it. Furthermore, as cervical cancer rates have decreased among white women, they have risen among Black women. For reasons that require no explanation, poverty increases vulnerability to mental illness. Of all groups in this country, Black women have the highest rates of admission to outpatient psychiatric services. It has been argued by health activists that most adult Black women live in a state of psychological stress.

Two out of three poor adults are women, and eighty percent of the poor in the United States are women and children. This means that women are the majority of the recipients of many health and nutritional programs sponsored by the federal government. Because Black women are disproportionately represented among the beneficiaries of these social services, they have been hurt most deeply by the cutbacks in the federal budget. When the cutbacks in Aid to Families with Dependent Children occurred, most of the women who lost AFDC also lost their Medicaid coverage. Federal cuts in the Maternal and Child Health Block Grant resulted, in almost all states, in the reduction of services offered in maternal and child health clinics, or in the curtailment of the number of people eligible to receive this care. As a consequence, almost a million people, most of whom are children and women of childbearing age, became ineligible to receive services at community health centers. This means, for example, that fewer Black women now receive prenatal care, a fact that has fatal implications, because babies born to mothers receiving no prenatal care are three times more likely to die in infancy than those whose mothers do receive such care. At the same time, federal funding for abortions has become virtually nonexistent, while the government continues to strongly subsidize surgical sterilization. This process is a vicious cycle, further entrenching poor people in conditions that make ill health inevitable. Standing at the intersection of racism, sexism and economic injustice, Black women have been compelled to bear the brunt of this complex oppressive process.

Afro-American women are twice as likely as white women to die of hypertensive cardiovascular disease, and they have three times the rate of high blood pressure. Black infant mortality is twice that of whites, and maternal mortality is three times as high. Lupus is three times more common among Black women than white, thus the funds channeled into research to discover a cure for it have been extremely sparse. Black women die far more often than white women from diabetes and cancer.

This cycle of oppression is largely responsible for the fact that far too many Black women resort to drugs as a means—however ineffective it ultimately proves to be—of softening the blows of poverty. Because of intravenous drug use in the Black community, a disproportionately large number of Black women have been infected with AIDS. Although the popular belief is that AIDS is a disease of gay white men, the truth is that Afro-Americans and Latinos are far more likely to contract AIDS than whites. This is true among gays, among IV drug users, among heterosexual partners, and among children. Black and Latino men are two and a half times as likely to get AIDS as white men. Latina women are nine times as likely as white women to contract AIDS. But the most frightening statistic is reserved for Black women, who are twelve times more likely to contract the AIDS virus than white women.

Four times as many Black women as white women die of homicide. In the meantime, under the Reagan administration, hospitals serving predominantly poor Black communities—including those with excellent trauma units, designed to treat victims of violence—closed down. Such was the case with the Homer G. Phillips Hospital in St. Louis, the largest teaching hospital for Black medical students in the country. On average in this country, there is one doctor per 1,500 people, but in central Harlem, there is only one doctor per 4,500 people.

A statement by the Public Health Association of New York City during the first year of the Reagan administration warned:

> The health of the people of New York City is actively endangered by the already imposed cuts and by the threatened cuts in funding for health care services and for medical care services. To express ourselves in clear language, so there is no misunderstanding: We are talking about dead babies whose death can be prevented; we are talking about sick children and adults whose illnesses can be prevented; we are talking about misery for older people whose misery can be prevented. We are speaking of these unspeakable things in a wealthy country and in a wealthy state, whose people deserve better. The malignant neglect of federal, state and local governments is literally killing people now and will kill and destroy the lives of many more in the future. We urge a massive infusion of federal and state funds to restore and rebuild services now, before the consequences of their breakdown demonstrate in even more tragic and dramatic ways the human and economic cost of this neglect.[2]

Outside of South Africa, the United States is the only major industrial country in the world that lacks a uniform national health-insurance plan. While this country is sorely in need of a national health-care plan, there has been an increasing trend toward the privatization of health care. As one author plainly put it, the principle of the Reagan administration was "Profits Before People, Greed Before Need, and Wealth Before Health."[3]

In urging the privatization of health care, the government has prioritized the profit-seeking interests of monopoly corporations, leaving the health needs of poor people—and especially poor Black women—to be callously juggled around and, when need be, ignored. For-profit hospitals often refuse outright to treat poor, uninsured patients, and they engage in the unethical practice of "dumping" welfare recipients on public hospitals, even when those patients are in urgent need of treatment. This was the unfortunate fate of Sharon Ford, whose baby became one of the many fatalities of a process that places profits before people's health needs.

Because the hospital emergency room is a major setting for medical treatment in the Black community, this pattern of the privatization of hospitals is having an especially devastating impact on Black people—and on Black women in particular. In 1983 only 44.1 percent of Afro-Americans receiving health care made visits to a private doctor in her or his office. On the other hand, 26.5 percent went to a hospital emergency room and 9.7 percent received treatment in an outpatient clinic. By contrast, 57 percent of white patients receiving medical care visited private physicians, 13 percent went to emergency rooms and 16 percent to outpatient clinics.

The degree to which private corporations threaten to monopolize health-care services is revealed by the fact that the Hospital Corporation of America, which controlled two hospitals in 1968, now controls almost five hundred and is a dominant force in the hospital business. Other such corporations are Cigna, American Medical International and Humana. Health-care workers—a majority of whom are women in the lower-paying occupations—have also suffered from this privatization trend, for corporate takeovers of public hospitals have frequently resulted in union-busting and a subsequent freeze on wages and cutbacks on benefits.

The only ones who benefit from a competition system of medical care are the rich, who will have to pay less for health care for the poor, and those providers who skim the cream off the medical market and leave the real problems to a diminished and even-more-inadequately-financed public sector. It is yet another example of the basic Reagan policy of serving the rich, encased in a Trojan Horse, this one labeled "cost containment," "deregulation," and "free choice."[4]

It is clearly in the interests of Afro-American women to demand a federally subsidized, uniform national health-insurance plan. We need subsidized programs that reflect the progressive experiences of the women's health movement over the last decade and a half, programs that emphasize prevention, self-help and empowerment.

One of the main obstacles to the development of a national health plan is the same unrelenting pressure placed by government on all social programs benefiting poor people, and people of color in particular—namely, the runaway military budget. Since 1980, the military budget has more than doubled, taking approximately $100 billion from social programs that were underfunded to begin with. Between 1981 and 1986, $1.5 trillion was spent on military programs. As the Women's International League for Peace and Freedom points out:

> Defense Department spending in 1986 was $292 billion, but the actual costs of the military in that year were over $400 billion if hidden costs like veterans benefits, nuclear warheads in the Department of Energy's budget, and the part of the interest on the national debt attributable to past military expenditures are taken into account.[5]

The budget cuts that have affected health and other social services are not, strictly speaking, cuts, but rather transfers of funds from the civilian to the military budget. Instead of providing poor people with adequate food stamps, the corporations that make up the military-industrial complex are awarded gigantic defense contracts. Ironically, forty-five of the top one hundred defense contractors who received more than $100 billion in prime-contract awards in 1985 later came under criminal investigation.[6]

As we examine the political forces responsible for the violation of Black women's health rights, it becomes clear that the increasing militarization of our economy is culpable in a major way. The politics of Black women's health are also directly influenced by the general assault on democracy in this country, which reached a high point during the Reagan years. It is not a coincidence that a government that would sabotage the rights of every citizen of this country by permitting the development of a secret junta controlled by the Central Intelligence Agency and the National Security Council also seriously infringed upon the health rights of black women and all poor people.

The Iran-contra Hearings revealed the extent to which we were rapidly heading in the direction of a police state. The CIA operatives involved used government and private funds to support the most reactionary forces in the world—from the contras in Nicaragua to the South African-supported UNITA in Angola. They were involved in gun running, drug trafficking, bombings, assassinations, and attempted overthrows of democratically elected governments.

The executive branch of the government during the Reagan years was dominated by corporate executives and by top military men. They continued to serve the monopoly corporations as they carried out the bellicose policies of the military. As they conducted undeclared wars in various parts of the world, they were responsible for the domestic war against poor people, one of whose battlefields involved the cutbacks in health services whose effects have been so detrimental to Black women.

Reagan's 1987 nomination of the ultraconservative Robert Bork to the Supreme Court was yet another offensive against the welfare of Black women and others who suffer from racism, sexism, and economic exploitation. As Senator Edward Kennedy so poignantly observed, "Robert Bork's America is a land in which women would be forced into back-alley abortions, Blacks would sit down at segregated lunch counters, (and) rogue police would break down citizens' doors in midnight raids. . . . " Fortunately, progressive forces joined hands and succeeded in blocking the confirmation of Judge Bork to the Supreme Court.

It is from the success of progressive campaigns such as this one, as well as from the important work of organizations such as the National Black Women's Health Project, that all of us who are concerned with remedying the deplorable state of health care in this country must glean important lessons. We must learn consistently to place our battle for universally accessible health care in its larger social and political context. We must recognize the importance of raising our voices in opposition to such backward forces as Robert Bork and the outdated conservatism he represents. We must involve ourselves in the anti-apartheid movement in solidarity with our sisters and brothers in South Africa, who not only suffer the ill effects of negligent health care but are daily murdered in cold blood by the

South African government. We must actively oppose our government's continuing bid for Congressional support of contra aid; we must not allow our sisters and brothers in Nicaragua, whose revolutionary strivings have made health care available to all of their country's inhabitants on an equal basis, to be defeated.

While we fight for these larger victories, we must also learn to applaud the small victories we win. As I opened with the wise words of Audre Lorde, so I would like to conclude with this passage taken from her book, *A Burst of Light:*

> Battling racism and battling heterosexism and battling apartheid share the same urgency inside me as battling cancer. None of these struggles is ever easy, and even the smallest victory must be applauded, because it is so easy not to battle at all, to just accept, and to call that acceptance inevitable.[7]

Footnotes

1. Audre Lorde, *The Cancer Journals* (San Francisco: Spinsters/Aunt Lute, 1980), p. 17.

2. Alan Gartner, Colin Greer and Frank Riessman, *What Reagan is Doing to Us* (New York: Harper and Row, 1982), p. 50.

3. Ibid., p. 48.

4. Ibid., p. 46.

5. "The Women's Budget," Women's International League For Peace and Freedom, 1986, p. 3.

6. Ibid.

7. Audre Lorde, *A Burst of Light* (Ithaca, N.Y.: Firebrand Books, 1988), pp. 116–17.

For the past several decades, black women have consistently had a twelve to fifteen percent poorer five-year survival rate from breast cancer than white women. While black women develop breast cancer less frequently than white women, more of us die from the disease—primarily because we do not receive adequate health care. Studies show that you can help reduce your cancer risk by stopping smoking, improving your diet and conducting regular breast self-exams.

In 1980, black lesbian poet Audre Lorde chronicled her reckoning with breast cancer in The Cancer Journals, *an acclaimed work that has become a cornerstone of feminist literature. In the following passage from her collection of essays,* A Burst of Light, *published in 1988, Lorde continues her story about living with cancer.*

Living with Cancer
Audre Lorde

June 7, 1984
Berlin

Dr. Rosenberg agrees with my decision not to have a biopsy, but she has said I must do something quickly to strengthen my bodily defenses. She's recommended I begin Iscador injections three times weekly.

Iscador is a biological made from mistletoe which strengthens the natural immune system, and works against the growth of malignant cells. I've started the injections, along with two other herbals that stimulate liver function. I feel less weak.

I am listening to what fear teaches. I will never be gone. I am a scar, a report from the frontlines, a talisman, a resurrection. A rough place on the chin of complacency...

So what if I am afraid? Of stepping out into the morning? Of dying? Of unleashing the dammed gall where hatred swims like a tadpole waiting to swell into the arms of war? And what does that war teach when the bruised leavings jump an insurmountable wall where the glorious Berlin chestnuts and orange poppies hide detection wires that spray bullets which kill?

My poems are filled with blood these days because the future is so bloody. When the blood of four-year-old children runs un-remarked through the alleys of Soweto, how can I pretend that sweetness is anything more than armor and ammunition in an on-going war?

I am saving my life by using my life in the service of what must be done. Tonight as I listened to the African National Congress speakers from South Africa at the Third World People's Center here, I was filled with a sense of self answering necessity, of commitment as a survival weapon. Our battles are inseparable. Every person I have ever been must be actively enlisted in those battles, as well as in the battle to save my life.

June 9, 1984
Berlin

At the poetry reading in Zurich this weekend, I found it so much easier to discuss racism than to talk about *The Cancer Journals*. Chemical plants between Zurich and Basel have been implicated in a definite rise in breast cancer in this region, and women wanted to discuss this. I talked as honestly as I could, but it was really hard. Their questions presume a clarity I no longer have.

It was great to have Gloria there to help field all those questions about racism. For the first time in Europe, I felt I was not alone but answering as one of a group of Black women—not just Audre Lorde!

I am cultivating every iota of my energies to do battle with the possibility of liver cancer. At the same time, I am discovering how furious and resistant some pieces of me are, as well as how terrified.

In this loneliest of places, I examine every decision I make within the light of what I've learned about myself and that self-destructiveness implanted inside of me by racism and sexism and the circumstances of my life as a Black woman.

> *Mother why were we armed to fight*
> *with cloud wreathed swords and javelins of dust?*

Survival isn't some theory operating in a vacuum. It's a matter of my everyday living and making decisions.

How do I hold faith with the sun in a sunless place? It is so hard not to counter this despair with a refusal to see. But I have to stay open and filtering no matter what's coming at me, because that arms me in a particularly Black woman's way. When I'm open I'm also less despairing. The more clearly I see what I'm up against, the more able I am to fight this process going on in my body that they're calling liver cancer. And I am determined to fight it even when I am not sure of the terms of the battle nor the face of victory. I just know I must not surrender my body to others unless I completely understand and agree with what they think should be done to it. I've got to look at all of my options carefully, even the ones I find distasteful. I know I can broaden the definition of winning to the point where I can't lose.

June 10, 1984
Berlin

Dr. Rosenberg is honest, straightforward, and pretty discouraging. I don't know what I'd do without Dagmar there to translate all her grim pronouncements for me. She thinks it's liver cancer, too, but she respects my decision against surgery. I mustn't let my unwillingness to accept this diagnosis interfere with getting help. Whatever it is, this seems to be working.

We all have to die at least once. Making that death useful would be winning for me. I wasn't supposed to exist anyway, not in any meaningful way in this fucked-up whiteboys' world. I want desperately to live, and I'm ready to fight for that living even if I die shortly. Just writing those words down snaps every thing I want to do into a neon clarity. This European trip and the Afro-German women, the Sister Outsider collective in Holland, Gloria's great idea of starting an organization that can be a connection between us and South African women. For the first time I really feel that my writing has a substance and stature that will survive me.

I have done good work. I see it in the letters that come to me about *Sister Outsider*. I see it in the use women here give the poetry and the prose. But first and last I am a poet. I've worked very hard for that approach to living inside myself, and everything I do, I hope, reflects that view of life, even the ways I must move now in order to save my life.

I have done good work. There is a hell of a lot more I have to do. And sitting here tonight in this lovely green park in Berlin, dusk approaching and the walking willows leaning over the edge of the pool caressing each other's fingers, birds birds birds singing under and over the frogs, and the smell of new-mown grass enveloping my sad pen, I feel I still have enough moxie to do it all, on whatever terms I'm dealt, timely or not. Enough moxie to chew the whole world up and spit it out in bite-sized pieces, useful and warm and wet and delectable because they came out of my mouth.

. . .

June 17, 1984
Berlin

I am feeling more like an Audre I recognize, thank the goddess for Dr. Rosenberg, and for Dagmar for introducing me to her.

I've been reading Christa Wolf's *The Search for Christa T.* and finding it very difficult. At first I couldn't grapple with it because it was too painful to read about a woman dying. Dagmar and a number of the women here in Berlin say the author and I should meet. But now that I'm finished I don't know if I want to meet the woman who wrote it. There is so much pain there that is so far from being felt in any way I recognize or can use, that it makes me very uncomfortable. I feel speechless.

But there is one part of the book that really spoke to me. In chapter five, she talks about a mistaken urge to laugh at one's younger self's belief in paradise, in miracles. Each one of us who survives, she says, at least once in our lifetime, at some crucial and inescapable moment, has had to absolutely believe in the impossible. Of course, it occurs to me to ask myself if that's what I'm doing right now, believing in the impossible by refusing a biopsy.

It's been very reassuring to find a medical doctor who agrees with my view of the dangers involved. And I certainly don't reject non-damaging treatment, which is why I'm taking these shots, even though I hate giving myself injections. But that's a small price balanced against the possibility of cancer.

November 8, 1986
New York City

If I am to put this all down in a way that is useful, I should start with the beginning of the story.

Sizable tumor in the right lobe of the liver, the doctors said. Lots of blood vessels in it means it's most likely malignant. Let's cut you open right now and see what we can do about it. Wait a minute, I said. I need to feel this thing out and see what's going on inside myself first, I said, needing some time to absorb the shock, time to assay the situation and not act out of panic. Not one of them said, I can respect that, but don't take too long about it.

Instead, that simple claim to my body's own processes elicited such an attack response from a reputable Specialist in Liver Tumors that my deepest—if not necessarily most useful—suspicions were totally aroused.

What that doctor could have said to me that I would have heard was, "You have a serious condition going on in your body and whatever you do about it you must not ignore it or delay deciding how you are going to deal with it because it will not go away no matter what you think it is." Acknowledging my responsibility for my own body. Instead, what he said to me was, "If you do not do exactly what I tell you to do right now without questions you are going to die a horrible death." In exactly those words.

I felt the battle lines being drawn up within my own body.

I saw this specialist in liver tumors at a leading cancer hospital in New York City, where I had been referred as an outpatient by my own doctor.

The first people who interviewed me in white coats from behind a computer were only interested in my health-care benefits and proposed method of payment. Those crucial facts determined what kind of plastic identification card I would be given, and without a plastic ID card, no one at all was allowed upstairs to see any doctor, as I was told by the uniformed, pistoled guards at all the stairwells.

From the moment I was ushered into the doctor's office and he saw my x-rays, he proceeded to infantilize me with an obviously well-practiced technique. When I told him I was having second thoughts about a liver biopsy, he glanced at my chart. Racism and Sexism joined hands across his table as he saw I taught at a university. "Well, you look like an *intelligent girl*," he said, staring at my one breast all the time he was speaking. "Not to have this biopsy immediately is like sticking your head in the sand." Then he went on to say that he would not be responsible when I wound up one day screaming in agony in the corner of his office!

I asked this specialist in liver tumors about the dangers of a liver biopsy spreading an existing malignancy, or even encouraging it in a borderline tumor. He dismissed my concerns with a wave of his hand, saying, instead of answering, that I really did not have any other sensible choice.

I would like to think that this doctor was sincerely motivated by a desire for me to seek what he truly believed to be the only remedy for my sickening body, but my faith in that scenario is considerably diminished by his 250-dollar consultation fee and his subsequent medical report to my own doctor containing numerous supposedly clinical observations of *obese abdomen* and *remaining pendulous breast*.

In any event, I can thank him for the fierce shard lancing through my terror that shrieked there must be some other way, this doesn't feel right to me. If this is cancer and they cut me open to find out, what is stopping that intrusive action from spreading the cancer, or turning a questionable mass into an active malignancy? All I was asking for was the reassurance of a realistic answer to my real questions, and that was not forthcoming. I made up my mind that if I was going to die in agony on somebody's office floor, it certainly wasn't going to be his! I needed information, and pored over books on the liver in Barnes & Noble's Medical Textbook Section on Fifth Avenue for hours. I learned, among other things, that the liver is the largest, most complex, and most generous organ in the human body. But that did not help me very much.

In this period of physical weakness and psychic turmoil, I found myself going through an intricate inventory of rage. First of all at my breast surgeon, had he perhaps done something wrong? How could such a small breast tumor have metastasized? Hadn't he assured me he'd gotten it all, and what was this now anyway about micro-metastases? Could this tumor in my liver have been seeded at the same time as my breast cancer? There were so many unanswered questions, and too much that I just did not understand.

But my worst rage was the rage at myself. For a brief time I felt like a total failure. What had I been busting my ass doing these past six years if it wasn't living and loving and working to my utmost potential? And wasn't that all a guarantee supposed to keep exactly this kind of thing from ever happening again? So what had I done wrong and what was I going to have to pay for it and WHY ME?

But finally a little voice inside me said sharply, "Now really, is there any other way you would have preferred living the past six years that would have been more satisfying? And be that as it may, *should* or *shouldn't* isn't even the question. How do you want to live the rest of your life from now on and what are you going to do about it?" Time's awasting!

Gradually, in those hours in the stacks of Barnes & Noble, I felt myself shifting into another gear. My resolve strengthened as my panic lessened. Deep breathing, regularly. I'm not going to let them cut into my body again until I'm convinced there is no other alternative. And this time, the burden of proof rests with the doctors because their record of success with liver cancer is not so good that it would make me jump at a surgical solution. And scare tactics are not going to work. I have been scared now for six years and that hasn't stopped me. I've given myself plenty of practice in doing whatever I need to do, scared or not, so scare tactics are just not going to work. Or I hoped they were not going to work. At any rate, thank the goddess, they were not working yet. One step at a time.

But some of my nightmares were pure hell, and I started having trouble sleeping.

In writing this I have discovered how important some things are that I thought were unimportant. I discovered this by the high price they exact for scrutiny. At first I did not want to look again at how I slowly came to terms with my own mortality on a level deeper than before, nor with the inevitable strength that it gave me as I started to get on with my life in actual time. Medical textbooks on the liver were fine, but there were appointments to be kept, and bills to pay, and decisions about my upcoming trip to Europe to be made. And what do I say to my children? Honesty has always been the bottom line between us, but did I really need them going through this with me during their final difficult years at college? On the other hand, how could I shut them out of this most important decision of my life?

I made a visit to my breast surgeon, a doctor with whom I have always been able to talk frankly, and it was from him that I got my first trustworthy and objective sense of timing. It was from him that I learned the conventional forms of treatment for liver metastases made little more than one year's difference in the survival rate. I heard my old friend Clem's voice coming back to me through the dimness of thirty years: "I see you coming here trying to make sense where there is no sense. Try just living in it. Respond, alter, see what happens." I thought of the African way of perceiving life, as experience to be lived rather than as a problem to be solved.

Homeopathic medicine calls cancer the cold disease. I understand that down to my bones that quake sometimes in their need for heat, for the sun, even for just a hot bath. Part of the way in which I am saving my own life is to refuse to submit my body to cold whenever possible.

In general, I fight hard to keep my treatment scene together in some coherent and serviceable way, integrated into my daily living and absolute. Forgetting is no excuse. It's as simple as one missed shot could make the difference between a quiescent malignancy and one that is growing again. This not only keeps me in an intimate, positive relationship to my own health, but it also underlines the fact that I have the responsibility for attending my own health. I cannot simply hand over that responsibility to anybody else.

Which does not mean I give in to the belief, arrogant or naive, that I know everything I need to know in order to make informed decisions about my body. But attending my own health, gaining enough information to help me understand and participate in the decisions made about my body by people who know more medicine than I do, are all crucial strategies in my battle for living. They also provide me with important prototypes for doing battle in all other arenas of my life.

Battling racism and battling heterosexism and battling apartheid share the same urgency inside me as battling cancer. None of these struggles is ever easy, and even the smallest victory is never to be taken for granted. Each victory must be applauded, because it is so easy not to battle at all, to just accept and call that acceptance inevitable.

And all power is relative. Recognizing the existence as well as the limitations of my own power, and accepting the responsibility for using it in my own behalf, involve me in direct and daily actions that preclude denial as a possible refuge. Simone de Beauvoir's words echo in my head: "It is in the recognition of the genuine conditions of our lives that we gain the strength to act and our motivation for change."

November 10, 1986
New York City

Building into my living—without succumbing to it—an awareness of this reality of my life, that I have a condition within my body of which I will eventually die, comes in waves, like a rising tide. It exists side by side with another force inside me that says no you don't, not you, and the x-rays are wrong and the tests are wrong and the doctors are wrong.

There is a different kind of energy inherent within each one of these feelings, and I try to reconcile and use these different energies whenever I need them. The energy generated by the first awareness serves to urge me always to get on with living my life and doing my work with an intensity and purpose of the urgent now. Throw the toys overboard, we're headed for the rougher waters.

The energies generated by the second force fuel a feisty determination to continue doing what I am doing forever. The tensions created inside me by the contradictions are another source of energy and learning. I have always known I learn my most lasting lessons about difference by closely attending the ways in which the differences in me lie together.

November 11, 1986
New York City

I keep observing how other people die, comparing, learning, critiquing the process inside of me, matching it up to how I would like to do it. And I think about this scrutiny of myself in the context of its usefulness to other Black women living with cancer, born and unborn.

I have a privileged life or else I would be dead by now. It is two and a half years since the first tumor in my liver was discovered. When I needed to know, there was no one around to tell me that there were alternatives to turning myself over to doctors who are terrified of not knowing everything. There was no one around to remind me that I have a right to decide what happens to my own body, not because I know more than anybody else, but simply because it is my body. And I have a right to acquire the information that can help me make those crucial decisions.

It was an accident of circumstance that brought me to Germany at a critical moment in my health, and another which introduced me to one holistic/homeopathic approach to the treatment of certain cancers. Not all homeopathic alternatives work for every patient. Time is a crucial element in the treatment of cancer, and I had to decide which chances I would take, and why.

I think of what this means to other Black women living with cancer, to all women in general. Most of all I think of how important it is for us to share with each other the powers buried within the breaking of silence about our bodies and our health, even though we have been schooled to be secret and stoical about pain and disease. But that stoicism and silence do not serve us nor our communities, only the forces of things as they are.

November 12, 1986
New York City

When I write my own Book of the Dead, my own Book of Life, I want to celebrate being alive to do it even while I acknowledge the painful savor uncertainty lends to my living. I use the energy of dreams that are now impossible, not totally believing in them nor their power to become real, but recognizing them as templates for a future within which my labors can play a part. I am freer to choose what I will devote my energies toward and what I will leave for another lifetime, thanking the goddess for the strength to perceive that I can choose, despite obstacles.

So when I do a reading to raise funds for the women's health collectives in Soweto, or to raise money for Kitchen Table: Women of Color Press, I am choosing to use myself for things in which I passionately believe. When I speak to rally support in the urgent war against apartheid in South Africa and the racial slaughter that is even now spreading across the U.S., when I demand justice in the police shotgun killing of a Black grandmother and lynchings in Northern California and in Central Park in New York City, I am making a choice of how I wish to use my power. This work gives me a tremendous amount of energy back in satisfaction and in belief, as well as in a vision of how I want this earth to be for the people who come after me.

When I work with young poets who are reaching for the power of their poetry within themselves and the lives they choose to live, I feel I am working to capacity, and this gives me deep joy, a reservoir of strength I draw upon for the next venture. Right now. This makes it far less important that it will not be forever. It never was.

The energies I gain from my work help me neutralize those implanted forces of negativity and self-destructiveness that are white america's way of making sure I keep whatever is powerful and creative within me unavailable, ineffective, and non-threatening.

But there is a terrible clarity that comes from living with cancer that can be empowering if we do not turn aside from it. What more can they do to me? My time is limited, and this is so for each one of us. So how will the opposition reward me for my silences? For the pretense that this is in fact the best of all possible worlds? What will they give me for lying? A lifelong Safe-Conduct Pass for everyone I love? Another lifetime for me? The end to racism? Sexism? Homophobia? Cruelty? The common cold?

November 13, 1986
New York City

I do not find it useful any longer to speculate upon cancer as a political weapon. But I'm not being paranoid when I say my cancer is as political as if some CIA agent brushed past me in the A train on March 15, 1965 and air-injected me with a long-fused cancer virus. Or even if it is only that I stood in their wind to do my work and the billows flayed me. What possible choices do most of us have in the air we breathe and the water we must drink?

Sometimes we are blessed with being able to choose the time and the arena and the manner of our revolution, but more usually we must do battle wherever we are standing. It does not matter too much if it is in the radiation lab or a doctor's office or the telephone company, the streets, the welfare department or the classroom. The real blessing is to be able to use whoever I am wherever I am, in concert with as many others as possible, or alone if needs be.

This is no longer a time of waiting. It is a time for the real work's urgencies. It is a time enhanced by iron reclamation of what I call the burst of light—that inescapable knowledge, in the bone, of my own physical limitations. Metabolized and integrated into the fabric of my days, that knowledge makes the particulars of what is coming seem less important. When I speak of wanting as much good time as possible, I mean time over which I maintain some relative measure of control.

In the following piece, another cancer survivor shares her story, offering courageous and triumphant words for black women confronting this disease.

On Cancer and Conjuring
Janis Coombs Epps

Words are to be taken seriously. I try to take seriously acts of language. Words set things in motion. I've seen them doing it. Words set up atmospheres, electrical fields, charges. I've felt them doing it. Words conjure.[1]

Cancer is a conjuring word. Perhaps that is why my doctor did not use the word cancer when explaining my condition. Rather she told me, "Your results indicate a gross malignancy on the lower portion of your colon." I couldn't believe what she was saying.

Is she telling me that I have cancer?

"Your tests indicate that the tumor is several centimeters and is located in the lower segment of the bowel," she continued, drawing a pencil sketch of the colon which to me looked like a curvy snake poised to strike.

Is she telling me that I have cancer?

I was only sure when she began asking questions about how often I had seen blood in my stool, and whether it was bright red or dark red. I was a thirty-three-year-old Black woman in my prime. I was sassy, and thought I was fine! I was a dissertation away from a doctoral degree and was a college professor. I applauded myself for owning my own home, and single-handedly raising two bright, beautiful children after a tumultuous divorce; I also had a steady boyfriend who treated me like royalty.

Now, some Black woman doctor no older than I was saying something about an operation that might save my life and tumors and malignancies and carcinomas.

But all I heard was the conjuring word cancer. Pictures of things dark and evil-spirited possessed me. Images of withered, skeletal fingers. Empty eyes in deep hollow sockets. Decay. Death. Cancer. I couldn't get the word out of my head. Over and over again I repeated the word silently. And every time I heard it, it was as if two great clashing cymbals collided next to my eardrum, and every vibration was a reiteration of cancer, cancer, cancer, cancer until the sound was small and weak and barely audible. But then the clash would come again crashing thunderously throughout my being. The word and its reality engulfed me. I sat motionless in the middle of my hospital bed with tears streaming down my cheeks. God had played a dirty trick on me. I had cancer and I was going to die.

As my doctor talked on, matter-of-factly, about "my disease" and the possibility that I might well have to have a colostomy, I became silently hysterical. The tears would not stop! The room was spinning! Every now and then I would catch a phrase—artificial anus—an incision from the colon through the wall of the abdomen. Inside I was screaming, trying to drown out her words. Perhaps if I did not hear them, their reality would go away. Surely God was paying me back for some terrible sin I had committed. I couldn't think of what it could be, but he knew how vain I was, how important it was for me to be considered pretty. And now this doctor was talking about my wearing a hideous bag for the rest of my life—a disgusting thing to be worn on the outside of my body to hold my bodily waste.

This lady can't be for real.

For the next few days I was in shock. Not the stupefied shock of silence, but the shock of mindless chatter that hides what is really on one's mind. For some reason it was important to me that I appear normal and in control (most likely because I felt so abnormal and out of control). When a visitor would ask, "How are you doing?" I could hear my voice, well-modulated and in control say, "Just fine. The doctor says that the tumor is malignant, but once it is removed I should be fine."

That is what my voice said. But the ticker tape inside my head was saying,

I've got cancer and I'm going to die, so get the f— out of my face asking me how I'm doing!

I was angry with the world and more than anything I wanted to be alone in my misery.

In fact, as I look back to that time, I am sure that I needed to be alone. Fundamentally, I am a loner anyway, although I am also a mother, daughter, sister, friend and teacher. I spend my free time engrossed between the covers of a book, or scribbling away madly in a notebook, or sitting mesmerized by a movie in a darkened theater. So the way I live my life is the way I chose to handle its tragedy—alone. Other cancer victims, like Audre Lorde, have said that "each woman responds to the crisis that (breast) cancer brings to her life out of a whole pattern, which is the design of who she is and how her life has been lived. The weave of her everyday existence is the training ground for how she handles crisis."[2]

Whenever I am in a crisis state I have a need to curl up in the fetal position and think—or not think. It is the way I heal myself. Being in a hospital was at odds with my own healing methodology; for hospitals don't allow for aloneness. Someone is always coming to take temperatures, test urine, take blood and give shots. Doctors make rounds, friends visit, families hold hands and love you. I needed time to myself to comfort me.

But how do you tell those who love you, who are going through their own pain at the thought of losing you, that at such a critical time you don't want their physical presence? You don't tell them. Instead you act pleased that they are there offering their support. You chat courteously with the hospital staff. You welcome friends—always smiling and talking, but never mentioning the word, cancer.

Secretly I wished they would all go away. That I could throw the flowers and the dish gardens through the hospital windows. That I could strut down that hospital hall with my hands on my hips and indiscriminately curse anybody who happened to get in my way. I needed to be loud and boisterous like drunk women I have seen standing in alley ways. I didn't need anybody's pity, and I needed to show myself that I was in charge of my own life. I wanted to point my finger and shake my head and shout that cancer didn't rule me. I was mad!

But cancer is a conjuring word with powers of its own. And it didn't care whether I was mad or not. It was out to get me. Either I had the operation, or I died.

I am told that the doctors wrestled seven hours in the operating room seizing and removing the power that cancer had over my colon. Still they were not sure. So radiation and chemotherapy were scheduled. "Not immediately," I heard them say. "When she has been released from the hospital and is stronger."

My memories of the six weeks I was hospitalized following the surgery are vague, partially due to the drugs I was taking and partially because I have chosen to forget. I can remember vaguely the sensation of hips numbed by numerous injections. I'd ring the bell for the nurse. "Is it time for my shot yet?" I'd ask anxiously. "Not yet. In a little while. Just hold on," the white-clad figure would say.

Please bring my shot. I can deal with the pain from the surgery, but I need the shot to anesthesize my brain, so I don't have to think anymore.

But that is all I did—think. I cannot count the number of times I feigned sleep so I would not have to talk with anyone. Excuses were made for my rudeness when I ignored family and friends. A psychiatrist was called in because my depression was so severe. He was a kind, sensitive man who told me in a quiet way that I must eventually accept and deal with the fact that I had cancer. I said, "I know you're right. I must plan for my life and for my death." But inside I thought,

You must be out of your mind if you think I'm going to accept this shit! You say I have cancer, I say I had cancer.

I think the real story of the healing process of my bout with cancer starts here—whether to allow the conjuring powers of the word CANCER to possess and define me. I could either live my life as a cancer victim, making all my decisions based on that reality, or I would press on with my life as I was accustomed to living it. If I could control nothing else in my world, I would at least control the way I thought.

From the moment I truly realized that I might die, or might possibly spend the rest of my days with a bag hooked to my side, I felt totally out of control—as if some force outside of myself was determining my destiny. Of course, that is always the way it is. We are never totally in charge. But when we are healthy we rarely consider the role of fate in our lives. We make our own decisions and take charge of our lives, so we think. After my operation it was clear that "the others" had wrestled control of my reality, so it appeared. I ate and got out of bed on their schedule, had to be helped to the bathroom, and I was told that I was not to walk the halls alone because I was too weak. I appeared to be a good patient, doing exactly what they asked. But all of the time I was going deeper into myself. For the six weeks I was hospitalized I did not look at a complete television program, I did not read a book; I did not thumb through a magazine. I simply lay there. It was my way of rebelling. "They" might control my physical reality, but "they" could not control the me that dwelled deep within.

I began to see a duality at work in my life. I could talk to everybody on one level and think my own thoughts on another level. I had stumbled upon a way to deal with the horrors that were happening to my body. I saw myself as being separate from my body. "Janis, we can't find out why your temperature is so high. Another operation may be necessary."

Fine. I'm not really here. This is just my body.

Janis, you're losing so much weight we may have to put a hole in your shoulder and feed you through a tube.

Hey knock yourself out. This ain't really me.

Janis, just to make sure that we got it all, you will have to take chemotherapy treatments for six months.

So what. This is just my flesh.

Most of the time I was scared, but I could deal with the fear by not defining myself as this cancerous bed-ridden specimen. The real me was unaffected.

Once I had worked out the distinction between my body and the real me, my greatest challenge became the thought of losing my children. Of all the things in the universe, I love my children most. So I made numerous bargains with God that if I was allowed to live to see them reach adulthood I would become the "perfect" person. My greatest fear was that my bargain would not be honored, and my children would not have me. I was sure that they would be loved and taken care of, but they wouldn't have me. They would not be privy to my thoughts, my ideas, my guidance. I knew that nobody could raise them like I could.

As my three-year-old daughter sat on my lap on Sunday during visitation hours, I became so choked up I could not speak. I could not leave her. She was too little to be motherless. My ten-year-old son was in the joke-telling phase of childhood, and seemed oblivious to my gloomy mood. He was simply happy that he and I could hug each other and spend some time together. He continued to tell one joke after the other and to laugh hysterically after each. As I half listened to "Why did the chicken cross the road? To get to the other side. Yuk! Yuk!" I knew that he would make it—even without me. He had my strength and sensitivity, and to my way of thinking he had been exposed to me long enough for me to be imprinted in every sinew of his character. I did not feel that I had, as yet, imprinted myself on my daughter in the same way. I couldn't let go. I had so much more love to give.

There is not much more to tell. I did not have to have the feared colostomy. But there was another operation, radiation and chemotherapy. But those were things that happened to my body, not to me.

In retrospect, I do not know how much of what I remember is colored by my understanding of my reality at the time. I live daily with the thought of death—that the silent thing will overtake me and I will be no more, but I am no longer afraid to say the word cancer.

It has been several years since my trauma—strong, healthy years. Years that I have watched my toddler turn into a little girl, a little girl who acts a lot like me. Years that have seen my little boy grow into adolescence and become more his own person. In some ways, I am more serene and calm and at peace with myself, having faced the reality of my own mortality. In other ways, I am more frenzied and anxious to get on with life.

I am thankful for the love and support of my mother, father and sister, and for my friends who always saw me as whole and complete—and for the cadre of Black doctors who not only took care of me, but continue to love me.

Cancer is indeed a conjuring word. But its power comes from our fear. I have faced death and I know when my time comes, whether I am stalked slowly by cancer, or hit swiftly by a Mack truck, I am clear. Those are things that might happen to my body, but my spirit will rise victorious.

Footnotes

1. Toni Cade Bambara, "What It Is I Think I'm Doing Anyhow," *The Writer On Her Work*, ed. Janet Sternberger (New York: W.W. Norton & Co.; 1980), p. 63.

2. Audre Lorde, *The Cancer Journals* (San Francisco: Spinsters/Aunt Lute, 1980), p. 9.

Despite all the stumbling blocks in their path, black women interested in becoming physicians have historically managed to achieve their goals. Perhaps their desire to comfort and heal can be traced back to the slave era, when black women passed their remedies and treatments from generation to generation.

In the following piece, a recent medical school graduate writes about several early black women doctors. Facing blatant racism and discrimination at every turn, these women nonetheless acquired the skills and training to improve the health of their community. Acknowledgement of their tireless efforts is long overdue.

Surpassing Obstacles: Pioneering Black Women Physicians
Melissa Blount

Black women have played a part in the medical profession since the Emancipation Proclamation was signed in 1863. The first black woman to receive a medical degree was Rebecca Lee, who graduated from the New England Female Medical College in Boston in 1864, only fifteen years after Elizabeth Blackwell became the first woman to graduate from an American medical school. Other early black graduates included Rebecca Cole, who received a degree from the Woman's Medical College of Pennsylvania in 1867, and Susan McKinney Steward, who graduated from the New York Medical College and Hospital for Women in 1870.[1] By 1890, according to a census, black women physicians numbered 115, or 2.6 percent of all women physicians.[2]

To be successful in this demanding career at that time, women needed superior education as well as family influence and support. Dr. Carolina Still Anderson studied at private schools before she entered Oberlin College in 1864 at age fifteen.[3] After she graduated from the Woman's Medical College in 1878, she applied to the New England Hospital for Women and Children for an internship. She was refused by the board of physicians "because of her race." The board of management, however, voted unanimously to instate her, and she was able to complete her internship.

Obstacles to Success

A major obstacle black women faced in becoming physicians was their difficulty securing internships. As Dr. Isabella Vandervall explained in 1917, the new law of compulsory internship presented "an almost insurmountable barrier to black women physicians." She told of her own struggles and humiliations in trying to obtain internships at various hospitals. The law, she said:

> ... casts a serious reflection upon those white people—democratic and philanthropic Americans—who lavishly endow colleges and hospitals and allow colored girls to enter and finish their college courses, and yet, when one steps forward to keep pace with her white sisters and to qualify before the state in order that she might do same services for her colored sisters that the white woman does for hers, those patriotic Americans figuratively wave the stars and stripes in her face and literally say to her: "What do you want, you woman of the dark skin! Halt! You cannot advance any further! Retreat! You are colored! Retreat!"[4]

Dr. Vandervall was angry because she could not acquire a license to practice in Pennsylvania. Similarly, Dr. Dorothy Boulding Ferebee, after graduating from Tufts University School of Medicine in 1924, encountered great difficulty in finding internship training. Only after she placed first in a competitive examination was she appointed to an internship in a government hospital.[5]

Making it difficult or nearly impossible for blacks to obtain residency positions was one way of excluding them from the medical profession. Generally, only black hospitals admitted Negro doctors seeking to complete their training. In a study conducted in 1927, only twenty-one of 1,696 hospitals employed black interns and of these, fourteen treated only black patients.[6] In addition, many black physicians had limited privileges at private hospitals. If surgery was indicated, black physicians had to turn their patients over to white doctors. Dr. Edna L. Griffin, who served Mexican and black patients in Pasadena, California, also recalls that the hospitals where she worked would either refuse to admit black patients or, if they were admitted, insist on keeping them in private rooms. This practice was seen as late as the 1960s.[7]

Besides the obstacles to obtaining residency posts, black women were discriminated against in appointments to administrative positions. Moreover, according to Mary S. Macy, "no colored medical women belonged to southern belt state medical societies"; she suspected that these organizations excluded colored women from membership.[8] Ms. Macy's suspicions were probably correct—the National Medical Association was established in 1895 because blacks were ignored by the American Medical Association. Barring black physicians from professional association membership prevented them from getting top positions since many hospital appointments were open only to members of the county medical societies. It was not until black doctors picketed the AMA's 1963 convention that things began to change.[9]

May Edward Chinn and Lena Edwards

Early black women physicians were very dedicated to their profession, expecting little in the way of monetary reward. A classic story of the struggles of black women is the narrative of Dr. May Edward Chinn.

Born in 1896, Dr. Chinn lived in poverty as a child, but her mother had an unwavering desire to see her daughter educated. With her mother's help, Dr. Chinn was able to attend Columbia University. Growing up in New York City during the Harlem Renaissance, Dr. Chinn wanted to study music. The attitude of a prejudiced professor, however, discouraged her from pursuing musical studies. After struggling through his class and learning that she would have to take five more courses with him, she decided to consider other fields.

Because of a childhood sickness and the scarcity of doctors in Harlem, she changed her major to the sciences. This was a high goal since, in 1920, there were only sixty-five black women physicians in the country. After receiving her degree from Columbia Teachers College, Dr. Chinn became the first black woman to graduate from Bellevue Hospital Medical College. She was also the first black woman intern at Harlem Hospital and the first woman ever to ride ambulances on emergency calls.

Because no private hospitals in New York gave black physicians admitting privileges, Dr. Chinn set up private practice with seven other doctors. Her patients included an order of black nuns and several prostitutes whom she charged minimal fees. She described how poor black women came to her with frostbite and pneumonia, their reward for standing in the cold and rain waiting for someone to pick them out of the crowd of maids lined up at 67th Street and Jerome Avenue. Of course, they could not pay her.

Because of conditions around her, Dr. Chinn chose to continue her education and obtained a degree in public health, so that she could "attack some of these problems on a bigger than one-to-one basis." Dr. Chinn also took up the study of cancer, looking for ways to detect it in its early stages, after her mother died of the disease. Because of her commitment to service, Dr. Chinn is something of a legend in Harlem to this day.[10]

Like Dr. Chinn, Dr. Lena Edwards was dedicated to serving whoever needed her help. After receiving her medical degree from Howard University in 1924, she went on to train in obstetrics and gynecology. She was teaching at Howard in 1960 when her son, a priest, convinced her to become a missionary to migrant workers in Texas. She took the job because she felt that "after God had given me six children and they had done so well, I was going to try to help somebody who had not had such an opportunity. Those of us who have shouldn't forget the fellow who has not."[11]

With this thought in mind and heart, she set out for the migrant labor camp. She was so appalled at the women's obstetrical problems and the high pre- and postnatal mortality rate that she helped to build a two-story clinic for mothers, donating 14,500 dollars of her own funds. After an article about Dr. Edwards appeared in *Ebony* in 1962, President Kennedy appointed her to the Federal Advisory Council on Employment Security. In 1964, she was awarded the Presidential Medal of Freedom by President Johnson. Like Dr. Chinn, Dr. Edwards has a list of honors, awards and accomplishments that fills several pages.[12]

Continuing Discrimination

Black women who entered the medical profession in later years continued to encounter problems. Dr. Dorothy Brown, a general surgeon in Tennessee, graduated from Meharry Medical College in 1948 and interned at Harlem Hospital. When she sought a residency at Harlem Hospital, however, she was refused, an incident demonstrating that much of the prejudice black women faced was due to sexism. To complete her training, Dr. Brown returned to Meharry, and even there had to prove her capability as a surgeon. She recalled one night when the chief resident had just completed the last of a series of emergency cases with her. When another suddenly came up, he told her he couldn't go on. She advised him to get some rest and said she would handle the case by herself. "Since that episode, my word to women students is that when you pass through the doors at seven or eight in the morning, you are not a woman, you're a doctor."

Dr. Brown later became chief surgical resident at Meharry, where, as part of her job, she operated on poor risk cases. An older patient who was diagnosed as having a ruptured appendix was dismayed to learn that Dr. Brown would be doing the surgery. He refused her services, saying that she was just a little girl and didn't know what she was doing. She bowed out and let the male assistants prepare him for surgery. "I just waited until he got to the operating room, then I operated on him. . . . I told him afterward."[13]

Researcher Dorothy Mandelbaum believes that people who come from poor families, as Dr. Brown did, have an inner urge that causes them to persist and overcome obstacles. She cites as an example, a black physician who had been invited to watch an operation, but was told by the doorman to go around to the clinic entrance. As she started forward, he tried to stop her and she threatened to have him arrested for assault if he persisted. She added, "You'd play a game with them after a while. You'd walk down the hall and somebody'd be running after you. . . and when you got to the elevator, you'd smile. That was my way."[14]

To become a doctor, a woman must have great determination. Dr. Yvonne Hines, a dermatologist, feels that "prejudice and racial discrimination are a means to keep minorities and women away from desirable positions." You must believe in yourself, she says, because people will try to "turn you around." An extreme example is that of a black woman physician who went to Marion County, Alabama to serve as the new director of their Public Health Medical Center in 1978. The Ku Klux Klan threatened her, burned a cross on her lawn, and finally set fire to her house when she didn't leave. Fearing for the safety of her children, she decided it wasn't wise to stay. As she was preparing to go, however, the local newspaper ran a page of petitions asking her to stay, since her dedication and clinical expertise were obvious. She did and had no future problems.[15]

Discouragement has not always been so severe. The family and teachers of Dr. Leona Edwards, a Phi Beta Kappa at Howard University, advised her not to set her goals too high. But she was determined to persevere and entered Howard Medical College in 1958.[16] Dr. Edwards stressed how women have been made to feel guilty for having a career and a family. Dr. Edith Irby, the first black to graduate from a white southern medical school, contended that "the major problem women doctors have probably is in having families and rearing children."[17] Dr. Edwards felt that if the extended training schedule had not existed when she was a resident, she might never have completed her training. The program enabled her to finish her training in twice the time it would normally take, allowing her more time to spend with her husband and son. Dr. Edwards has seen some women quit to save their marriages and after all those years they "wind up as a lab assistant or something—what a waste!"[18]

Many women don't even make it that far. Dr. Marion Fay, president and dean of the Woman's Medical College in 1964, blamed high school counselors for not encouraging black women to enter medicine.[19] "The idea that medicine and matrimony can't mix is presented as an established truth. A realistic picture needs to be presented," she said. Carol Lopate summed it up when she explained, "The scarcity of female as well as male medical students from lower class and rural areas is not only a result of inadequate finances, but also a lack of stimulation and encouragement in the home and at school."[20]

Moreover, many black students cannot finance a medical education. Grants have not always been available and blacks have been affected disproportionately by government cutbacks. "Sex and color used to have a lot to do with it, but not any longer. The problem is mainly economic and educational deprivation," commented Dr. Elizabeth Davis of Harlem Hospital.[21]

Breaking the Last Barriers

Black women have traditionally entered such primary care specialties as pediatrics, psychiatry and internal medicine, where they encountered little resistance. But if a woman tried to enter a male-dominated specialty like surgery, few positions were available. Slowly, this has begun to change. Dr. Jeanne Sinkford, for example, became one of the few black women dentists at a time when women made up less than one percent of the total. She graduated at the top of her class and went on to become the first woman associate dean of Howard University's College of Dentistry.

Because the number of black dentists has been decreasing since 1930, Dr. Sinkford has encouraged black women to consider this profession. She has advised students that "it takes a lot for a woman to be in a top position, particularly in a male profession. You have to be better to be accepted as equal. Once your colleagues accept you as a competent person, they don't mind your being there."[22] Dr. Hines, the dermatologist, echoes her sentiments: "Once you know your stuff thoroughly, they can't touch you."

Dr. Clotilde Dent Brown is another woman who broke into a male-dominated field. Dr. Brown was the first black woman to become a colonel in the U.S. Army. She found that her sex handicapped her more than her race, but she was determined to succeed.

"A Negro woman can make whites respect her abilities," she said. "People who scream prejudice and give up could never have made it anyway."[23]

Dr. Angela Ferguson, one of many black women researchers and an authority on sickle cell anemia, has received certificates of merit from the AMA for her work.[24] Black women have also begun to secure top positions in administration. Dr. Mildred Bateman became the first black to head a state mental health department in the United States. Dr. Helen Octavia Dickens was named director of obstetrics and gynecology at Mercy Douglass Hospital in 1948 and became chief of obstetrics and gynecology at Woman's Hospital in Philadelphia in 1956.[25] Dr. Jane Cooke Wright, a highly respected surgeon and researcher in cancer chemotherapy, was named associate dean of New York Medical College in 1967.

Black women have made enormous strides in medicine and shall continue to do so. We must learn from the past while dealing with the present. The more we strive to accomplish as individuals, the more obstacles we will overcome.

Footnotes

1. "Dr. Rebecca Lee, First Woman Medical Graduate," *Bulletin of Medico-Chirurgical Society of the District of Columbia*, 6 (1949) : 3.

2. L.M. Holloway, "O Pioneer!" *Philadelphia Medicine*, 71 (1975): 407–411.

3. M.J. Jerrido, "Early Black Women Physicians," *Women's Health*, 5 (1980): 1–3.

4. I. Vandervall, "Some Problems of the Colored Woman Physician," *Woman's Medical Journal*, 27 (1917): 156–158.

5. J.L. Brodie, "Dorothy Boulding Ferebee, MD," *Journal of the American Medical Women's Association*, 15 (1960): 1095, and J.H. Roy, "Pinpoint portrait of Dr. Dorothy Boulding Ferebee," *Negro History Bulletin*, 25 (1962): 160.

6. B. Van Hoosen, "Opportunities for Medical Women as Interns," *Medical Woman's Journal*, 34 (1927): 138–139.

7. H.K. Branson, "The Doctor from Meharry," *Medical Woman's Journal*, 52 (1945): 36–37 and "The Plight of the Black Doctor," *Time* , 92 (1968): 46–47.

8. M.S. Macy, "The Field for Women of Today in Medicine," *Woman's Medical Journal*, 27 (1914): 49–58.

9. "The Plight of the Black Doctor," op.cit.

10. G. Davis, "A Healing Hand in Harlem," *New York Times Magazine* (22 April 1979), pp. 40–68.

11. S.A. Scally, "Dr. Lena Edwards: People Lover," *Negro History Bulletin*, 39 (1976): 592–595.

12. "Lady Doctor to Migrant Workers," *Ebony*, 17 (1962): 59–68.

13. E. Levy and M. Miller, "Dorothy Brown: A Doctor for the People," *Ms.*, 6 (1978): 65–68.

14. D.R. Mandelbaum, *Work, Marriage and Motherhood*, (New York: Praeger, 1981), pp. 69–70.

15. F. Sihora, "Three Strikes is Not Always Out," *Ebony*, 34 (1979): 44.

16. J. Robbins, "More than a Mother," *Redbook*, 33 (1969): 90–91, 134–137.

17. "Edith Irby Revisited," *Ebony*, 18 (1963): 52–58.

18. J. Robbins, op.cit.

19. "Outstanding Women Doctors," *Ebony*, 19 (1964): 68–72.

20. C. Lopate, *Women in Medicine*, (Baltimore: Johns Hopkins University Press, 1968), p. 49.

21. "Outstanding Women Doctors," op.cit.

22. "Howard's First Lady of Dentistry," *Ebony*, 23 (1968): 103–108.

23. "The Colonel is a Lady," *Ebony*, 24 (1968): 100–108.

24. "1962 Medical Women of the Year," *Journal of the American Medical Women's Association*, 18 (1963): 81–88.

25. "New Day, New Doctor," *Ebony*, 19 (1964): 27–35.

In January 1989, in a special issue on the health of black Americans, the Journal of the American Medical Association reported the following distressing statistics: While representing about twelve percent of the nation's population, blacks comprise only six percent of the total U.S. medical school enrollment, five percent of medical school graduates, five percent of postgraduate trainees, three percent of physicians in practice and two percent of medical school faculties. Of the nation's 585,597 physicians a mere 3,250, or less than one percent are black females, according to the AMA.

After a steady rise in the 1970s, the number of black applicants to medical schools peaked in 1981 at about 2,600. Since then there has been a steady decline in the number of black applicants and black students admitted to U.S. medical schools. Several factors, including drastic cutbacks in federal aid and affirmative action programs, the deterioration of urban schools, an increased interest in other careers, perceptions of racism and the mercenary image of the medical establishment, have made medicine a less attractive career choice for blacks.

At the same time that blacks are steering clear of medicine, there is an increasing demand for black physicians. In the face of AIDS, soaring infant mortality rates and the scourge of crack cocaine, more black physicians than ever are needed to provide quality care for urban communities whose residents have historically received substandard treatment and lacked adequate access to medical care.

To successfully complete medical school, one needs strong will, determination and sustained support from many quarters. For the black female who chooses medicine as a career there can be many challenges, but also many rewards, as the following article illustrates.

On Becoming a Physician: A Dream Not Deferred
Vanessa Northington Gamble

I felt great comfort as I walked down Peach Street. I had spent so much of my life on this narrow street of well-maintained rowhouses in West Philadelphia. My mother's family had owned a home here since 1928. After my parents separated, my sister, my mother and I had come here to live with my grandmother for two years. Until I was an adolescent, I spent every weekend here. My grandmother, Cora Northington, was a short, chubby woman with a hearty laugh. She was a storefront minister and a medium who held seances every Friday evening in her home. She also gave private readings. People in the neighborhood who had problems sought out Mother Northington for her advice. "Nanny, there's a lady to see you," my sister and I would announce, embarrassed. We did not believe in spirits and certainly did not think that they could offer guidance and protection to the living.

Whenever I had troubles, I too would come visit my grandmother. I would tell her my problem and she would offer me stern advice, strong arms, and plenty of good food. "I love to see a child eat," she would say. I listened, especially when it came to sweet potato pie. After spending time with my grandmother, my burdens always seemed lighter.

As I walked down Peach Street on this winter day to visit my sister, I was very troubled, but both my grandmother and mother were gone. My mother had died only two months previously. I now found myself depressed and plagued with self-doubt. I wondered whether I was going to be able to finish medical school.

A neighbor called to me. I knew most of the residents of the street. As a child, I had played under their watchful eyes. My achievements had become a source of pride for them. When I had graduated from college, the neighbors had taken up a collection to give me a communal gift. The elderly woman who summoned me had been a friend of both my mother and grandmother and I had known her all my life. She wanted to know how I was doing. I lied and told her that all was well. She knew better and started talking to me about the importance of faith. "I remember when you were a little girl and you'd be playing in the street and your grandmother would say, 'My baby's going to be a doctor when she grows up.' I didn't believe her, of course. But your grandmother certainly did believe that that was going to happen." She wanted me to remember how firmly my mother and grandmother had believed in my dream of becoming a physician. I was not to lose that faith. I needed her reassuring words. They felt warm, welcoming and familiar. I pictured my grandmother, sitting in her rocking chair, telling me, as I had heard so many times, "Sugar, everything will be just fine." I could also hear her pointedly saying, "Spirits *do* protect loved ones."

I think often of this story. It explains to me the essence of how I, a black woman from an inner-city neighborhood of West Philadelphia, beat the odds and achieved my dream. I had unwavering family support. My mother and grandmother cherished and fought for my dream. When they were gone, there was always someone in my life who carried on their work. I was reminded of my dream and never lost sight of it.

My mother, Carrissa Northington Gamble, had always held before me and my sister visions of a better life. She raised me with the belief that, despite any roadblocks, the path to my becoming a physician would be made clear—even if she herself had to remove the obstacles. My mother was a beautiful, vivacious woman. My sister and I were the center of her life. She was not, however, an overly indulgent parent. She enforced a strict code of conduct which included, "I don't want any babies brought into this house!" She believed that my sister and I should be able to take care of ourselves. "I'm not raising any ornaments," she would proclaim. She also let us know that she would help us in any way she could. "As long as I have a dime, you and Karen each have a nickel," she reassured us.

My mother's oft-spoken motto was, "My kids are going to make it." This motto was translated into action, especially when it came to education. She once used her savvy to con the school system into approving my transfer to a junior high school outside of my assigned district. She did not want me to attend the one in the neighborhood because she thought it academically inferior. This was at the height of the civil rights movement.

Initially, my request to attend the school with the better curriculum was denied. "That's okay," my mother told the principal. "My lawyer will see about it." My mother did not have a lawyer, but I got my transfer.

I decided at the age of six that I wanted to be a physician. I do not exactly remember how my dream came about. I think I realized that medicine was a high-status, financially rewarding profession. As I saw it, medicine was the pinnacle of success in American society. And my mother and grandmother had always encouraged me to be ambitious and shoot for the stars. Also, if I could become a physician, my family could escape West Philadelphia. I wanted to buy them a big house with lots of land.

Medicine would also fulfill my need to be independent. I saw my mother go through a series of marginal, low-paying jobs such as catering assistant and clothes presser. I also saw her involved with men, including my father, who were not very dependable. I remember her anxiously waiting for the child support check which often did not come. "Vanessa, go down to Nanny's; she has a ham waiting for us so we can have something for dinner." I did not want to be like my mother—I wanted to be able to support myself. My mother's brother once articulated this necessity to me. "You go on and get an education and become a doctor. I don't want you to be like your mother—having to depend on some guy. If a man doesn't treat you well, I want you to be able to say bye-bye blackbird."

Regardless of the origin of the dream, throughout childhood and adolescence I led my life with the single-minded determination to become a physician. I asked for, and received, toy chemistry sets and microscopes as Christmas presents. I worked as a student volunteer in a hospital. I voraciously read science books and biographies of physicians, all of whom were white. Nonetheless, I found inspiration in the stories of women physicians such as Elizabeth Blackwell, the first woman to graduate from an American medical school, and Emily Dunning Barringer, New York City's first woman ambulance surgeon. Their struggles and achievements told me that I too could reach my goal. I was never sidetracked by the fact that I did not see a black woman physician until I was fifteen.

My dream received universal support and encouragement. No one questioned or ridiculed it. Friends of my mother would proudly say, "Vanessa is going to be a neurosurgeon like Ben Casey when she grows up." My family physician, Dr. Maceo Morris, also supported my goals. Dr. Morris, an elderly black man, would say, "You're going to be a doctor. Don't let anyone tell you you're going to be a nurse."

I was not a wide-eyed dreamer. I knew that grit and talent were not enough. This fact became traumatically clear when I saw a former classmate nodding out on the corner. I knew that he was as bright as I and once had as much promise as I. In elementary school, he and I used to compete against each other for the best grades. He was now a junkie and I was working to become a doctor. The episode made me realize that despair and poverty of the spirit were abundant in my community and how incredibly lucky I had been to have been raised on such a caring, loving street.

I took a giant step toward my goal during my years at the Philadelphia High School for Girls, an academically prestigious magnet school. At Girls' High, I enrolled in advanced science courses and joined the Future Physicians of America Club. I also took four years of Latin because I thought that all doctors needed to know it. When I graduated in 1970, I was class president, a *summa cum laude*, and the winner of the Latin prize.

The years at Girls' High were significant. I became a staunch believer in its distinctly feminist ethos—"A Girls' High girl can do anything." The school taught us that we should not set limits on our lives because we were female. I also discovered that I could excel in an academically rigorous, predominantly white environment. I had also obtained unassailable credentials to enter college.

I chose to go to Hampshire College, a new, experimental school that was scheduled to open in Amherst, Massachusetts, in September 1970. Hampshire's innovative, interdisciplinary curriculum attracted me. Besides, the college appealed to my pioneering spirit. I would be a member of a college's first graduating class. Today, I chalk it up to youthful idealism.

I almost did not make it to Hampshire. Three weeks before I was to enter, my mother tried to kill herself. I was sleeping and heard the doorbell ring. I thought that it was part of my dream. Then I heard a glass break and woke up to find my father and a family friend carrying my mother's limp body out of the door. "Vanessa, pills." I was left alone, not knowing whether she was dead or alive. My mother recovered, but I do not know what precipitated the crisis. Perhaps a failed relationship. Perhaps the stress of raising two children on her own. I thought it was because I was going to leave home. Though my mother demanded that I go to college, I nonetheless realized that my foundation in life would be more unsteady. I was not going to be able to lean on my mother as much as I had in the past. I was going to have to be more self-reliant.

Once in college, I almost did not stay. During my first semester, my mother tried to kill herself again. My guilt was overwhelming, but my family continued to insist that I stay and I did. They thought that my mother's depression would worsen if I left school because of her. My mother's psychological burdens eventually did lighten and my life at college became less difficult. Throughout these crises, my mother constantly spoke of her hope that I would become a physician. Our dreams had become inextricably linked.

At Hampshire, I gained a new perspective on American medicine. I began to view medicine in its broader context as a system that reflected the social, economic and political views of the wider society. In addition to my medical school requirements, I took courses in medical sociology, medical economics, public health and comparative health systems. This growing interest in the social aspects of American medicine was reflected in my senior project. I wrote a history of the infamous Tuskegee Syphilis Study. The study, conducted by the United States Public Health Service from 1932 to 1972, allowed more than four hundred poor black farmers to go untreated for syphilis without their knowledge. Their participation in the study

directly contributed to the deaths of several of the men. I was outraged. I learned that medicine, considered a neutral clinical science
by many, reflected the racist views of American society. It was a lesson that I was not to forget.

Although Hampshire had a non-traditional curriculum, I gained
admission to several medical schools and decided to attend the University of Pennsylvania. I wanted to continue my work in social
medicine, and Penn's M.D.-Ph.D. program would allow me to go to
medical school and complete graduate work in the social sciences.
The most compelling reason, however, for my return to Philadelphia
was personal. My mother needed me. After winning her battle with
mental illness, she faced a new foe—breast cancer.

I was painfully aware of the havoc that breast cancer could
wreak. Two years earlier, in 1972, it had killed my grandmother. I
was the one who had brought her disease to the attention of my family. "Nanny, what is that," I asked, pointing to the large ulcer on her
left breast. "Nothing, sugar." I knew better. I had seen her adminis-
tering salve to the wound. I told my mother. My grandmother was
reluctant to seek treatment, but eventually relented. I don't know
why she hesitated, but the diagnosis was the one that she feared. I
watched the chubby, strong woman become a thin, frail invalid.

A few months after my grandmother died, my mother found a
small lump in her right breast. She was forty-three. She had a radical
mastectomy and started chemotherapy. It was not her first encounter
with cancer. At the age of twenty-nine she had had a hysterectomy
for cervical cancer. When I saw her in her hospital bed after her
breast surgery, she looked so vulnerable. I waited before I walked
in. She was talking to a doctor, a psychiatrist, it turned out. After he
left, she and I had a long conversation. Her mood was better than I
had expected. She said that she was not going to let this disease
knock her down. The woman who had twice tried to kill herself, now
adamantly embraced life. She wanted to live. She had an excellent
prognosis. None of her lymph nodes were positive for cancer and no
evidence of metastasis was found. Despite her good spirits and
rapid recovery, I felt an obligation to return home. My mother was
alone now. My grandmother was dead and my sister was off to college.

I entered the medical school at the University of Pennsylvania
filled with mixed emotions. I was proud that I had gained admission
to a prestigious Ivy League school. I was even closer to my dream. I
looked forward to the opportunity to continue to study the social
aspects of medicine. I also felt an attachment to the University. I had

been born in the Hospital of the University of Pennsylvania and as a teenager I had worked as a candystriper there. My mother had had her surgeries there.

Hopeful expectations and longstanding ties, however, were counterbalanced by ingrained hostility toward Penn. The University coexisted uneasily with my childhood neighborhood—each viewed the other as a threat. Penn saw "the community people" as a menace to its status as a bastion of higher education for a predominantly white, affluent population. No welcome mats were put out for the black people who lived around the campus. University City sought to differentiate itself from West Philadelphia. The people of the surrounding community viewed Penn as a threat to its boundaries and dignity. I grew up hearing rumors that the University planned to expand by demolishing all the houses in my neighborhood. I also heard stories about how badly black people were treated at the Hospital of the University of Pennsylvania. I myself had not yet witnessed such behavior. However, I knew that by enrolling in Penn, I would be torn between these two worlds.

Medical school rocked my dream of becoming a physician. Instead of feeling closer, it seemed more elusive. The problem was not academic. I did well in my classes and in my clinical rotations. I even received honors in several. The uncertainty flowed from personal waters. For the first time in my life, I had to face the fact that not everyone believed that a black woman could be or was qualified to be a physician. "Oh, you'll get into medical school because you are a black woman," a white male college classmate—and medical school aspirant—had once told me. I would gain admission not because I had excelled in college, but because I would fit the affirmative action plan. I was at Penn not because of my credentials, but because I was a special admit. I was taking a place that could have been occupied by a white male. I began to question whether I would ever be a welcome member of the club.

The atmosphere at Penn was certainly less hostile than that which greeted Nathan Francis Mossell, the first black student to graduate from its medical school. As he walked into class in fall 1879, students stomped their feet and hissed, "Put the damn nigger out." Letters protesting his admission were also sent to the administration. On one occasion, as Mossell walked by a river near the University's campus, some students attempted to push him in. No, things for me were a bit more subtle. "Let me introduce the student doctors," the resident announced. He proceeded to address the three white male medical students as "Dr." and me by my first name.

One of the most painful reminders of my insecure status occurred during my junior clerkship in internal medicine. Wearing a lab coat and carrying a stethoscope, I walked into a patient's room at the Veterans' Administration Hospital. The patient, an elderly white man, had been admitted for evaluation of a high blood calcium. I walked into his room and introduced myself as a student doctor. I proceeded to ask him questions about his medical history. Later, the white male intern came out of the patient's room. "You know what that guy asked me," he laughingly announced. "'Why didn't that girl clean up while she was in here?'" My being mistaken for a maid became a joke on the ward team, all of whom, other than myself, were white and male.

The next morning on rounds, the attending physician said, "Let's go see Vanessa fluff up some pillows." I did not find the episode humorous. I was angry. I was shaken. Despite my difficulties, I had begun to define myself as an aspiring physician and expected others to see me as one. I might not be welcome in the club, but they were going to have to let me in because I would be qualified. This incident shook my self-confidence and threatened to undermine not only my professional identity, but my personal one. I had spent so much of my life in pursuit of becoming a doctor. Now, it became very clear that my race and gender would overshadow my credentials, achievements, white jacket and burning desire to become a physician. I recall thinking that if I had been a white woman, at least the patient would have mistaken me for a nurse.

Although the episode angered me, I said nothing to my colleagues. I suffered in silence and even joined in their joking. I was afraid to confront them and show my anger. I did not want to jeopardize my status as a medical student. I thought that it was more important to get a good evaluation from this rotation.

I told the story to Dr. Helen Dickens, an older black woman physician. She was an obstetrician and gynecologist who was the associate dean for minority affairs at the medical school. She was responsible for there being more than twenty black students in my class of 160. Seven of us were black women. Dr. Dickens felt it was her responsibility not just to get us there, but to keep us there. Her door was always open. She had attended medical school nearly fifty years earlier and had been the first black woman admitted to the American College of Surgeons. Dr. Dickens was a short, plump woman in her seventies. She reminded me of my grandmother. She too provided me with comfort and encouragement. She told me that when she had first applied to Penn in the early 1940s for postgraduate training in obstetrics and gynecology, the medical school was not receptive to her admission because "she would not enjoy herself." A group of prominent black Philadelphians who were pushing for her appointment, informed the medical school dean that she was not coming there to enjoy herself, but to learn. She was eventually accepted.

I told Dr. Dickens that, at times, I was made to feel as if I were inferior to my classmates and that I didn't belong there. She looked at me sternly and said, "The way I always figured it, is that for me to have gotten from where I started to where I am, I had to be better than they. You should start thinking that way." I tried to, but it was not always easy. During troubled times, I continued to receive support and encouragement from my mother. She helped as best she could, but I was now part of a white, professional world with which she had no experience. However, she always made sure that I ate and had some change in my pocket. I would come home to find my refrigerator and freezer stocked and a few dollars on the kitchen table. My mother had picked up a new trade. She called herself a certified public accountant. She was a numbers writer. Once when she was hospitalized at University Hospital, I came into her room and found her calling in her numbers to her bookie. I was appalled. "Mommy, I'm a medical student here," I said despairingly. "How do you think that you're getting through?" she responded. She won that argument.

I also received enormous help from faculty and friends from Hampshire and I visited Amherst as much as possible. It became my haven. The community there firmly believed in me and my dream. My college advisor, hearing that I was having a difficult time, once sent me a letter reassuring me that I had everything it took to make it through medical school. Hampshire was also the only place where I felt free to talk about my anxieties and insecurities about being a black woman medical student and not fear that that would be used to undermine me. I prized the acknowledgement that there I would always be a special person.

During medical school, I also got to see firsthand that medicine did reflect the views of a racist American society. I saw black people ridiculed because of their dialect. One hospital even kept a list in its emergency room of "humorous" examples of black dialect and folk medicine knowledge. I discovered that older black people were more often referred to by their first names than their white counterparts. I often heard inferences made that black mothers cared less for their children because they brought them to clinics, not private physicians' offices. I found out the stories that I had heard from my neighbors about black people and University Hospital were true.

Most times when I saw racism in medical school, I remained silent. I was afraid to speak out. Occasionally, I would make a sarcastic comment. For example, one time a resident was describing the medical problems of an uncooperative, noncompliant, poorly educated patient to the ward team. "You know, he's your typical West Philadelphia patient." The group laughed. "Excuse me, but I've lived in West Philadelphia all my life and I don't know what a typical West Philadelphia patient is. Would you care to enlighten me?" Stony silence answered my inquiry. However, I felt slightly vindicated. I had made my point and had let him know that black people are not homogeneous.

Once, during my first semester, my anger turned to rage. Gross anatomy was probably the most intense course of the first year. Not only was there the emotional uneasiness involved with the dissection of a human body, there was a great amount of material to be memorized. Anatomy lab groups were composed of six students. My group had only five. One student had dropped out of medical school the first month. We were shorthanded, but we made do. By Thanksgiving, our stress level peaked. Finals were fast approaching and another member of our group decided that he was not going to come to lab anymore. He, however, changed his mind after about two weeks. When he returned, he decided that he wanted to dissect the part of the body that I had been assigned. He did not even approach the other group members. I did not step aside. He continued to badger me. I asked him to leave me alone, politely at first, then angrily. My anger rose because he started talking about how *his* father had been an alumnus and donor to the medical school and that he deserved to be treated better. The implication was that *my* father was not an alumnus and that I should not have the same privileges as he. I snapped. I told him once again to leave me alone. He didn't. "If you don't get out of my face, I'm going to slap you." He kept it up. I slapped him. I instantly regretted my action. I feared suspension. I was afraid that my dream of becoming a doctor had come to its end. Fortunately, the episode blew over and there were no repercussions. Afterward, however, I kept my anger inside. I could not afford another eruption.

My medical school years were most deeply affected by my mother's battle with breast cancer. The optimistic indications of her initial surgery proved false. Her cancer reappeared three years later during my first year of medical school. This time it had spread to her lungs and there was to be no extended period of remission, but slow, unremitting progression of the disease. University Hospital became a nexus for both our lives. It became an essential component of her struggle to live. This is where she would be hospitalized several times and receive numerous cycles of chemotherapy. For me, the hospital was central to my medical education. I would take many of my clinical rotations there. Within the wards of University Hospital, I played two parts—daughter and medical student. Over time, tensions developed between these two roles.

Despite any anxiety I had about my status as a black woman medical student, I was able to use my position to ensure that my mother got the care and respect that she probably would not have received had she been the usual black clinic patient. I learned that the white jacket did bestow on me certain power. I asked residents to recommend oncologists. "If a member of your family had cancer, to whom would you take them?" Several recommended Dr. Peter Cassileth because of his clinical and interpersonal skills. I contacted him and he graciously accepted my mother as his patient. My mother, who was on Medicaid, was thus able to receive her medical care from one of the top oncologists at the hospital. Whenever I accompanied her to the emergency room, I always wore my white jacket—even if I were not on a clinical rotation. I wanted to make sure that we were not treated in the condescending, rude manner that the ER staff used with other patients.

For most of my life, my mother had been my guide. Our roles were now reversed. I used my burgeoning medical knowledge to help her navigate the complex and mysterious world of medical oncology. I explained to her all the procedures and treatment she would undergo. I usually accompanied her when she came to the hospital for chemotherapy. My presence made her less anxious; at least I understood what was happening. It also made her proud. Her daughter was a student at a major medical center!

I also found personal support within the medical community because of my position. Medical school friends would go visit my mother whenever she was hospitalized. Residents would ask me about her progress and how I was faring. An oncology fellow once said, "This is going to be very hard on you. Do you have someone to take care of you?" The concern, at times, came from people I did not personally know. I once wheeled my mother down to radiology for her chest x-ray and was waiting for the radiology resident to give me the reading. I put the film on the viewing box. It showed that the cancer had almost completely taken over her lungs. "A patient of yours?" "No, my mother." He turned to me, eyes full of sorrow. "I'm so sorry."

Although my identity as a medical student was beneficial for my mother's medical care, it came with a price. There were times when my two roles—daughter and medical student—clashed. A few physicians found it easier to talk to me about my mother's condition as if she were one of my patients. They used cold, clinical language. "Her latest biopsy shows progression of the metastasis." One of her x-rays was once shown at a radiology conference that I was attending. For teaching purposes, the most clinically interesting x-rays of currently hospitalized patients were presented. Names of the patients were not revealed, but I knew from the medical history that it was my mother's radiograph. On the verge of tears, I left the conference. I did not need to be around for the disinterested discussion of this patient's prognosis.

Most crucially, my being a medical student robbed me of my faith. Throughout my mother's illness, she and my family steadfastly believed that she was going to get better. They were able to use their conviction to help them cope with her disease. Unfortunately, I could not share in their hopefulness. I saw the objective clinical data and knew that she was going to die.

Throughout her illness, my mother's spirit remained indomitable and she fought back vigorously. She tenaciously held onto life and never wallowed in self-pity. One morning I called her when she had nausea and vomiting because of her chemotherapy. I called back later. No answer. Worried, I went over to her house. She was fine. "Oh, I went out. I didn't feel like sitting here feeling sorry for myself," she said, explaining her absence. My mother's feistiness and courage were unsurpassed. But slowly, the beautiful, vivacious woman became bedridden and dependent on an oxygen tank.

My mother died December 8, 1977, at University Hospital. She was forty-seven. Five days before her death, she acknowledged to me for the first time that the end was near. The two of us sat in her bedroom, she on the bed, I on a chair. We discussed her financial affairs and her funeral. "My wig is over there." "Your wig?" "You're not going to bury me bald-headed are you?" My mother, whose hair had fallen out because of her chemotherapy, was vain to the end. During the years of my mother's struggle with breast cancer, I had slowly adopted the stance of the medical professional—detached and unemotional in the face of a patient with a terminal disease.

That is how I coped with my mother's dying. My medical student facade fell on this night. Crying, I looked at my mother. "Mommy, are you going to be here for Christmas?" Christmas had always been my family's most joyous and favorite holiday. The fear that she would not be alive to celebrate it gripped me. "Vanessa, don't do this to yourself." "Mommy, I love you." I got up and lay on the bed with her. She held and comforted me as I unleashed years of grief. I was once again a daughter.

My mother's death, although not unexpected, shattered my life. I lost the remaining person whose life-long love, faith and hard work had brought me to the brink of my dream. I lost my sense of family. I felt guilty because my connection to the medical profession had not saved her. I felt regret because I would never buy her or my grandmother that great big house with all the land. I felt devastated because they would not see me graduate. "How do you know that they won't see you graduate?" a friend asked.

A depression so enveloped me that I did not know whether I would even make it to graduation. I found it hard to work and began to doubt whether I wanted to be a physician. The dream which my mother and grandmother had so fought for and believed in began to slip away. My friends rallied and convinced me that if I gave up my dreams then grandmother and mother would truly be dead. Their legacies had been to give me the love, support and nurturing that I needed to pursue my life's goal. I could not let their work come to naught. Gradually, with a lot of help from my friends, I got back on track.

Graduation Day. One of the happiest days of my life. I thought that because my mother and grandmother were dead I would have no one with whom to celebrate. I told my best friend. Since she does not stand on rituals, I thought she would see my point. "What do you mean, you're not going to graduation. You'd better get your butt there. We have plans to be there." She was right. Friends and family came from afar to see me achieve my dream. I waited expectantly on the wings of the stage to hear my name called. "Vanessa Northington Gamble." I walked regally across the stage to get my medical school degree from the dean. "We did it," I said to Mommy and Nanny. I knew they were there and would always be with me. I too had come to believe in spirits.

During her medical internship in the late 1970s, the author of the follow-ing piece was invited to participate in a research project on collaborative health care. The goal of the project was to develop strategies to improve interactions between patients, nurses and doctors. The passage is from a journal the author kept during the study.

All names have been changed to protect patient confidentiality.

Doctor's Journal: Healing from the Inside Out
Lorraine Bonner

August 15

I had an interesting conversation with Ms. Moses yesterday in my office. Ms. Moses had been my patient for a little over a year, when she had been admitted to the hospital delirious, with a fever over 104 degrees, terribly sick. She is a black woman in her fifties, a teacher in a preschool, who had always been very healthy. She turned out to have systemic lupus, a rather mysterious disease of unknown cause, which, although it can be controlled with medica-tions, is usually a chronic condition, flaring up and receding during the life of the person who has it.

Ms. Moses did well, responding rapidly to the medication, and over the past year we have been gradually reducing the dose. She is a very religious woman whose husband pastors a small Pentecostal church in our neighborhood. She told me yesterday that she'd been having some insomnia, waking up early in the morning, which is often a sign of depression. I asked her what she did when she woke up like that, and she said that she thought about various scriptures that were meaningful to her, and that they often helped her get back to sleep. I told her that I thought that was very good and we both agreed that drugs were not necessary.

There was a different quality to her visit yesterday. For a long time it had seemed that problems of her family life, or job, or other people's problems had always had a central place in what she told me when she came in. Yesterday, everything in everyone else's life was all right, and we could really talk about her.

I decided to take a chance. I said, "Now this may sound a little strange, but you know me, I'm a different doctor, with strange ideas. Is there any way that you can see anything good about your lupus? Any benefits it has brought you? Any way in which it has had a positive impact on your life?"

She laughed in my face. "Positive? Benefits? You sure are a strange doctor!" But we talked about it some more, and she agreed that it was a basic principle of her religion that bad experiences always contained some good, although she had never thought of her own experience in that way.

I said I could see that she hated her lupus, that she was very angry about the sickness, pain and limitations it had brought to her life, but that her lupus was a part of her right now, in some way, and that it didn't seem to me to be healthy to have nothing but negative feelings about something that was a part of oneself. Had she gotten to know herself better through the experience of illness? Did she have a new insight into life? Did she have a growth in her understanding of giving and receiving, she who had spent her whole life giving to others, now suddenly having to receive help? Could she appreciate her lupus as a gift?

She became quite thoughtful as we talked. These ideas were new and yet somehow familiar. What had this to do with healing? Should she give thanks for her lupus as a gift from God, a blessing in disguise? Or should she reject her lupus, calling on God to take it away? She said she'd think some more on it.

October 1

My neighbor, Rose Merritt, who is about thirty-two, has been very sick. She has kept my daughter after school for the last few years, and her daughter and my daughter are best friends. Three or four weeks ago, when school started, I dropped by to see Rose, and to make the after-school arrangements. She was in bed in the back room. It was unusual for her to be in bed, and I thought that her face looked a little swollen, but she didn't seem to be uncomfortable, and she said that she felt all right.

I hadn't seen her up and around after that, and my daughter said that Rose stayed in bed most of the time. Her sister Mary was staying with them, and I told her, and Rose's husband Jack, that I would be glad to see Rose medically, at no charge, if they wanted me to.

Rose and Jack are evangelists, at times traveling across the country holding revivals and faith healing meetings. At home, they devote most of their time and energy to the church, living on whatever the Lord provides them. When I offered to see Rose, Jack told me that she was waiting on the Lord to heal her, that she believed that she would be healed by faith. I said that I thought that was very beautiful and that I could respect that belief, and if they did ever change their mind and decide to take medical action, to let me know and I would do whatever I could.

A few days after we had this conversation, a friend of theirs called me at home to ask me if the police could be called to make Rose go to the hospital. I said I didn't think so, and the call made me worry a little more about her condition.

Yesterday, I went to pick up my daughter, and I spoke to Jack about Rose. He was very distressed, almost sick with worry. He had healed people himself through the grace of the Lord's power, but he also knew that the Lord's plan is beyond our understanding, and that at times it seemed to make more sense to pray and take medicine than to pray and not take medicine. He loved his wife and her faith was extremely strong, he told me, but the minute she said the word, he would take her to the hospital.

He told me that he appreciated my offers of help, and that he would like me to see her sometime, but that he needed to clear it with her first. As we were about to leave, he came back out from Rose's room and said she would see me.

I was shocked when I went into her room and saw her. She had total body edema, the most extensive I'd ever seen. Her arms and legs and face were swollen tight and her abdomen was stretched out before her as if she were about ten months pregnant. She was having trouble breathing. Her eyes had a wild look in them as she looked at me, and I wondered, touched to my depths, if she were dying.

At first, I guess, she must have thought I had come to persuade her to take medicine, and I think that some of the wildness in her eyes was a reflection of a fear that some of her precious energy might have to be expended defending herself from me. But as we talked, and she realized that I had come to listen to her, she relaxed, and the look in her eyes became more peaceful and direct, even happy. But at times, that wild look of deep suffering would flash back over her face.

She said that she was on a faith walk. She was already healed, she told me, but it was just not manifest to the "natural eye." Her major problem, as she saw it, was that her relatives wanted to "gang up" on her and force her to accept medical attention, preventing her from living out this test of faith. It was so important to her that she be allowed to carry this experience through to the end.

She talked a lot about faith and confidence in God. She said, "What if I went to the doctors and the doctors said I was incurable? I'd have to turn to God in the end then, right? Well, I'd like to turn to God in the beginning."

She said she wasn't against medical science, her children all went to the doctor for their checkups and their shots; she wasn't stupid, but this illness was different. This illness of hers was sent by God. It was a test of her faith, and she was so happy that she had confidence in her God.

I asked her if she could see going to the doctor, accepting medical help, as part of God's plan. The doctor has knowledge and skill as part of God's grace; the doctor is, in a way, God's agent. She nodded, she knew that argument. It had to be just God, she told me. It had to be very clear, crystal clear, that her healing had come from God. She knew the doctors could draw the fluid off her right away, but she didn't want that. She would wait. She had confidence.

She started to tell me that since her childhood she had felt chosen for some great manifestation of spiritual power, and that this illness, this test of her faith, was something sent from God to instruct many people. Her face took on its happiest and calmest expression as she told me this. I could feel her deep joy at having been chosen. She felt very special and positive about her illness: it was a gift, a blessing. I was struck by the easy way that she said that, a concept with which I struggle daily. I thought about my recent conversation with Ms. Moses about the meaning of illness and wondered if some lesson had been prepared for me in this meeting with Rose.

In the past few days, she said, she had begun to have cravings—a craving for milk, and also she'd been craving clay. I asked her some more about this, and she said that when she began to crave the clay, some friends had gone to a health food store, and by some miracle, a special shipment of especially high quality eating clay was due in from Germany within a few days. She had gotten some of it, and was eating it, a few spoonfuls a day. She had the jar brought to me and I tasted some. It was rather sanitized and antiseptic, not like the dense eating dirt I'd tasted before, straight from the ground, but with that same power to remind one that we are, in our substance, of the earth. I told her I thought the cravings were good, a positive sign, and that she was right in listening to her body and doing what it asked of her. I said that I was very impressed and inspired by her strength and spirit, and that I believed her when she said she had already been healed, and that I especially believed her feeling that she had been chosen for some special manifestation of God's will. I thanked her for telling me all that she had, and told her that I was ready to help her in any way that I could.

She said that I had already helped her a lot, just by listening to her. She said she felt stronger for my support. I knew that inside I felt a lot less certain than she did, and that a part of me still wondered if she would live or die, but I could see that she felt stronger, and I in no way wanted to violate her.

October 2

Yesterday afternoon Jack called me and said that Rose had decided to go to the hospital. I went over to their house to examine her and to arrange transportation. The history of her illness was that she had started getting sick last spring, with swelling of her ankles and shortness of breath, and that over the next six months, the swelling had progressed to her entire body. She said, too, and Jack and Mary confirmed, that at times she was delirious, and I guessed that this may have been because she was just not able to breathe well enough to get all the oxygen she needed for her brain to work. Most of the time, though, she was quite clear, and she told me the story of her illness coherently. She said that about two years ago, she had noticed a "growth" in her abdomen, which she felt was connected with this illness. It had moved around, she said, and had seemed to grow. It had been four or five years since she had any sort of examination. She'd had no pain.

Her blood pressure was over two hundred, twice as high as it should have been; her pulse over one hundred; and she was breathing at a rate of thirty-five or forty breaths a minute, when normal is more like eighteen. Looking back into her eyes, I could see evidence of extensive disease of the blood vessels, such as might be present with longstanding, uncontrolled diabetes or high blood pressure. I could hear her breath moving clearly through both lungs, although she could not fully expand them, and her heart sounded regular, without any murmurs or other abnormal sounds. Her abdomen was distended and rock hard. Her extremities were massively swollen and tight. Her nervous system seemed to be functioning properly, although she was weak and couldn't walk. I guessed that she weighed close to three hundred pounds.

They had no insurance and were not on Medi-Cal. I called the hospital where I usually practiced and asked how to have her admitted. They said she would have to leave a large cash deposit or else go to the county hospital. I said, no, she wasn't going to the county hospital, and she didn't have any money: how was it to be done? The person I was speaking to had to speak to her superior. I would have to say that she was "non-transferable." Fine, I said. She's definitely non-transferable. I guess I was naive, but I hadn't realized that people were still being turned away from the hospital because they had no money.

It is hard to have her there in the hospital, to have to acknowledge simultaneously the two world views. What was the meaning of faith, of "waiting on the Lord?" If you had to go to a doctor, did that mean that the doctor was stronger than God? God wouldn't have given us the intelligence to develop medicine if He hadn't meant for us to use it. How was one to know His intention?

Faith is a heavy number. When one sees this hard, cold, tangible, physical world, and these hard, tangible, physical bodies that we have, what is it that gives one the knowledge, the certainty, that there is more to existence than that, whether one calls that "more" God, or Allah, or the transpersonal plane, or the astral world or whatever? How do I know that? How do I know there is more? It seems to me to be as direct an experience as the experience of the wetness of water, and yet it is called faith by the rest of the world and gets second-class treatment. It doesn't seem as regular and predictable as the physiological kind of healing, yet at times it seems much more powerful. Why had Rose been able to heal others, but not herself?

Rose was disappointed at having to come to the hospital. I asked her about her change of mind, and she said that in talking to more experienced ministers, she had come to accept their counsel to go to the hospital. I sense a kind of defeated quality in her, yet she is brave and continues to affirm that the Lord's will will be made manifest. I really don't know what the outcome will be.

October 6

Rose is fairly stable now, after a few anxious days. Two days after I admitted her, she went into a coma, and I spent a frantic day trying to find out why, checking every possible cause, getting nowhere. So much is wrong with her body, so many tests are abnormal that it is hard to find out what specifically made her go from lucidly discussing spiritual philosophy to complete unresponsiveness twelve hours later. I finally decided that she was septic, infected from the usually harmless bacteria that normally live in the intestines, released now into her bloodstream by the swelling and excess fluid in her body. I started her on an antibiotic at the end of the day, and it began to look as though her coma was lightening.

We've gotten enough fluid off her body now to really be able to examine her, and it is clear that there is a big, hard mass in her abdomen. It is hard not to think that it might be cancer. I find myself reflecting again on the purpose or potential fruitfulness of illness. I have told Rose and Jack that it might be cancer, and they are content. This is their work, this is their test, this is the will of their Lord. I think that God must be pleased with them for the way they are bearing His witness. Rose especially has no fear. There is a kind of radiance to her, a joy at being found worthy of such a test. Her confidence grows daily.

After she began to come out of the coma, her urine output stopped. I ordered a scan of her abdomen, which showed that the flow of urine between the kidneys and the bladder was completely blocked by this mass, a huge tumor that appeared to arise from her pelvis. I don't think we have much else to offer her except surgery.

October 8

The radiologist did a needle biopsy of the mass in Rose's belly; the tissue was hard and gritty, and the pathology report came back suggestive of cancer. The surgeon disagrees, and it is certainly true that she has enough other things wrong with her—her diabetes, her high blood pressure, the compression of the internal veins by the tumor—to explain most of what is going on without the need of any additional causes. Yesterday her blood count dropped suddenly, and I had to give her a blood transfusion, with no idea of where the bleeding was. At least now she's making urine again, although I don't know whether both or only one of her kidneys are functioning, and her mental status is clear.

Her family is completely in favor of whatever medical intervention is necessary, and I don't think there will be any problem with them consenting to surgery. Her husband is quite cheerful. It is as if, for the rest of the family, although not for Rose, it was important to do "everything possible" on the worldly level before resting on the Lord. Having done so, they are now content.

Still, for Rose, there is an element of her experience which she does not understand, although she does not say what it is. Why should the righteous suffer, Jack asked me, when the wicked can get healed every day? I see Rose wrestling with this contradiction, and I know she will raise it to a higher level and develop a new awareness of the Lord. Perhaps, if she had not gotten sick, or if she had gotten sick and been quickly healed, she might have grown full of pride, feeling she knew the Mystery, feeling she had the Lord at her beck and call. Perhaps this illness, more than any other that I have witnessed, brings forth the truth that this life in which we are engaged, if it has any purpose and meaning at all, is far more complex than we can know. Last night when I visited Rose, she was cheerful and relaxed, talking about her religious experiences and visions. For a while she was speaking in tongues, an ecstatic flow of rhythmic syllables. Explaining the meaning of it, she said that ordinary language is just not adequate to describe the soul's vision of the Divine. I feel privileged to witness such faith. What I am coming to see is that the mind cannot comprehend this greater reality, that the mind is too small, too young, too limited, bound by this yes-no, front-back, good-bad world of the physical to even begin to understand. Yet, for some of us, as for Rose, there is a sense of a bare brushing of the fingertips against the edge of something that is more essential to our lives than air or water. It is strange to think that mental understanding, which we regard as our highest faculty, is superseded by some other faculty whose name we do not even know. What is this attitude, this knowledge that transcends understanding, and what is its relationship to empowerment and healing?

October 15

Yesterday Rose went to surgery. After all the work, all the hope and fear, all the waiting and prayers, what was found? An enormous fibroid tumor of the uterus! A completely benign and common condition, which, had it not grown to such a large size, need not have threatened her life at all, and, even more importantly, would not continue to threaten her health once removed.

After the difficult course of her illness, and all the frightening things that had happened, for the Lord to have let us all off with only a fibroid was nothing short of miraculous.

October 17

I saw a young black woman in my office yesterday. She had a cold. She was dressed as if for work and when I asked her if she'd taken any time off for her illness, she said no, she hadn't. I said, "Sister, you know viruses only catch you when you're weakened in some way, when your resistance is down, you're tired or not eating well or your mind is in conflict and turmoil."

She said, well, yes, she had been running a lot lately, and feeling bad. She started crying then, and began telling me about the difficulties of her life: she was a single parent with three children to support, working hard, perhaps too hard in a job that paid well but was far from her inner spirit. She was not, she said, "happy inside."

She told me that she had gone to college as an art major but had left to marry. I told her that she should take some time off from work and give some thought to her life, the direction she was taking, what she really wanted to do—if she really wanted to get at the root of her illness and not just treat the symptoms. I took notes for her as she talked, listing the areas that seemed important to her: her education, her career, her family, the expression of her artistic potential, and I told her that it was essential that she take some time that was hers and hers alone, where she could be by herself and take care of her own needs.

I hadn't even examined her, but it felt like this was the most important part of treating her cold, and when I told her that this was what I thought illness was all about, and that she should say she appreciated her cold, she did, laughing. I examined her then, saw no reason to suspect anything other than a virus, and gave her a recipe for a home remedy. She had cried a lot and said that she felt much better.

Somehow it seemed strange to me that I should be able to reach this level because of a cold. I wondered what made her receptive to the idea, or if it was something about me and the way that I presented it that made it through to her. Why had it worked this time?

It made me think of another patient, Ms. Miller, an old lady who is in the hospital now, who was hearing voices and wanted to stay at home. She finally did end up in a nursing home, did fairly well for awhile, then started going downhill again. Everything is negative. Nothing that anyone does for her is any good. There is absolutely nothing, *nothing* positive or pleasant in her life. The pillows put too much pressure on her head. The blankets are too heavy. Every day I come to see her, and I ask her how's she doing. "Terrible," that's how she's doing. The nurses, she says, won't come when she calls. They don't talk to her. When I try to talk to her about her medical condition, she switches the conversation to how much she needs some bobby pins for her hair. I try to make her comfortable when I come to see her, to help her change positions; I don't think she's even once thanked me for anything I've done. She never thanks the nurses for their care. I've tried to get her to think back on her life, to happier times and pleasant memories, but she cuts those conversations off. She'd rather concentrate on the present with all of its unpleasantness and pain. I've never known anyone so addicted to feeling bad. She reminds me, in a way, of other addicts, of alcoholics and people who abuse other substances. There can be a self-destructive quality that directly contradicts longevity. I feel frustrated by it and wonder what my role is, if Ms. Miller's health care is to be truly collaborative. She is locked in this struggle between life and death: well, aren't we all? She's not sure to which side she wants to throw her energy, but the very act of deciding is itself an act of life. Yet, what is it that is so seductive about this misery? What chains her to her pain? Is it the same thing that makes me feel so impotent when I want to live to the fullest of my power? Is it a kind of fear?

October 29

Ms. Miller died yesterday. She had terminal pneumonia, but she really died of total failure to cooperate. Her autopsy proved nothing: she didn't have cancer or heart disease; she might have lived forever if she had just agreed to do it. She was one of the hardest patients I have ever cared for.

It's not hard to be a technician as a doctor, it's not hard to roll up your sleeves and put on gloves and work. There's nothing really hard about that, especially after you've had some experience. What is hard is fear, your own fear and the patient's fear, and pain, all the old buried pain that we all carry around with us that we hope never to see again. What is hard is to see in that other person all that enrages us about ourselves, all of our own shortcomings and failures, carried out to their natural end in illness and despair.

If I were going to rewrite the Golden Rule, I would include in it some invitation to love oneself, too, and perhaps that is what collaborative health care needs most: the kind of love that cuts through the pain and fear and reaches to the very heart. The heart is steady, and the mind, always questioning, can learn from that: here's the sun coming up, and the poor old battered earth turning all gold and green again, every morning, every spring: that's real longevity. It doesn't make any sense to feel one way or another about it: it just is. All you can do is pay attention.

TWO: TELL THE WORLD ABOUT THIS

Roots
Lucille Clifton

call it our craziness even,
call it anything.
it is the life thing in us
that will not let us die.
even in death's hand
we fold the fingers up
and call them greens and
grow on them,
we hum them and make music.
call it our wildness then,
we are lost from the field
of flowers, we become
a field of flowers.
call it our craziness
our wildness
call it our roots,
it is the light in us
it is the light of us
it is the light, call it
whatever you have to,
call it anything.

The sexual abuse of children is one of the country's most frequent and widespread crimes, affecting as many as twenty-five percent of female children before they reach the age of thirteen, according to the Federal Bureau of Investigation. Gail Wyatt, a researcher at the University of California at Los Angeles, cites studies that suggest that black females, primarily between the ages of nine and twelve, are more frequently victims of sexual abuse than white females. Most abuse occurs in the home and is perpetrated by someone known and trusted by the victim such as a family member, neighbor, babysitter or minister. To compound the problem, only one to ten percent of the incidents of incest and childhood sexual abuse are reported.

Many black women are no longer suffering in silence from the abuse they have suffered. They are purging themselves of their pain by talking to counselors, joining support groups and sharing their experiences with others in plays, poems and essays.

The author of the following piece is representative of the black women who are reclaiming their lives by shattering the silence around sexual abuse in the black community.

I Call Up Names: Facing Childhood Sexual Abuse
Andrea R. Canaan

Dear Mother,

I began to choose to live during the summer of 1982. In October of that year I was thirty-two years old. It was exactly twenty summers after it all began.

I turned.

I faced the direction past. I understood it was a detour to forward, an echo of present. I believed this way led to a livable future.

I decided to stop fading, becoming silent, still. I decided to remember the bright promise I had at three and five and eight and eleven...

I decided to live in the arms of a woman who taught me, helped me to remember that I had been a child then.

I had forgotten, I believed myself a woman, responsible, guilty, to blame.

Everyone had treated me like I was a woman, responsible, guilty, to blame.

"What do you feel?" my lover asked. "What do you think about it all?"

I blinked in confusion. "Feel about it? Think about it all?" I felt nothing. I thought nothing about it all. I sat inside her blazing eyes seeing and hearing an example of what I could feel, what I could think. I saw grief for the child I had been. "It was not your fault," she said.

Her words struck me in a true place like a hammer perfectly put to a nail. I knew she spoke the truth. In her arms I was safe for the first time since I was eleven.

He was a Methodist minister. You taught me to call him godfather, even though he was not. He paid our bills, bought our food and clothes. He gave you money. He gave me money.

I washed the floors, changed the beds, dusted the furniture, ironed the clothes inside the big house on the avenue; where the clothes, the floors, the beds, the furniture were never dirty to begin with.

I was the child they never had, a servant girl, an arrangement. I was a little black girl from the Magnolia Project.

James Arthur Daniels was at least thirty years older than my eleven years. He abused me emotionally, sexually and physically. It started just before my twelfth birthday. This abuse lasted nearly a decade.

When I was fifteen James Daniels raped me for the first time. I mean full penetration, his penis in my vagina and in my ass. Before that, he used his fingers, his hands and objects like bottles. He used his mouth once but he hated my female taste.

I did not believe it was rape. I believed that I was bad, that I had seduced him. I believed that I deserved the pain, the ripping, his bruising hands, his sharp teeth.

It was not a mirage. It was not my imagination or a dream. I was not crazy. I did not make it up. None of it is made up.

I did not dream the loss. I did not make up the guilt, force my separation from God, my church, my community. I did not imagine the shame, the judgement, the cold silence and distance. That I was placed apart and blamed is real.

By 1987, after years of therapy, authentic loving and a decision to live sane and whole, I believed that I was finally finished with James Daniels. I believed that I had gotten over your selfish and self-centered response to my telling you about how he'd abused me. I believed that after twenty-five years I could forgive and/or let go of those who left me unprotected, those who blamed me, those who judged a child guilty of her own abuse.

What I found as I attempted to complete this work, was yet another layer of abuse just beneath nearly a decade of James Daniels.

I had also been abused by two women.

One of them was you.

The other was Henrene Baker, the teacher I met at church camp.

I kept the secret.

I kept it even from myself, even when the knowing stood between me, a slow death and an informed lie.

I remember your abuse of me, Henrene's abuse of me in snatches. I jump back, away, as if scalded, as if hexed, as if my memories lie and all the lies are truth.

As the memories come I shake my head in disbelief and despair. Not my Mama. My Mama loved me, sacrificed her entire life for me. She loves me best.

I put my hands out, try to stop the images, the memories, the dreams, the deep in my heart knowing. I pray they are lies, an illusion. I have tried everything to avoid seeing my cancellation, myself willingly sacrificed in your eyes.

Mother, you sexually abused me when I was a child. You allowed my sexual abuse for nearly a decade. You cut my lifeline at eleven for a pittance. You snatched my childhood. You betrayed me. You bound my child devotion to you, to your care and protection, even at the expense and death of mine.

As I came to know this, began and continue to remember this, I was terrified that you would not believe me, that you would reject me.

I was sure you would judge me, call me whore, slut, bastard, ungrateful, good-for-nothing, unworthy of my birth. I knew that you would translate this deepest betrayal of me into your pain, your need, your burden.

There is still a place in me that wants you to hold me, to comfort me, to say that you were/are sorry, that you were wrong, that it was not my fault. There will always be that place even though I am letting go of you. I am letting go of you and taking care of me because you did not. For most of my life, I have mothered myself.

I am writing to you because I have come to a place beyond fear. I move toward a cleansing and fueling anger that will end my grief.

I will not hold secrets. I will no longer keep the silences or the unsaid rules. I am embracing the doe-eyed girl I was at eleven. I am holding me. I tell me it was not my fault. I am honoring my courage and strength during those nightmare years. I am so grateful to my-self for saving my life until this time when I can remember, name and become myself. I tell myself that it is over; the lies, the tearing and bruising, the betrayal, the hate, that particular death wish, is over.

In the name of the Goddessses and Gods known and unknown, named and unnamed,

In the name of my foremothers and forefathers known and un-known, named and unnamed,

In the name of my brothers and sisters, my friends and my lovers, my daughters and sons, those who died so young and those who are yet living,

I pray that I continue to break the cycles of madness visited man upon woman, man upon man, woman upon woman, woman upon man, father upon daughter and son; mother upon son and daughter, kin and neighbor against each other. I pray these truths will afford my daughter no betrayal at my own hand, nor any betrayal that I know of and will not stop,

I call up my names: Woman who has been born in the arms of a woman and welcomed home. I shout truth teller, silence breaker, life embracer, death no longer fearing, woman reunited with her child self. I sing woman who is daughter, sister, lover and mother to her-self. I hum woman planter, gatherer, healer. I drum woman warrior, siren, woman who stands firmly on her feet, woman who reaches in-ward to her center and outward to stars. I am woman who is child no longer, woman who is making herself sane, whole.

It is done.

So let it be.

Blessed be.

Confronting years of pain and silenced emotions, the following author writes of being sexually abused by her minister father. Her courage informs and strengthens us all as we work toward healthier lives.

A Daughter Survives Incest: A Retrospective Analysis
Linda H. Hollies

There has been a gigantic mountain in my life since the age of twelve or thirteen. This mountain could not be moved, and it was too overwhelming for me, a child, to attempt to climb. I didn't have the faintest idea that a mountain could be chipped away at, or even tunneled through. So, what did I do with this mountain? I tried to ignore it! I was positive that no other individual could have a mountain like this in her life. This type of mountain didn't have a name; it was never mentioned in my world. The mountain didn't have a face; it appeared in the night, simply as an ugly mess. Now, if it had no name or face, how could I describe it to anyone? If I didn't talk about it, maybe it would just go away.

My father brought this mountain into my world, for you see, I am the victim of incest. He was a very angry man. He was called "Thor, god of thunder" by his children. He yelled, screamed and hurled insult upon insult at us. His demeanor was seldom pleasant, either at home or away; he was a strict disciplinarian and quick to whip with the handy strap. He was emotionally, physically and mentally abusive to me and my seven siblings; his behavior toward my mother was the same. I cannot remember one kind or encouraging remark my father ever made to me; my accomplishments were usually belittled or ignored.

The act of incest alone is enough to cause one psychological trauma and lifelong emotional damage, but when coupled with heavy theological ramifications, one is in double-trouble! My father was the assistant pastor of the small, family-type, Pentecostal church I was raised in and where God's love was constantly preached; respect for parents was another favorite topic. But the most popular theme was the sinner and the sinner's abode in hell. Well, I had problems. I could not love this man who came into my bedroom and did unmentionable things to me; I could not believe that God could love me and yet allow this to continue. I surely had no respect for my father as a parent. Therefore, I was a sinner, right?

Another dynamic at play was the fact that my father found scripture to justify the liberties he took with me (the story of Lot and his two daughters, who had sex with him after they made him drunk, to perpetuate his lineage). Now, if this was a Biblical injunction, sanctioned by scripture, why was I threatened and physically abused when I was told not to talk about this to anyone, and especially not my mother? Of course, my father had an answer: "Your mother has had one heart attack, and if she really doesn't understand the Bible, this might kill her"—a typical threat. I did not know that this was just another lie, but I did know that I didn't want my mother to die. What would happen to me then?

Now, when I was growing up, there were no "Just Say No" programs, no television coverage, no Oprah Winfrey show—there was no one to talk to about this mountain that I faced. I wondered what I had done to invite this invasion of my person, this assault against what I had been taught was good and decent behavior? Was I really going to hell? I could not receive any clarification or reassurance because there was no one to talk to about this ugly mess. I felt I should love my parents because "this is the first commandment with the promise of long life," and I surely wanted to live long. What was I to do? Ignore the mountain? Try to push it out of my mind? Pray about it? Have faith? Would it disappear?

As I have since learned, my rationalizations were indicative of someone raised in a dysfunctional family: don't talk about the issue; don't feel; be loyal to the family and do not allow outsiders to know what's going on. I knew outsiders should not be brought into this mess, but why couldn't my mother see, hear, tell and know what was going on? Couldn't she notice my anguish—intuit my grief— how could she not be aware of my pain?

My mother was a "total woman." She was always well-groomed, in a starched house dress, and she would never wear curlers or sleepwear around the house. She was a good cook and an immaculate housekeeper. She was the "perfect" wife; whatever her husband said was *law!* She related to all of us as the woman who carried out her husband's orders and commands. My siblings and I went almost everywhere she went, because my father was "too much of a man" to babysit! He was "too saved" to allow her to use any form of birth control, and she was "too saved" to disobey. She never made any decision without consulting him. Although we spent a great deal of time with her, she was not emotionally available to any of us; seldom did she smile or display affection toward us, except for the perfunctory good-morning, good-bye, hello and good-night kisses that my father demanded from all of us. She was repressed, afraid of conflict and rejection and never knew what "living" was all about. Her husband would not allow her to work because that might incite rebellion—against her role as wife; her function was to be mother to his children.

As I reflect on the experiences and traumas of my childhood, I am amazed and grateful that I have sanity today, but I realize that I have the natural instincts of a survivor. The atmosphere in our home was perhaps similiar to a slave labor camp, with father as master and mother as general overseer. There were no loving relationships; we related to my father out of fear and to my mother out of respect. My father used the word love to justify his cruel behavior—"it's because I love you that I must whip you." I recall the one time he asked me if I loved him and I honestly replied, "No." He tried to slap the "hell" out of me. "Little saved girl, you *must* love your father and respect him as well!" I was an adult, married and pregnant with my first child, when I challenged my mother and heard her say to me, for the very first time, "I love you." And they were my primary caregivers, nurturers, protectors from the outside world? From them I was to learn trust and intimacy?

I married my childhood sweetheart immediately upon graduation from high school. He was shy and introverted and had a horrible relationship with his parents. He was just what I needed, a man who was an emotional mess, who wouldn't make too many demands upon me. We were together long enough to have two sons and to make life miserable for each other. He is a decent human being; I simply refused to be "wife." My earliest prayer was to never be like my mother, the "total woman."

The most significant incident in this lifelong struggle involved my sister, Jacqui. She was "my" baby. She is three years younger and I looked after her (as a matter of fact, with mother's constant pregnancies, I looked after all of my siblings and my mother as well). After I moved out of the house, my father approached my sister to molest her. The same pattern and the same threats were involved, but my sister didn't accept this "strange" behavior. She called me.

I approached my husband, who was somewhat aware of my personal history. I had explained to him why I would not visit my mother, except when my father was at work, and why I would not allow my sons to stay overnight. When I told him about the situation, we went to see an attorney. His advice was to consult with my mother, have a warrant sworn out and have my father arrested. My husband even told my mother that we would move into her home and take over financial responsibility. She absolutely refused. However, she did confront my father and the molestation of my sister ceased.

I felt relieved for Jacqui, but I became very angry with my mother as I thought about her behavior when I finally told her what was going on with me at the age of sixteen. This was after enduring three years of hell alone, not having a big sister to turn to and not trusting that my mother would believe my word against my father's. She was wise enough to set my father up—she walked in and caught him in the very act. He cried, asked forgiveness, and of course she forgave him. When I asked to move out-of-state in order to reside with my brother, she replied, "You have to stay here. Your father loves me, nothing will happen to you again!" When the molestation and rape resumed, there was no reason to return to her. My back was against the wall. My mother was no protection for me; she could not provide the emotional nurturing I needed for growth and development.

After the break-up of my first marriage, I was a single parent, a working adult and enjoying a measure of success, yet the mountain was still in control. My sense of worth was steadily diminishing; nothing covered my deep sense of shame. The "filth" of my secret was eating me up and there was no one to confide in. I desired intimacy, but I was afraid to allow anyone, male or female, to come close to knowing me. I had no experience in relating in honest relationships. The demands that I placed on myself to "be perfect" did not allow for leisure, nor did I have the patience with others who wouldn't or couldn't measure up to my specifications.

I was a very unhappy woman. I remarried. This time I selected a man who was twelve years my senior. He, too, was from an unstable home and had been in a bad marriage and was an active alcoholic. Once again I selected a man who would need me and yet was emotionally unavailable to me. To further complicate matters, we had a daughter.

My sons did not prevent me from working long hours (my job was in the steel mills), as long as I provided the monetary benefits, but having a daughter meant to me that some major lifestyle changes were necessary. So, I went back to school to complete degree requirements, and to get a professional position so that I would have quality time to spend with my little girl. My husband's insecurities caused him to challenge this desire for additional education, and since I refused to compromise (or to be controlled), I left him, moved to a city miles away, and enrolled.

While living with a friend and her family, I began to attend church services at the United Methodist Church. Their theological stance was broadly based; their "God" was not so restrictive. And in this setting I again considered my personal relationship with God. This God loved me, just as I was; this God invited me to come and receive the abundant life. This was appealing to a survivor—I wanted to know what "authentic" living was all about. But the mountain was still there, and I was not able to talk to anyone. I still hated my father; I went to talk with him and apologized for hating him all those years. He did not understand my pain nor my anger. Forgiveness was supposed to follow my repentance, but I never felt forgiven, for I honestly could not forgive him! Most importantly, I could not forget! But this newfound relationship with God and a new community were too delightful to turn my back on. Once again I felt that if I could just pray correctly and ignore this mountain, it would go away.

Finally, the burden of carrying this secret became too much, so I went to the pastor to "confess." With much emotion, I told my story and he listened attentively, after which he advised me to "agree with him in prayer." When I left, I had two secrets: one from my childhood, and the newly found secret that my "new" relationship with God did not perform the miracle of wiping my memory clean or restoring love for my father within my heart. The fault/blame had to be mine; this was the only logical conclusion. The mountain was yet in control.

Where was the peace in my life? My other endeavors, such as working with the Christian Education Department and the young adult ministry in the local church, completing university requirements and reuniting with my husband after two years did not bring release from the mental and emotional bondage to the mountain. The cycle continued—better jobs, more material gains, even professional positions and recognition—but the shame and humiliation which caused me to doubt my self-worth and faith remained.

The Christian experience challenged me to grow and expand my horizons. I felt "called," but I did not feel worthy and I certainly was not ready. I decided to continue to work in the church, but I would keep my full-time, well-paid position as supervisor at General Motors. On the other hand, I was getting more and more involved in the life of the local congregation. Could God actually require more? Besides, my father was a minister and I had no trust in him. Would I be accepted/trusted if the story of the mountain was known? For surely I had a great part in the mountain, right? If I was going to minister to others, I had to look good—to act as if I had it all together and had *most* of the answers.

At the age of forty, I met Dr. Lee M. Jones, a United Methodist pastor. He challenged me to attend seminary and to allow God full use of my time, talents and gifts. But this man did not know my story! Unfortunately, Dr. Lee was in my life for only two months, as he and his family were transferred to the East Coast for another assignment. His wife, my husband, he and I all discussed this matter of seminary and spent time in prayer together. My husband, surprisingly, was open to this new idea and did not oppose me at all. So, in September 1984 I entered Garrett Evangelical Theological Seminary. My daughter and I moved to Evanston, Illinois, and rented an apartment; my husband remained in our home and visited on his off days. This was one of the most exciting periods of my life. New knowledge, new people, new avenues for expressing ministry!

I had heard of clinical pastoral education, or CPE, but I could find no black students who had taken it. The school required a full battery of psychological tests as well as two counseling sessions. God, the mountain will show up! I will not pass these tests, for I am determined to be honest—well, as honest as I can be. I will talk about an abusive father, but I won't say that I was sexually abused. I won't look so bad. I passed! I'm going to take CPE!

I wanted a female supervisor because I felt she would understand better, and I applied to one center where I knew a female would supervise during the summer. I was accepted. Beth Burbank was relatively young and fairly reserved, but she was aware of mental abuse issues as her mother had a history of psychotic breaks. It was not my issue, but I decided to give it a chance and work toward moving the mountain.

My goals were to risk being vulnerable; to work on a personal statement of theodicy; to learn how to relax and have fun; and to come to terms with my own mortality. Supervision was not easy for me. I couldn't open up and be honest with Beth. She related that she had never supervised a northern Black woman before, so I wanted to "look good" to this white woman. And I wanted to impress her because I had shared with her that CPE just might be the vehicle for my ministry.

The group experience was so powerful for me. When I finally established a trust level with the group and the process allowed me to risk letting them know about my mountain, I did share—I told of my experience as a child and young adult, with no emotions being expressed. "It happened, I survived." The youngest woman in the group told me that she felt my pain and said that I didn't have to be strong. Then she gave me permission to cry. This was a breakthrough! This experience began my grieving process over a lost childhood and innocence; over the rejection by both parents and the lack of love and trust in my life. Finally I was able to place blame where it belonged—on my father, not on myself. I was also able to experience anger freely for the first time. Because our family's church had equated anger with sin, there was never a way for my siblings or me to have an open or positive expression of anger. As children, the admission of anger had been cause for a whipping.

One day Beth was sharing "story theology" with us and read Psalms 139, which is her favorite passage. As she read verse 13, "For you have formed my inward parts; you have covered me in my mother's womb," the word "formed" seemed to swell within my head. I could actually see myself as a dot sitting on the head of a pin in my mother's womb. I began to watch the forming, shaping and becoming of "baby" Linda. God seemed to be a mockery to me at that instant as never before. Overwhelmed, I jumped up and ran from the group into the women's toilet. Beth concluded her remarks to the group and found me sitting in a stall, crying. When she inquired what was wrong, I replied, "nothing." When she questioned why I had run out of the group, I replied, "I don't know." Beth then asked, "Linda, are you angry?" I replied, "Of course not!" I could not conceive of anyone who would admit to being angry with God. Beth managed to talk me out of the stall, and that day, in the toilet, we had one of our best supervisory sessions. She taught me about anger, constructive and destructive. I realized authentic anger that day. I claimed my anger. I chipped at the mountain. The mountain moved.

After only one quarter of CPE, I learned more about myself than I had ever known. I became vulnerable, took risks and grew because I was cared for and accepted, with my faults and limitations, by my peers and supervisor. I entered into therapy after the quarter, for I wanted to learn more and to continue this growth. The time had not fully come that I could explore all of my issues. Beth pressed me to seek therapy.

I wanted a Black, female, feminist therapist but could not find one. I did find a white feminist pastoral counselor, working on a Ph.D. in pastoral psychology at Garrett-Northwestern, and we worked well together. I continued chipping away at the mountain. But I didn't want to touch my mother and her part in my pain. I wanted to lay all of the blame on my father. I wanted to keep the pretense that my mother cared and that she really could not have known the horrible trauma I had undergone. The therapist suggested that we role play. "Tell your mother that she failed you. Tell her that she was a poor mother for not protecting you." My mind rebelled. The words would not come. No. My mother was not the issue.

My father died in 1981 and I thought that with his death the mountain would lose some of its hold on me, but I did not find that to be true. I needed my mother. I wasn't ready to *know.* All of my adult life I had attempted to "buy" my mother's love, as well as that of my brothers and sisters. I refused to confront my mother. But growth demands risk-taking. Removing mountains requires digging into everything around them. My unrealistic expectations of my perfect mother had to be faced.

June 1985 found me living in Lansing, Michigan, and assigned to my first pastorate. Again, my husband was remaining behind for a while, so I asked Mother to travel with me and stay for a couple of weeks. In the middle of her second week with me, I asked the question that I needed an answer to and her response was: "I thought it had started again, but I didn't want to know. I needed your father to love me." How sad. How pitiful.

After this confession, all of my illusions were destroyed. I knew that my mother had sacrificed me for what she hoped and wished was love. I refused to see my family for almost a year. I remained in therapy, but found a white, female psychiatrist. I worked on becoming whole: I worked on "cutting the ties" to my family so that I would never need them in the sick, dependent manner I had experienced; I worked on understanding how I was more like my parents than I was different. On April 26, 1986, I had a dream that my mother was trying to join my father. I knew she was going to die. I had to work on saying appropriate good-byes. I never accomplished this.

On May 16, 1986, my mother had a massive brain stroke; she remained in a coma for twelve days. All the siblings agreed to stop life-support systems and my mother died May 30th. I did not grieve. I was too angry. She was only fifty-nine and had never experienced life. To wait for death is to die by slow torture. To do nothing is to rot. I saw in my mother's death the story of many black women, wives, mothers, sisters and daughters. They exist in an empty place, a vast interior of emptiness.

I knew that if I did not continue to chip away at the mountain, I would be in trouble. So, in May of last year I resigned from the church to take a rest, both mentally and physically. I also tried to immerse myself in "doing" so as to escape the inescapable grief. I realized that as long as my anger remained, the grieving could not begin.

In September 1986, I began a residency in clinical pastoral education at the Catherine McAuley Health Center in Ann Arbor, Michigan. I was very much in touch with my anger, because it would not allow others to reach me. I had shut down again because I did not want to hurt. I did not fully comprehend that I had to hurt in order to stop the hurt. My goals were centered around being open to feedback on the impact of my anger on relationships and to understand what purpose my shutting down and closing myself off to feedback served. I had much trust in the group and in the process to see me through what I knew would be stormy times.

I have grown to understand and to accept that the mountain will always be a part of my history—there is no magic "memory eraser." I have come to accept the strength of being a survivor, as well as the negative aspects, which prevent me from knowing what real living is all about. I have accepted as a gift the grace of God that allowed me to come through this situation with the determination not only to help myself, but to reach out to others with mountains in their lives they cannot name. Those things in my life that I have worked so hard to hide, tried so desperately to keep secret, have produced some of the greatest "stuff" with which to do ministry. Sharing my story gives hope to others and it also reaffirms the value of who I am.

The greatest gift I have received during this year has been another woman with the story of incest. One day in group, as I struggled not to break down under the weight of knowing that my primary caregivers were not capable of giving me care, this Catholic nun gently reached over and touched my hand. Who knows at what point of discouragement and despair the simplest act of love may reach a soul and turn it again to the light? This simple act of love taught me that my family of origin might never be there for me, but in the providence of God many others have been sent to reach out and touch my life with love, concern, compassion and care.

Many truths have come together for me during this intense one-year journey. I realized that my whole life had been lived in grayness. I realized that my mother had only given me birth, for she did not know how to teach me about life; for no one had been there to teach her. I have experienced "the New Birth." I'm learning ways to express my anger so that it is constructive. I have learned how to share and to be vulnerable.

I am committed to learning as much as I can about myself and how to be a mountain-mover so that I can be an example for my sister, for my "mothers," and for my daughters. I have gone through the pain of reconciling with both my parents this summer. I am able to say that I love both of my parents. My anger at the pain they caused me has not dissolved the love. I hate what my father did to me as a child. I hate that my mother was not willing to leave him or capable of doing so when confronted with the truth of my situation. I hate that she had a "poor me" attitude and a victim's stance in life. I hate that he was a sick man and abused me, my sister and my mother.

My mother was a woman with hopes, dreams, and aspirations before she elected to become a wife and mother. My often unfounded expectations of her kept us at a distance for many years. I wanted her to be perfect for me, but she was human. She lived the life she chose though often she was sad, disappointed and hurt. She wanted her own prince charming and never got him. She wanted a perfect daughter. She never got that either. She was a failure as a mother, but this was not her number one priority in life. She chose to be a wife. I am grieving for my mother. I miss her terribly and I love her.

From my father I have gained my love of knowledge and excellence; a love of good clothes and grooming habits, and an outgoing personality. Yet I realize that I have a mean, rebellious streak that is just like him and a deep-seated anger that will feed on itself if left unchecked. My father is who and what he was. There is no changing my past. I cannot make him better or different.

I now understand that many of our actions and reactions today are based on early experiences with our parents that we continue to transfer to significant others, mates, children as well as to work, church and social relationships. Adult awareness gives us the power to change our mental tapes and to re-parent ourselves in a different manner. Every occasion in life is one from which we can learn. Our lives begin with loss, the loss of the security of our mother's womb. To be able to truly cut the cords that bound me to both parents has been the first step toward living my life in its fullness.

In the United States, a woman is battered about every eighteen seconds, according to the FBI. Violence in the home injures four to six million women each year. In addition to the fear and financial constraints that dominate most battered women's lives, racial and cultural issues often make it more difficult for black women to leave abusive relationships.

Thanks to increased awareness in the black community, a growing number of abused black women are seeking help in support groups and battered women's shelters, and using the criminal justice system to end the violence in their lives. They are standing up for the healthy, nurturing relationships they rightly deserve.

The following article is excerpted from the book Chain Chain Change: For Black Women Dealing with Physical and Emotional Abuse.

Love Don't Always Make It Right: Black Women and Domestic Violence
Evelyn C. White

Several years ago, a black woman left her husband. The woman, a singer, had traveled all over the world with him, stayed in luxurious hotels and to all observers seemed to live a glamorous and exciting life. But in reality, this woman was being abused by her husband. For nearly twenty years she had lived under his complete domination and control, never knowing when she might be threatened or physically assaulted. One night after suffering another of his beatings, the woman decided she'd taken enough abuse. With thirty-six cents she walked out on him and started a new life.

That woman was Tina Turner. Today she is a world-famous Grammy Award winner and one of the most successful singers in the music industry.

If you've been involved in a violent heterosexual or lesbian relationship for a long time, or seem to end up with one abusive partner after another, you might think that it's all your fault or that you're just unlucky when it comes to love. Neither is true. Like Tina, you haven't done anything to make your partner abuse you, nor is it your "luck" that's the problem. There are many traditions that support violence against women. The abuse you are suffering is being experienced by millions of other black, brown, yellow, red and white women all over the world.

Unlike earlier times, domestic violence is no longer considered just a "family matter"—something to be endured by women like yourself behind closed doors. It is now recognized and treated as a serious social and criminal problem that is rooted primarily in the acceptance of male dominance over women. Many people, including police officers, social workers, judges, attorneys, counselors, ministers, teachers, writers, nurses and doctors are working to increase public awareness of domestic violence and to change the systems that contribute to your abuse.

Images and Expectations of Black Women

In 1928, black American writer and folklorist Zora Neale Hurston wrote an essay, "How It Feels To Be Colored Me." Today, more than half a century later, her words are still very much needed to help black women overcome the destructive images and unrealistic expectations that contribute to the physical and emotional abuse in our lives:

> I am not tragically colored. There is no great sorrow lurking behind my eyes. I do not mind at all. I do not belong to the sobbing school of Negrohood who hold that nature somehow has given them a lowdown dirty deal and whose feelings are all hurt about it. Even in the helter-skelter skirmish that is my life, I have seen that the world is to the strong regardless of a little pigmentation more or less. No, I do not weep at the world—I am too busy sharpening my oyster knife.[1]

The image of black women as long-suffering victims can keep us passive and confused about the abuse in our lives. Not only does this stereotype affect our intimate relationships, it impacts our daily experiences as well.

In a contemporary parallel to Hurston's essay, noted black feminist scholar Barbara Smith points out, "It is not something we have done that has heaped this psychic violence and material abuse upon us, but the very fact, that because of who we are, we are multiply oppressed."[2]

And who are we? Abolitionist Sojourner Truth, educator Mary McLeod Bethune, choreographer Katherine Dunham, playwright Ntozake Shange, opera singer Leontyne Price, civil rights heroine

Rosa Parks, Olympic champion Jackie Joyner-Kersee, politician Shirley Chisholm, activist Angela Davis and academician Barbara Jordan are all part of our stellar black female heritage. Yet too often are the images of black women reduced to the big-bosomed slave "mammy" or the wigged and high-heeled streetwalker with equally stereotypical "evil," "domineering" and "bitchy" images in between.

The often repeated response that black women are honored in our communities is far too simplistic. It does not address the reality of the many hardships that go along with being black and female. For instance, according to the most recent FBI statistics, we are at a greater risk of being raped than any other group; fifty-seven percent of us raise our children alone; because of the job discrimination we suffer, our children are likely to spend more than five years of their childhood in poverty, compared to only ten months for white children. We have been "honored" to endure these and other burdens that have often prevented us from participating fully in life. And we have done so, not because we like being burdened, but because sexist, racist and homophobic social systems have given us little choice.

The images and expectations of black women are actually both super- and sub-human. This conflict has created many myths and stereotypes that cause confusion about our identity and make us targets for abuse. Like Shug Avery in Alice Walker's *The Color Purple,* black women are considered wild but also rigid and "proper." We are unattractive but exotic, like Vanessa Williams, the first black Miss America who was later dethroned.

We are passive but rabble-rousing like political activist Flo Kennedy. We are streetwise but insipid like Prissy who "didn't know nothing about birthin' no babies" in *Gone With the Wind.* We are considered evil but self-sacrificing; stupid but conniving; domineering while at the same time obedient to men; and sexually inhibited yet promiscuous. Covered by what is considered our seductively rich but repulsive brown skin, black women are perceived as inviting but armored. With all the mixed messages about us, society finds it difficult to believe that we really need physical and emotional support just like everybody else.

The Abused Black Woman—What's Love Got To Do With It?

Abused women have a tendency to put everyone else's needs before their own. Because of our cultural history, this conditioning in black women is particularly strong. Perhaps more than others, an abused woman is likely to hold traditional views about love, romance and relationships. You make a commitment to your partner and have a big investment in the relationship. You expect your partner to protect and provide for you physically, emotionally and perhaps even economically. Abused women usually give above and beyond the call of duty to their relationships.

Thus, when you are assaulted by the person you love, your beliefs and expectations about your relationship are shattered as well as your body. Many abused women liken the experience to having the rug pulled out from under their feet. There have probably been many good times in the relationship. Despite their violent behavior, abusers can be loving and are sometimes greatly admired within their community. Consequently, the abused woman faces conflicts both in her home and in her heart.

In order to get things back on safe footing you are likely to work harder—to cook better meals, to be more understanding or to pay more attention to your partner. But it is batterers who are responsible for their behavior, no matter how much they have conditioned you to believe that it is your fault. It is important to realize that no amount of good cooking, housekeeping, love, attention or self-blame will stop abusers from striking out when their tension level builds up. It is their responsibility to learn how to deal with their stress in a healthy way instead of using violence. In short, you didn't cause the abusive behavior, and you can't cure it.

Yes You Can

You might wonder if it is really possible to learn to free yourself from an abusive relationship. There are thousands of formerly abused black women who are today living without violence in their lives. They are a testament to your ability to get free, too.

To begin the process of ending violence in your life, it is essential that you tell someone you are being abused. It is impossible to change your situation or for others to help you if you do not admit there is something wrong in your life. As difficult as it may be to accept that your partner is abusing you, you must stop denying or minimizing the reality of your situation. Domestic violence is not to be taken lightly. It increases in frequency and severity unless there is some type of intervention. Look at it this way: If a stranger punched you out, slashed your car tires or pulled a gun on you, you would probably tell somebody about it. Your partner's violent behavior should be revealed, too. You don't deserve or have to be a sacrificial lamb.

Telling friends or trusted family members about your abuse can be a positive first step toward getting the help you need. You might also consider sharing your experiences with a black church leader in your community. After a long history of silence, many members of the clergy are beginning to confront the real issues of domestic violence and its destructive impact on black families. Some black churches are even affiliated with shelters for battered women or provide meeting rooms for support groups.

In the past two decades, a network of battered women's shelters have opened to assist abused women. Many of the shelter workers have made special efforts to respond sensitively to the insights and experiences of people of color. Shelters provide immediate safety and protection from the man who is abusing you and/or your children. Most of them offer counseling and support groups in which you'll meet other black women like yourself who can help you make independent decisions about your future life.

You can begin to put an end to your personal abuse by learning to love yourself in all your dimensions as a black woman. Learn to recognize your own self-hatred. Take an honest assessment of what you do and do not like about yourself and evaluate how many of your feelings are based on white beauty standards or symbols of success. How often do you greet other black women you might pass on the street? Do you bypass blacks in stores, banks, offices or other professional settings because you assume we are less competent in our jobs than whites? Do you seek out the black women in your community who appear to be improving their lives or do you assume they think they're "better" than you? Have you ever considered that other black women might really value having you as a friend? Remember the emotional scars in all of us run deep. They go back as far as our history in this country and none of us will recover from the damage overnight. But we cannot begin to overcome the insecurities and self-hatred that contribute to the abuse in our lives until we take an honest look at why these feelings exist.

It is not selfish to nurture yourself as you have nurtured so many others. Go back to school, take a vacation, exercise, get a medical check-up, pursue the employment you are really interested in and believe you are qualified to do. So much of our black beauty and ability has been camouflaged by poverty, nutritional deficiencies, and excessive physical and mental despair. Even baby steps toward putting yourself first will help to rid your life of domestic violence.

Changing your patterns and your relationship will involve pain, fear and lots of hard work. Some days you may feel lonely, depressed, angry and overwhelmed by it all. You may get sick of calling the police on your partner, listening to attorneys or spilling your heart out to a counselor. You may start wondering if any of your efforts are helping at all and might be tempted to just throw in the towel and live with things the way they are.

It is important to remember that no police officer, judge or counselor has the absolute power to stop your partner from abusing you. Not one of them can do more for you than you can do for yourself by taking the steps that will make you believe that you are a caring, gifted, valuable, unique and beautiful black woman who deserves and can have a loving, non-abusive relationship.

Footnotes

1. Zora Neale Hurston, "How It Feels To Be Colored Me," in *I Love Myself When I Am Laughing* (New York: The Feminist Press, 1978), p. 153.

2. Barbara Smith, introduction to *Home Girls* (New York: Kitchen Table Press, 1983), pp. xxxiv-xxxv.

Historically considered the backbone of health care providers in the black community, midwives have made enormous contributions to the well-being of black women. As the following piece reflects, traditional black midwives did more than just bring children into the world. They brought a vibrant world of wit, wisdom, courage and compassion to all the lives they touched.

Thank You Jesus to Myself:
The Life of a Traditional Black Midwife
Linda Janet Holmes

Black women have a long and rich history as midwives in this country. These grassroots midwives, who are frequently called "grannies," have provided midwifery care to large segments of women across racial categories and geographic regions for more than a hundred years. Their greatest contributions, however, have been in the South where they waited on countless black women in childbirth. Particularly when racism, economic deprivation and rural isolation made access to medical care difficult or impossible to obtain, the midwife was a primary source of care. By the 1960s, when the majority of "granny" midwives in other ethnic groups had been replaced by medically-based hospital practices, there were still hundreds of black lay midwives practicing in the deep South. Some of these women had midwifery lineages that extended as far back as slavery.

It is important to differentiate between traditional black lay midwives, modern lay midwives and nurse-midwives. Traditional midwives in all parts of the world tend to acquire their skills empirically. Southern black midwives frequently followed their grandmothers, mothers or other senior midwives in the community as part of their preparation for becoming a midwife. Traditional midwives also are frequently "called" in a spiritual sense into their practice and may be strong personal bearers of spiritual wisdom and/or may integrate spiritual practices into their birthing practices. In addition, midwives who are traditional usually are sensitive to and supportive of culturally specific rituals surrounding pregnancy and birth.

Nurse-midwives are recognized for their formalized training. They are registered nurses who are required to complete a standard course of training that usually includes extended rotations within medical settings. While the modern lay midwife is similar to southern black lay midwives in that her practice is usually home-birth oriented, many modern lay midwives are younger and are politically active in the birth alternatives movement. (Some women's organizations and midwife groups are now arguing that women should have greater opportunities for direct entry into midwife education without having to be registered nurses first.)

While modern lay midwives practice legally in several states and nurse midwifery practices continue to proliferate, state health departments have been successful in efforts to eradicate many black lay midwifery practices. In the past, these midwives have been easy targets for elimination. For the most part, even on the local level, independent midwifery organizations simply did not exist. Even their clients—potentially their greatest advocates—were anxious to take advantage of recently gained access to hospital-based obstetrical care. For example, in the 1960s, access to Medicaid and the gains of the civil rights movement made it possible for significant numbers of black families to receive long-denied hospital care. For many, the midwife came to be viewed as an "old-timey" symbol of the past and the choice of last resort. Interestingly, while a new wave of primarily white and middle-class consumers were beginning to have an impact on increasing birth options, these groups never successfully championed the cause of the black lay midwife. Meanwhile, many of the black midwives realized that "the longest part of that road was behind them" and they were ready to "sit down some." For whatever the reason, the demise of the black midwife did not generally evoke organized protest from midwife clients, broad-based consumer groups or the midwives themselves.

In 1981 I went to Alabama to tape-record interviews with midwives whose practices had been dramatically affected by a 1978 Alabama law which stopped the issuance of any new lay midwife permits. When this law was passed, all of Alabama's practicing midwives were black women. According to the only available statewide listing, there were more than a hundred midwives who had official permits to practice in 1976. When I began this project, however, most of these midwives had retired, been forced out of practice or died. Mattie Hereford was an exception. In 1981 she was still an actively practicing midwife. I interviewed her at her home in Huntsville, a major northern Alabama city. A mother she attended in childbirth later told me Mattie had the power to simply walk in the room and alleviate her pains. Indeed, Mattie Hereford was the kind of person who could just swallow you up with her warmth. We ended our first day together eating watermelon alongside the road.

Linda: When did you decide to become a midwife?

Mattie: Well, I tell you Linda, when I decided to become a midwife, it was in '51. Before that, I had been practicing, but I was just a helper. I loved sick people and loved to be around them ever since I was eight years old, when I was just a kid. In the neighborhood—we lived in the country—anybody'd get sick, I'd go see about 'em. See if I could give them some water, do something for them. Carry them something from my mama's house. Running back and forth to see if my mama had what they needed. And that's the way I got started, I guess.

But at first, I didn't know anything about babies cause mama never did teach us nothing about 'em. I knowed she'd had this baby, this big stomach, but we children didn't know what it was all about. They would tell us that these babies, they'd get 'em out the creek. The biggest whipping I ever got was because I was looking under a branch in a stump for a baby. Cause I fell in there. Like to drown myself cause I got scared.

I was looking in the stump for this baby, knowing it come out of the creek, see. But there was a branch down around the house and I went to peep over in this stump, just like I'm looking in that bag, looking for a baby. And there was a possum with three little possum babies in there and it scared me. I fell back and almost drowned. And a first cousin of my aunt, he come in there and got me.

I got a real whipping for that. My mama said, "What was you looking for?" I didn't tell her what I was looking for. I said I was just looking. She said, "What you-all doing down there?" I said we went down for some sweet gum. I didn't tell no lie. We had been looking for sweet gum. But I was interested when I saw that stump to look for this baby. It wound up being a possum!

Well, and then I grew up. Still didn't know about babies until I got married. I was sixteen years old when I went on and got married. That was in nineteen hundred and fourteen. People would send for me then about as much as they do now. Tell Matt to come. She don't know I'm sick. Go tell Matt. Didn't have telephones, you know. And if I see a doctor come out, or a midwife, I'd take off. If I had a chance,

I'd take off and go sit and start delivering people. Octavia Moore, I practiced under her for seven years. I delivered twenty-seven babies that I don't have no record for. I just wanted to see it done and be with her to help her. She was an elder woman. She wasn't as old when she died as I am. She was in her seventies. But she was kind of swelled up with arthritis—rheumatism was what we called it back then. She would tell me often, she'd say, "I want you to learn because I won't be able to do it by myself. If you learn, you can carry it on. You come in and be with me." When she be in the neighborhood, they would send for me. She would say, "Go tell Matt," night or day, "Go tell Matt to come over here on such-and-such a place." So that's the way I started.

Linda: What do you think is the most important thing that you learned from her?

Mattie: Tying and cutting the cord. I see the baby coming, I'd support that baby with my hands so it wouldn't come too fast and tear the mother. You see? I support that baby's head and ask the mother to just take it easy for a while and rest. And, then when the urge come to push, I say you push on down when you have another contraction, another pain, that's what I call it. Wasn't no contraction. Before the midwife got there, I'd always get a rag or towel or something, you know. There wasn't many towels, then, but I would get something clean and take care. Wipe the baby's eyes.

Linda: What do you think that midwives do to keep the mother from tearing when she delivers?

Mattie: Well, one thing I do, Linda, I don't let the mother push too hard as the baby's coming into the world cause pushing too hard would rush the baby too fast and that'll cause the mother to tear. And as I said, when that baby's coming into the world, if you support that baby's head and give the mother a chance to rest, why, she'll open up more easier and let the baby's head slip out.

Linda: What do you do if you do get a small tear or a little nick that doesn't require stitches?

Mattie: I just tell the mother to be careful and don't sit on the commode too hard. Just take her time and it'll clear up. I say, bathe yourself off good with warm water and Ivory soap. Put a little Vaseline on it. That's the way I do them.

Linda: Did the older midwives do anything else? Some of the midwives have been telling me about some of the other things that people used to do.

Mattie: They would use a little lard and a little sugar. Sometimes they'd get a drop of turpentine and put it in the solution and mix it up together and put in on a white clean rag. That turpentine would draw the soreness out. I don't know what the sugar would do. And that lard would keep the cloth from sticking to you. Cause if you grease it, it ain't gonna hardly stick.

Linda: Did the older midwives ever make their own cord dressing?

Mattie: You know what, good question, Linda, cause I wouldn't have thought about it. They would ask for thread. Now that was when my mama was having us. You know, I was very curious and I would always try to sneak around. I know there was an old midwife. I was a kid when that woman would come into my mama's bedroom. The machine was sitting in my mama's bedroom. And she would ask her, where's the thread, the white thread? And I could always tell her. My mama would tell her, say ask Mattie.

Linda: How old were you when you started officially being a midwife?

Mattie: I was about, I was fifty-something years old, fifty-eight or something when I started. I was no young woman when I started. At first, I helped a doctor out. He had patients on the farm out there where I lived. Well, there were about eighteen families on that farm. Anytime anyone got sick and went to the boss man and told him that they wanted a doctor for so and so, he'd tell 'em, well go tell Matt. Get Matt and let Matt stay with 'em until the doctor get there. Well, now I did that for eight to ten years before I came to be a midwife. Didn't care what was the matter, night or day, people would come and get me. I would provide all the care I knowed how. They'd be real sick. I'd carry some camphor or something like that, I'd always have medication at my house, cause I had children, and every time some of the neighbor's children got sick, they'd come by saying tell Matt to send me so and so, such a child is sick. Well, I would do it, I couldn't keep no supplies in, cause I had to supply the whole neighborhood, you see.

Linda: How much did you get paid for delivering babies?

Mattie: Just twenty-five dollars a delivery. If it were twenty babies coming out at one time, it's just twenty-five. And, Linda, I didn't get that sometimes. One time I delivered a girl her baby she paid me and I told her, I said, do you know what? What Mama Matt? I said, your daddy never paid me for you. She said, Mama Matt, you got to be kidding. I said, it's the truth. I don't have to lie.

Linda: Did she offer to pay you or not?

Mattie: No, her daddy paid me. And I said, you don't have to do this. He said, oh yes, it's worth it to me. That you brought her into the world. I said, no, I didn't. Her mother brought her into the world. He said, I'm certainly glad you brought it up cause I forgot. I said, no you didn't.

Linda: Some of the midwives I've talked to, they don't know how many babies they've birthed. They have no idea. Do you know how many babies you've delivered?

Mattie: Eight hundred and thirty-nine up until last Friday. I know that.

Linda: What years were you the busiest?

Mattie: I believe it was in '67, cause I was delivering babies coming and going. In one week, I delivered seven babies from Tuesday morning before day 'til Friday night around twelve o'clock. I value all of them. Even though some of them owed me. I didn't feel too bad because when I would deliver a baby, peoples didn't have much money. I'd say, well the Lord did something to make somebody happy today.

Linda: What would you do for a mother who said she was having problems with a child who was teething?

Mattie: Well, there was a big wide leaf plant called a burdock. We'd dig that up and get the roots of it. And we'd peel that burdock. And we'd take it and cut it up in little bitty chips. Then we would get a needle and thread and we'd string it, just like a string of beads, 'nuff to go around the neck. And too, we'd use, they call it a rice button. That was a plain white button, not a pearl button. And if the baby had one tooth, we'd put that button around that. Another tooth come, we'd put another button. That's the way they did it.

I had a sister with a fifteen-month-old baby that had pneumonia. Dr. Turner couldn't get her fever down, and she was just sick and losing weight. Everything they'd give her to eat, she'd throw it up. My sister called me down there one night. Sent her husband after me. And I went down there with some quinine and some of my husband's snuff. I mixed it up with some lard and turpentine and half a teaspoon of camphor. I mixed all that up. Then I took an an old pillow case and tore it half in two, and made a wide band. I took that iron and scorched that rag all the way, just scorched it. Next, I put my mixture all over that thing. I wrapped it around the baby and sewed it around her. And when the doctor come back, that baby was eating like a little pig. He said, what a surprise. Said, you know Mary, I'm glad I changed the medication. She said, doctor, I have to tell you the truth. Matt cured this baby. Matt come over her last night and cured this baby.

I told you, I never had a doctor to come in my house to nary child I got, 'cept when they had a broken arm or broken leg. The only time they went to the doctor, I had one daughter, my second daughter, she had worm spasms and I carried her to the doctor. Started having them spasms on a Sunday and I was at church. And if I had been at home when she'd had that spasm, I'd a went out there in the field somewhere and got some cockleburs.

Linda: What's a cocklebur?

Mattie: Oh shit, Linda. A cocklebur, honey, is a weed that grows and it has a bud on it and you can walk through that and it'll stick all over you. Well, I'd got some of them and made a tea. Then, that would've stopped her. I did make the tea. You know, people wasn't able to get doctors all the time. They didn't have money from one end of the crop to the next or all through the year like we have now. So we just had to do the best we could, me and all the rest of 'em.

Linda: Did the midwives use any kind of teas to make the labor pains harder?

Mattie: Yeah. Black pepper tea. I let them give me some with my first one. They give me a lot of tea. They had me pushing and pulling on me, and when I wasn't having nothing but just false contractions, they kept ahollering. Look like the water ought to break. But she ain't bearing down, honey. And I was so tired when the time come for me to bear down, I didn't. I didn't have the strength to bear down. So, I learned myself how to be a midwife.

Linda: So, by the time you had the second baby...

Mattie: I knowed all about it. But you know, I ain't never had but one baby on the bed and the doctor take it. I always had my children on the floor.

Linda: What about a cord around the neck?

Mattie: I don't worry about that. If I can get my fingers between, up between there to reach that cord, I can reach that cord and pull that cord enough to slacken it. Then that baby will come on out. Cause I've had it with them around the neck twice, just double around there. But if I ever get it slacked enough before the baby come on out, why it's just gonna come out all right.

Linda: What was one of your most difficult births?

Mattie: My hardest one to deliver, you mean? I had a baby that come breech. I tried to get a doctor in and the people, they had a telephone, but they was on an eight-party line. Couldn't get through to nobody. And I went back in the house, went back to the bed, and I said to the mama, I still can't see nothing but his butt. So she prayed and I prayed. I said this baby's coming. I said you just bear with me, and with God to help me, this baby's going to be alive. Sure 'nuff, it was. I pushed that baby and kept mashing on it just like it was butter. I kept pushing. And you know, finally, I put my hand up in between her baby's butt and her. I got a little foot. And when I got that, honey, when I got that...

Linda: Hallelujah, right?

Mattie: Thank you Jesus to myself! And so finally that little butt slipped back.

Linda: Did you pull that foot out?

Mattie: Uh-huh. Pulled that foot out and that little old butt jumped back over there and directly here come the other foot. And the doctor had done told me one time when I called him about how to deliver when they come foot foremost, and that other foot come on out. I got up on the bed with her, in between her legs and pulled directly, just straight out. And here come that baby's butt and here come the head. And he hollered. And honey, I was a glad creature. I jumped out of that bed, got on my knees and said thank you Jesus. I had to go down cause He said every knee shall bow. And I know if I ever needed Him, I needed Him then. Cause I didn't want that baby to die and I didn't want that patient to die.

Linda: Now, the triplets.

Mattie: That was a big woman. I told her that I thought she was going to have twins, 'cause I done delivered thirty-two in that family. And when the first one was born, I looked at the little thing and I knowed there was more. I said there's another. She said, God I wasn't looking for but one. I said, you ordered one, but you're buying two. And then the next one came. So she got up and I put a pad on her, keep her from, you know, losing her waste on the floor and all. Then we got up and drank coffee and ate donuts. So she's sitting there in the chair and she said, I sure have the pains. So, I got her back in bed. And I looked in there and here come the other little bitty head. I had a bed full of babies.

Linda: What about the afterbirth? What did they do with the afterbirth in the olden times?

Mattie: Burn it up. Now they want you to wrap it up and just throw it in the garbage. But I don't want the dog to get it, so I still burn it up like in the old days.

Linda: When you were having babies, did you stay in bed for a long time?

Mattie: Nine days. And, keep the curtains down.

Linda: Did the white folks do that or just the black people?

Mattie: I don't know whether the white people did it or not. Of course, you know, wasn't many midwives that delivered many white babies at that time. But my eighth delivery was white. Now I done delivered more white babies for these last ten years. I have got eight deliveries coming up now and I ain't got but one black. I think it's because the white people got the insurance. And a lot of them claim they've had such a bad deal with the doctor.

Linda: Finally, was the midwife considered an important person in the community?

Mattie: No, not too much. Now, I wonders about that myself because I am very important to people. You know they say, there's Mattie Hereford, she's the midwife. I know I am important, because I feel it, you know, to myself.

. . .

Mattie Hereford died one year after this interview.

President of Planned Parenthood Federation since 1978, Faye Wattleton has been a militant advocate for women's reproductive freedom and a passionate defender of choice for all women. In this piece she addresses the burgeoning crisis of teen pregnancy in America, and outlines strategies for ensuring that black teens have access to the contraceptives and comprehensive sex education that will improve their chances for an independent and productive life.

Teenage Pregnancy: A Case for National Action
Faye Wattleton

In 1983 a twenty-five-year-old woman with a nine-year-old daughter gave the following testimony before Congress:

> In the tenth grade, my girlfriends and I were all sexually active, but none of us used birth control. I had hopes of a career and I wanted to go to college. One day my mother said, "Towanda, you're pregnant." I asked her how she knew. She said, "I can just tell."
>
> My mother wouldn't even consider abortion. I had nothing to say about a decision that would alter my entire life. A few weeks after the baby was born, my mother said, "You'll have to get a job." The only job I could get was in a bar.
>
> I spent two years dealing with the nightmare of welfare. Finally I went to the father of my child and asked him to take care of her while I went back to school. He agreed.
>
> I am now making some progress. I went to business school and I now have a job working in an office in Washington. But my life has been very difficult... I had ambitions as a child, but my hopes and dreams were almost killed by the burden of trying to raise a child while I was still a child myself.

This young woman's story is relived around us every day. The United States has the dubious distinction of leading the industrialized world in its rates of teenage pregnancy, teenage childbirth and teenage abortion. According to a study of thirty-seven developed nations published by the Alan Guttmacher Institute in 1985, the teen pregnancy rate in the U.S. is more than double the rate in England, nearly triple the rate in Sweden and seven times the rate in the Netherlands. Throughout the 1970s, this rate rose in the U.S., while it declined in such places as England, Wales and Sweden. Each year, more than one million American teenagers become pregnant; about half of these young women give birth.

Teen pregnancy is both cause and consequence of a host of social ills. The teenagers likeliest to become pregnant are those who can least afford an unwanted child: those who are poor, those who live with one parent, those who have poor grades in school and those whose parents did not finish high school. As the National Research Council points out, teen mothers face "reduced employment opportunities, unstable marriages (if they occur at all), low incomes, and heightened health and developmental risks to the children... Sustained poverty, frustration, and hopelessness are all too often the long-term outcomes." Compounding the tragedy is the fact that children of teenage mothers are more likely to become teen parents themselves. The burden is felt by the entire society: The national costs of health and social service programs for families started by teenagers amount to more than nineteen billion dollars a year.

Media accounts have tended to represent teenage pregnancy as primarily a problem of the black community, and implicitly—or explicitly, as in the case of the 1986 CBS Special Report on the "vanishing" black family by Bill Moyers—they have attempted to blame the problem on the so-called degeneracy of the black family. Such distortions of fact are particularly dangerous because they coincide all too neatly with the insensitivity to blacks and the blame-the-victim ideology that the Reagan administration so disastrously fostered.

High rates of teen pregnancy actually are as all-American as apple pie. Even when the figures for "nonwhite" teens were subtracted from the calculations, the rate of teen pregnancy in the U.S. in 1981 (83 per 1,000) far exceeded the teen pregnancy rates in all other major industrialized nations. In England and Wales, our closest competitors, the rate for teens of all races was just 45 per 1,000.

The fact of the matter is that teenage pregnancy rates in the U.S. have a great deal more to do with class than they do with race. The majority of poor people in this country are white, and so are the majority of pregnant teenagers. In a report published in 1986, the Guttmacher Institute examined interstate differences in teen pregnancy rates. It found that the percentage of teens who are black is relatively unimportant as a determinant of overall state variations in teenage reproduction. It is states with higher percentages of poor people and of people living in urban areas—whatever their race—that have significantly higher teen pregnancy and birth rates.

Teen pregnancy is as grave a problem within many black communities as are poverty and social alienation. One-third of all blacks, and one-half of all black children, live in poverty. And today the pregnancy rate among teens of color is double that of white teens. One of every four black children is born to a teenage mother. Such patterns can only intensify the problems already facing the black community. Disproportionately poor, blacks are disproportionately affected by the social and economic consequences of teenage pregnancy.

We need only to look to other Western nations to recognize both the cause of and the solutions to our teen pregnancy problem. American teens are no more sexually active than their counterparts in Europe; and teenagers abroad resort to abortion far less often than do those in the U.S. There is a major cause for our higher rates of teen pregnancy and childbirth: the fundamental discomfort of Americans with sexuality. Unlike other Western societies, we have not yet accepted human sexuality as a normal part of life. The result is that our children, and many adults as well, are confused, frightened and bombarded by conflicting sexual messages.

Most parents recognize their role as the first and most important sexuality educators their children will have, providing information and sharing family values from the time their children are born. Nevertheless, many parents are unable to talk with their children about such sensitive issues as sex and human relationships. Schools do not fill the gap. Only seventeen states and the District of Columbia mandate comprehensive sex education. As a result, many teenagers are abysmally ignorant about their reproductive functions.

The mass media, particularly television, only exacerbate the problem. Many teenagers spend more time in front of the television than they do in the classroom, and their sexual behavior in part reflects what they have learned from this thoroughly unreliable teacher. Nowhere is it more apparent than on television that America suffers from sexual schizophrenia: We exploit sex, and at the same time we try to repress it. Programs and advertisements bombard viewers with explicit sexual acts and innuendo. One study indicates that in a single year, television airs 20,000 sexual messages. Yet rarely is there any reference to contraception or to the consequences of sexual activity.

A substantial number of teens believe that what they see on television is a faithful representation of life. Many believe that television gives a realistic picture of pregnancy and the consequences of sex. And large numbers of teens say they do not use contraceptives because they are "swept away" by passion—surely a reflection of the romanticized view of sex that pervades the mass media.

Network executives, though they apparently have few qualms about exploiting the sexual sell twenty-four hours a day, have the hypocrisy to claim that good taste forbids them to carry ads for contraceptives. Some of the networks recently decided to accept condom ads, though not during prime time, and those ads promote condoms only as protection against AIDS, not against pregnancy. It should not surprise us, then, that America's youth are sexually illiterate, or that sixty-seven percent of sexually active teens either never use contraceptives or use them only occasionally.

We have not failed to resolve this problem for lack of majority agreement on how to do it. A 1988 Harris public opinion survey done for Planned Parenthood found a strong consensus about both the severity of the teen pregnancy problem and how to solve it:

- Ninety-five percent of Americans think that teenage pregnancy is a serious problem in this country, up 11 percent from 1985.

- Seventy-eight percent of parents believe that relaxed discussions between parents and children about sex will reduce unintended teen pregnancy.

- Eighty-nine percent endorse school sex education.

- Eighty percent support school referrals of sexually active teens to outside family-planning clinics.

- Seventy-three percent favor making contraceptives available in school clinics.

School-linked clinics that offer birth control as part of general health care are growing in number in many areas of the country. Community support and involvement are crucial to their development, to insure that the programs are consistent with community values and needs.

Clearly the vast majority of Americans, regardless of racial, religious or political differences, strongly supports the very measures that have proven so effective in reducing teen pregnancy rates in other Western nations. Unfortunately, an extremist minority in this country has an entirely different outlook on sexuality—a minority that has a level of influence out of all proportion to its size. Eager to cultivate the anti-family planning, anti-abortion fringe, the Reagan-Bush administration and its cohorts in Congress sought to whittle down Federal funds for domestic and international family planning, limit sex education in schools, eliminate confidentiality for birth control and abortion services and block the development of school-linked clinics. These vocal opponents object to everything that has proven successful elsewhere in the industrialized world. Their one and only solution to the problem of teenage pregnancy is, "Just say no!" But just saying no prevents teenage pregnancy the way "Have a nice day" cures chronic depression.

There is nothing inherent in American life that condemns us permanently to having the highest teen pregnancy rate in the Western world—nothing that Sweden, England, France, the Netherlands and Canada have been able to do that we cannot.

Parents must talk with their children about all aspects of sexuality—openly, consistently and often—beginning in early childhood. Every school district in the country should provide comprehensive sex education, from kindergarten through twelfth grade. Community groups need to support the development of school-linked health clinics. The media must present realistic, balanced information about relationships and the consequences of sex. Television, in particular, must end the restrictions on contraceptives advertising. Government—at the local, state and federal levels—must live up to its obligation to eliminate any financial barriers to family-planning education and services and to foster a community environment in which our children can flourish and aspire to a productive and fulfilling life.

But we must also recognize that the teen pregnancy problem cannot be solved through sexuality education and family-planning services alone. If our efforts are to succeed, society must provide all our young people with a decent general education, tangible job opportunities, successful role models and real hope for the future.

It is only by placing such a comprehensive national agenda at the top of the priority list that our society can protect the creative and productive potential of its youth.

In the following piece, eighteen-year-old single parent Mikeil Shaw and her mother, Wanda Brock, share their personal experiences and offer invaluable insights into the challenges of teen pregnancy in the black community. The interview was conducted by journalist Marsha R. Leslie.

In a Family Way:
Notes from a Black Teenage Mother
Marsha R. Leslie

Marsha: Why did you become sexually active so early?

Mikeil: I was a freshman in high school and on the drill team. In the ninth grade I became popular and got more attention from the boys. I would say I became sexual because of peer pressure—to satisfy the guy and because so many girls were talking about it. I felt they would call me a nerd if they knew I hadn't done it. Every time I turned around, that was all they were talking about. At first I was really strong, then I gave in to the pressure. I was really scared, but then I did it anyway.

Marsha: Do you think teenage pregnancies occur more among black girls than other populations?

Mikeil: Most black girls don't get abortions. When white teenagers get pregnant their parents force them to get abortions. So, it obviously looks like the black population is having a lot of kids. It also comes down to money. A lot of lower-class white girls have their babies. Higher-class whites tell their daughters that they're not raising any grandbabies and that the daughter's got to get out of their house. So they get abortions.

Marsha: What about the threat of AIDS? Aren't teenagers fearful of getting AIDS?

Mikeil: They feel they can't get it. Teenagers don't think about it much anymore. When we first heard about AIDS, it was the big talk. But now, it's like we know about it, but we don't care. We only think about the pleasure of it (sex). The attitude of my generation—all they care and talk about is—"Who's gettin' who?"

Marsha: What do you think will make them care and change their attitudes about AIDS?

Mikeil: If someone that we know personally got AIDS, someone young, in our generation, then, maybe . . .

Marsha: Did your sexual partners use contraceptives or was that your responsibility?

Mikeil: I guess they felt it was mine. The only thing I basically knew how to use was the condom. I knew that other contraceptives existed, but I didn't know how to use them.

Marsha: What were your feelings when you found out you were pregnant?

Mikeil: I found out I was pregnant in October 1988. I conceived in August. I went that long before I even knew I was pregnant.

I thought about myself a lot. I was on the drill team, danced and went to parties. I thought I didn't want to have a baby, that I was too young to have a baby. I was depressed and confused.

Marsha: Did you consider having an abortion?

Mikeil: Yeah. I had basically made up my mind to have an abortion, but I was scared.

Marsha: What did the baby's father think of the pregnancy?

Mikeil: He wanted me to have the baby. I remember calling him and telling him I wanted to have an abortion. I can still hear him crying on the phone. He had gotten a girl pregnant before and she had an abortion. He wanted me to have his baby and wanted us to be together forever.

He went out and got himself two jobs and was going to school to get his GED (General Equivalency Degree). We were going to be married. His birthday was May 14 and mine was June 11. We wanted to wait until we were eighteen so no one would have any say over us.

Marsha: Why didn't that happen?

Mikeil: LeRoy, my baby's father, passed away on New Year's Eve, before the baby was born. He committed suicide. He was a depressed person. He was a confused person in a lot of ways and he kept it all inside.

One time when I was with him, he tried to take some pills. I thought it was minor. We went to the hospital and they pumped his stomach and he was fine.

But this time, on New Year's Eve, he got a gun and shot himself in the head.

Marsha: If he wanted you to have the baby and had so much to live for, why do you think he killed himself?

Mikeil: That's the question I ask myself every single day. Why did he do it when he knew the baby was on the way? Nobody knows. He was depressed a couple of days before he did it. I could tell that something was not right. The day he did it, I talked to him. He sounded so much better. He sounded the opposite of what he felt, I guess. He was so cute that day. He told me to put the phone to my stomach so he could talk to the baby. I still don't know why he did it. That's the question that's always in his mother's and my head.

Marsha: Would you say your relationship with LeRoy was different than with your other sexual partners?

Mikeil: Yes. Because with my baby's dad I would say I loved him or felt that I loved him. With him it was different than the first time I did it. I wasn't scared anymore. His ways made me feel better. He wanted me to enjoy myself and not just him. He wanted it to be good for us together.

Marsha: What was your mother's reaction to your pregnancy?

Mikeil: When I conceived, my mom was in a drug rehabilitation center for cocaine addiction. I called her. She guessed right off and asked, "What are you going to do?" She didn't scold me. But she told me she didn't believe in abortions. She said that she got pregnant three times and had all three of her kids.

My mom got out of the rehab center in November and told the people there that she had to be home for her pregnant daughter. So, I felt the baby was helping my mom... that my mom was going to do better. She was home and going to church for about a month up until December. When LeRoy died, she was there for me for about two days and then she left. . . . She's here now. She still has problems. But I think my son helps her an awful lot.

She keeps LeRoy for me when I'm in school or want to go out. I don't even have to ask her. I know that taking care of him is helping my mom with stuff.

Marsha: Being a parent is a tremendous responsibility. How has parenthood affected your life?

Mikeil: It's not just Mikeil any more. I can't go anywhere. *We* go somewhere. It's like that now. It's harder because sometimes I forget. I'm still young and haven't gotten my kickin' out. I still have a lot of fun I haven't finished. But then I have to think of LeRoy. I have to turn down a lot of things in order to be there for my son. I have to be there for him. It's Mikeil and LeRoy now. I have to finish school for LeRoy, so I don't have to tell him we have to wait 'til the first of the month for the welfare check. I have to finish so my son can have things.

Welfare and me are not friends. I just got on it this month. I struggled with that, but I had to get on it. But it won't be for long. I'll get a job and there's a day care at school. I'll work half the day and go to school the other half.

Marsha: What are your future educational plans?

Mikeil: My plans are to get my high school diploma and then go to a community college and study child psychology.

Marsha: If you could have anything for your son, what would that be?

Mikeil: Just his dad right now . . . for him to have a father figure.

Marsha: What about in the future? What would you want for him?

Mikeil: A lot that I didn't have . . . a Bill Cosby Show-like thing. I know it's a fantasy world. But I want LeRoy to have everything he wants and needs. Not in a spoiled way. But so he won't have to wait 'til the first of the month. I want to show him that he'll have to work for things just like I have to work for things for him.

Marsha: What advice would you give other teenage girls?

Mikeil: Wait to have kids. It's no fun. And, if you do, take it a day at a time with pregnancy and raising your child. You'll have a better attitude toward your baby and yourself.

Marsha: What advice would you give to boys? What would you tell your son, for example?

Mikeil: That sex is a part of life. But if you're going to have sex, care about the person and use protection, even if the girl says she's on birth control pills. These young guys don't know how to be a father. They don't know what they're doing.

Marsha: What are the benefits in having LeRoy?

Mikeil: He's benefitting me a lot, because I have to think about him. I braid hair and get twenty dollars. I can take the money and go to the movies or I can take the twenty dollars, give it to my grandmother to keep so I can buy diapers for LeRoy. Those are the kinds of decisions I have to make. I always have to go with the decision for LeRoy. Having him is making me more independent and helping me to save money.

I love my son very much. Without him, I don't know where I'd be. He's just an infant, but he helps his mother. He helps me day by day—every day he's in this world with me.

When his dad died, my first response was that I'd have to kill myself too, to be with him. And then I didn't want to, because I could feel my son move inside me. Then I realized, "Oh, I have something to live for."

My baby makes me want to go to school. I could have dropped out and gotten my GED, but I don't want that. I want to show my son my high school diploma so he can see that I finished. He's my motivation and inspiration each day he's here.

In a Family Way: Part Two

Marsha: What was your reaction when you found out your daughter Mikeil was pregnant?

Wanda: I initially expected it. I had a gut feeling. She wanted an abortion at first. But I told her I don't believe in abortions. I think that every person should have their chance to live; that every person that is born or conceived was meant to be. God controls everything, I feel. I'm just religious. I feel that the baby was supposed to be here.

Marsha: Did you think about the impact of a child on your daughter's life?

Wanda: Not at that particular moment. I've always explained to them —my girls especially—the impact of teenage motherhood . . . what it would do to your self-esteem. You feel that you have to accept second best, especially if the father is not around. In Mikeil's case and in my case, it just happened that way.

Marsha: Did you tell your children about sex?

Wanda: Not so much with Mikeil, because when I approached her, she didn't want to hear it. That was when she was eleven. Then in 1982, I went to prison. When I went to prison and was away from her, she couldn't understand. She was a baby when I separated from her dad, so I had clung to her. It really had a big impact on her when I went away. Then my father died. That was somebody else taken away from her. And then LeRoy. There have been periods in her life when she's had someone close just zapped away. I think the losses have bombarded her and given her negative feelings about herself.

Marsha: Why did you go to prison?

Wanda: Welfare fraud. I think it affected Mikeil. I think that in some way she got pregnant as a way to hurt me, because she's angry at me for going to prison. We haven't talked about it, but I think the time will come.

Marsha: Would you say that your mother, Mikeil's grandmother, has been one of the stabilizing influences in her life?

Wanda: My mom is very stable. I lack stability and I realize that.

Marsha: Did your mother have children when she was young?

Wanda: My mom had her first child when she was fifteen. By the time she was twenty-one she had four. But my mom was married. She was married to my dad for forty-seven years. She had nine kids altogether—the first when she was fifteen and the last when she was forty-two. By the time I was seventeen I had two children.

Marsha: Why were you sexual so early?

Wanda: I don't know. When I came to Seattle, I was thirteen. So, it was a big culture shock for me. I had gone to segregated schools and lived in segregated neighborhoods. In Seattle, I talked and dressed differently from everyone else and I suppose I just wanted to be a part of things because I felt like an outcast. At that age, your peers are very important to you. So, boys became more important to me than anything.

I also came from a dysfunctional family. My dad was an alcoholic and I played the role of the scapegoat child. My wall of defense was to become a drug abuser myself and an unwed mom. Boys became important because they made me feel needed, wanted, loved and petted.

My mother and I were not close at all. My two sisters died when they were young, so I grew up primarily with my brothers and my dad. Men just became more significant in my life than females. So, what can I say? The male rulership had been instilled in me.

Marsha: How do you break the cycle of teenage pregnancy, parenting and poverty among black women?

Wanda: I think the best way to break the cycle is to raise your self-esteem.

Marsha: How do you do that?

Wanda: I think the answer is counseling and education. They are the keys to breaking the cycle. I think you can raise your self-esteem if you face your feelings and try to deal with them. For example, I know I have low self-esteem and I think all my children do to a certain extent. I think that if we can just get on top of the situation and realize that we're okay the way we are and get support for getting better, we'll do okay.

We need more support from each other. We used to have family meetings a lot and I want to get back into that. We need to praise one another and help each other find solutions to our problems.

People like myself, who've had the ups and downs—teenage pregnancy, teenage motherhood, drugs, prison, jails—we're down as far as you can get. It takes us a little longer to stroke ourselves and rebuild our self-esteem.

I was watching a television show last night and they said something about being a parent that really made me start thinking. They said that in order for us to win our kids' love, we have to first win their respect. I think that over a period of years, my kids lost their respect for me. So it's going to take some time to build it back up.

Marsha: Are you in a drug rehabilitation program or are you fully recovered?

Wanda: No, I'm recovering. I think a person recovers for the rest of her life.

Marsha: Mikeil said that teenagers aren't concerned about pregnancy or AIDS. Why do you think that is?

Wanda: It goes back to self-esteem. If you care about yourself, why wouldn't you care about getting AIDS? I can understand those feelings. When so many other things have gone wrong in your life and you see no future, you really get to a point where you don't care, you just give up.

Sometimes I feel like, "Oh God, what's the use of living?" Then I think there are a lot of reasons and myself is one. Right now I'm really taking a good look at Wanda and what God has given me. If I use what He gives me, instead of those things that I'm not supposed to use, things will be okay.

*On July 3, 1989, the U.S. Supreme Court upheld parts of a Missouri stat-
ute that barred abortions from being performed at public facilities, by public employees or through the use of any public resources. Many believe
that the ruling is a severe threat to the landmark 1973* Roe v. Wade *decision that gave American women a constitutional right to abortion.*

*While religious and cultural pressures have historically kept many
black women from the forefront of the reproductive rights movement, a
growing number of black women are becoming active in pro-choice efforts. For example, the National Black Women's Health Project sent thirteen busloads of people to a massive abortion rights march held in Washington, D.C. prior to the Supreme Court decision.*

*Because of economics and their lack of access to adequate health care,
women of color will clearly suffer the most by a tightening of restrictions
on abortions.*

*In the following piece, the author writes of her illegal abortion in the
early 1960s and advocates the right of every woman to safe and affordable
abortions.*

Abortion: A Matter of Choice
Judy D. Simmons

Abortion is a great equalizer of women. Whatever their age, class or
race, women tend to walk the same way after ending a pregnancy.
They sort of hunch their shoulders, fold their arms rather protec-
tively across their upper bodies, and take small steps. Of course,
they're pretty woozy when they come out; most stay in the recovery
room only long enough to get conscious and unsteadily upright. Nobody wants to spend a lot of time sipping tea and eating cookies in
the clinic, any more than she hangs around the dentist's office after
oral surgery or looks forward to a chummy tete-a-tete following an
audit by the Internal Revenue Service.

Aborting a pregnancy isn't the high point of a woman's day.
Nor, however, is it the melodramatic tragedy, social cancer, mortal
sin, legislative crisis or genocidal master plan that various segments
of the American public represent it to be. Women have been preventing and aborting pregnancies as long as they've been women. Afri-

can queen and pharaoh Hatshepsut, who reigned in Egypt between 1500 and 1479 B.C., invented a method of birth control. Numerous African women enslaved in the United States aborted pregnancies rather than bear children into slavery or give birth to the products of slave masters' rapes, notes Paula Giddings in her book, *When and Where I Enter*. A sixty-seven-year-old woman I know who has lived in a number of places in this country told me that every town she was ever in had its abortionist, and everyone knew where to find him or her. Abortion has been either legal or not a matter of public-policy intervention in many nations for ages. Like so many things one deals with in life, abortion is an uncomfortable but not uncommon experience. In the case of a girl we'll call Renee—a fifteen-year-old with a troubled home life, some emotional deficits and little practical awareness—abortion is a necessity, a mercy and a chance to build a better life.

These were my thoughts a few years back as I sat in a Westchester County, New York, women's clinic waiting for Renee to emerge from the inner sanctum where the abortions are done. These thoughts are a good deal more reasonable and coherent than the ones I had when I ended my first pregnancy in 1963. At that time, abortions were illegal in the United States. I traveled to Tijuana, Mexico, from Sacramento, California, where I lived and went to college. I can remember having one clear idea: If the place looked and felt like a butcher shop, I'd come home and let the pregnancy come to term. I had heard about the coat-hanger and knitting-needle abortions that were the standard methods for poor and nonwhite women before the 1973 *Roe v. Wade* Supreme Court decision that legalized abortion; and I had read about women being rendered sterile or dying as the aftermath of "back-alley" abortions. My thoughts at that time were sheer, simple fear and an awful sadness. A phase of my life was ending—an innocence, if you'll allow me that. Deciding to *have an abortion* went against every dream I'd had since I was seven or eight and found out how interestingly babies are made.

I was always a dreamy girl. As a preschooler I dreamed that I flew around heaven with a blue-eyed, blond-haired Jesus. I dreamed —until I actually did it at seventeen—that I'd be reunited with my father, who had divorced me and my mother when I was five. From the time I went from Rhode Island to segregated Alabama when I was seven, I dreamed I'd escape the red-clay dust, the gnats, the slop pails and the prejudiced white folks and get back up North to be Somebody.

Naturally, the deepest dream was that I would marry an intelligent, handsome, God-fearing man, be his divine helpmeet, have six children (to compensate for my only-child loneliness, I guess) and live happily ever after. To me, love, sex, marriage, children, goodness and happiness were all wrapped up in one romantic religious package that automatically came in the mail when you were old enough. Finding out that this wasn't so, in a scant three months of 1963, emotionally devastated me.

As I waited for Renee I pondered the similarities and differences in our abortion situations. In the twenty-odd years gone by between the two experiences, abortion has been legalized in the United States —that is an obvious difference. What's not so obvious, perhaps, is the psychological difference that makes. Renee didn't have to contact what amounted to an underground network and have a password (a previous patient's code name) to make her appointment. She didn't have to fly far away from home, family and friends and cross a national border feeling as if she had a flashing neon sign on her forehead saying ABORTION. She didn't have to fear being arrested when she went for a post-abortion checkup if the doctor decided to help some lout of a prosecutor polish his reputation by meddling in a personal matter that should never be part of the legal system.

Renee wasn't totally ignorant about the procedure and what to expect following it. I thought I'd have terrible cramps and bleed to the point of hemorrhage. Imagine my surprise when I returned to the hotel, fell asleep and woke up feeling wonderful, with only the discomfort of being famished from not having eaten all day. I then proceeded to eat the most delicious fried chicken ever sold by a restaurant. Relief is a great flavor-enhancer. If there's one cause I might take up the gun for, it's that girls and women should always be able to get safe, legal, caring, "sunshine" abortions. No one should be subjected to the terror of clandestine activity in addition to the other stresses that usually surround a decision to abort.

The similarities between Renee's experience and mine are an old story. Renee was impregnated by a man ten years her senior who said he was going to marry her. My "fiance" was thirteen years older than I. Renee's seducer was in an authority position—a security guard at her junior high school. Mine was my thirty-one-year-old languages professor (white and, it later turned out, gay). Renee was hungry for love and protection to make her feel wanted and worthwhile. So was I. Like most young girls—indeed, like many people in the United States—Renee imposed fantasy on reality, acting on the assumption that what she felt and wanted to happen was really what was happening. So did I. But it ain't easy, especially when you're a teenager whose awakening glands can make you think mud looks like fudge and smells like perfume.

The similarity between Renee and me that makes me angry is that adult women never talked to us *realistically* about being a woman, lover and mother. When I spoke with Renee the day before she went for the abortion, she showed no awareness of why her mother might stay married to Renee's tyrant of a stepfather, who was making advances toward Renee and terrorizing the family with physical violence, meanness about money and refusal to allow them visitors and telephone calls.

The kid wasn't anywhere near ready for parental responsibility, as far as I could tell. When I told her that the pretty cribs she saw on television cost upwards of four hundred bucks, her eyes got big. She told me that if she gave birth she'd have to go live with an aunt whose daughter, also a teenager, had recently had a baby. When I asked her why her aunt would want another teen with a child in the house, and where the money would come from to support them all, Renee just looked overwhelmed. Then I asked Renee why a twenty-four-year-old man who already had small children and lived with a grown woman would seduce a scrawny, underdeveloped child like Renee and not even protect her.

Renee's answers to these questions revealed that she'd been acting her age, playing the appropriate early teen games of get a boy to lie to you, compete with the other girl, send messages through friends, play hide and seek with parents. But Renee was the only teenager in that game, a vulnerable kid who feels she's unloved and unwanted by both her parents. *Where are the people who are supposed to supervise and protect this young girl?* I wondered. Renee's mother and aunts clearly didn't have any greater hopes for her than that she follow in their stunted footsteps of early motherhood, broken relationships, undeveloped skills and enforced dependence on men who may extract a high price for their support.

I know a woman who had her first child out of wedlock at thirteen, another at seventeen, then got married and had two more kids before her husband left her. The woman was very nearly crazy with bills and parental responsibilities. When she suspected that her sixteen-year-old daughter might be messing around, she responded to my query about a heart-to-heart mother-daughter discussion of responsible sex and birth control with a haughty "I'm not going to talk to her about those things. She'll think I'm condoning sex." Condoning sex! Did this woman's mother "condone" her having sex and a baby at thirteen? "My mother? Hell, no." Did that stop her from doing both? "I don't care. If my daughter's going to mess around, she'll just have to take the consequences." I ran screaming into the night.

Why, why, generation after generation, do we send young girls out ignorant? Sure, I remember comments from women such as "You better take care of yourself" and "You lie down with dogs, you get up with fleas," or "Girl, it's hard to be a woman." These are vague warnings indeed when the lust tide of puberty rises; when the guys are so sleek, sweet, masterful and full of smiles; when the experimental necking and petting sets the heated sap to running; when the first real manly hand touches your breast, and you feel a strange, silky saliva slide down your throat and discover a new reason for panties to get wet. Don't grown women remember what it's like to be fresh meat and jailbait? You have to beat dudes off with a stick. Sometime, somewhere, somebody's gonna get ya.

In theory, it's fine to say that men have an equal responsibility to protect against pregnancy and disease. In fact, God bless the child who's got her own, and God helps her who helps herself. Giving young girls a chance to develop their intellectual and spiritual possibilities, protecting them with supervision, information and devices as necessary, schooling them in the realities of sex, mating and motherhood counter the pervasive fantasies and compelling hungers of body and soul—all this is women's work, women's responsibility, women's mission. 'Cause we're the ones who get jammed up.

I don't know why so many women are reluctant to give their daughters of the flesh or spirit a shot at a better life. In my meaner moods I think it's because the adult women are deeply jealous of the younger girls' freshness, their very possibilities. Misery loves company. And, I suppose, some women think that women must sacrifice themselves on the biological alter—it's our punishment for tempting Adam in the Garden.

A conversation with my close friend Gigi gave me another thought: Maybe good, loving mothers are afraid that if they talk to their children about the down sides of motherhood and mating, their children will feel that Mother doesn't love or want them *really* and fall into a Freudian soup of neuroses. Or, said another friend, maybe mothers are embarrassed to discuss "intimate" things with youngsters since some inference may be drawn about Momma's own experience.

There may be another, sadder reason that some women don't prepare girls for the worst as well as the best. For many mothers and wives, filling those roles is the only identity they have, the only status they hold. If they start thinking about what they could have done in addition to or instead of tying themselves down so early and completely, they might feel very wasted. Few people volunteer to think that they've sold themselves short in life.

It's been said ad nauseam that we human beings use very little of our potential. One of my basic values is that more aware, skilled people participate in world affairs to rescue us human beings from the thieves and thugs who run everything for their own private or class interests. We shouldn't volunteer for slavery and exploitation, but that's just what we do when we place sexual and emotional gratification ahead of education and economic viability. We cannot teach our children what we ourselves don't know, and we cannot protect them if we have no personal and social power.

Obviously, I'm not as concerned about an embryo's right to life as I am about a child's quality of life, and the things that destroy it. What about war—nuclear and otherwise—social injustice and the irrevocable death penalty? What about the bombing of children in Libya, the slaughter in the Middle East and South Africa, or the United States government's devoting a hundred million dollars to sustain and heighten violence in Nicaragua? What about classism and racism, which condemn children to falling down elevator shafts and out of windows in slum houses, or poor nutrition, lousy medical care, police brutality and unemployed, crazed or simply juvenile parents? What about the feminization of poverty that results from too many girls and women having children before developing intellectual coping skills and economic positioning, whether or not there are husbands present?

Perhaps we can moderate the notion that becoming a mother means one has done something intrinsically special and sacred. Every species of animal and plant I've heard of reproduces itself. It doesn't take a creative genius or intellectual giant to have sex and reproduce other human animals, although it may take both to rear the human animal into a decent human being in this complex perilous time. It's the rearing that separates the women from the girls, not the birthing.

Had I been clear about these things when I aborted my pregnancy, I wouldn't have substituted the role of "tragic abortee" for the rejected role of "mother," nor punished myself for going against the prevailing notion that becoming a mother should be the crowning fulfillment of every woman's life. Biologically speaking, what I aborted at eight weeks wasn't a cute, cuddly baby. Between eight weeks and nine months anything could happen: spontaneous abortion, a car accident, the world blowing up, a thalidomide distortion —you name it. There's no guarantee that pregnancy means getting a perfect reflection of oneself in a lovely little package. Of course, chances are that I would have had a healthy baby, but my point is that it was foolish and unnecessary to torture myself with guilt over an *assumption*, a hope, a fantasy, that the embryonic cells might have become another Dr. Martin Luther King, Jr. They might also have become Charles Manson, or have never become a fully developed human being at all.

My decision to abort was quite practical as well. At the time, I was living with three roommates in Sacramento, financed by student loans and part-time jobs. The jobs I'd had—waitress, telephone magazine sales, nannying and civil-service clerkships—were dead-end enough to convince me I'd never make it into financial comfort and an advantaged lifestyle if I didn't get a degree, and certainly not if I were supporting and rearing a child. Plus, it had been understood from the day I was born that I would get a bachelor's degree at least, if not a master's. It would disgrace the whole family if I came home with a big belly, no degree and no husband. Out-of-wedlock wasn't fashionable or respectable in 1963. Having a child and releasing her or him for adoption was out as far as I was concerned. No kid of mine was going to wander the planet without my knowing its circumstances.

Furthermore, I was a child of divorce who had longed to have my father around, or to have my mother replace him with a stepfather. I thought—probably still think—that being wanted and loved by both a woman and an man is advantageous for a child's balanced development. (Maybe this idea is just my last romantic notion—certainly other parenting arrangements have worked well for many.) Although conventional wisdom emphasizes that boys need fathers, I think girls also need the consistent, nonsexual attention of a loving, committed man to help them understand male culture and to develop other aspects of their being than women tend to evoke. I did not and do not want the sole responsibility of rearing children. For me, it's just too much.

I think it's very important for girls and women to give themselves the chance to develop more than their biological and emotional abilities. This doesn't mean not being mothers and wives, but rather being other things as well. The world is profoundly in need of the "feminine" characteristics—empathy, cooperation and conciliation, nurturing and sharing.

Women cannot affect human affairs beyond the personal and familial by being only mothers and marginal survival workers. The hand that rocks the cradle does not, in fact, rule the world—it just rocks the cradle. Harriet Tubman, Sojourner Truth and Mary McLeod Bethune didn't educate and free enslaved Africans by just rocking cradles. Women didn't get the vote, found Planned Parenthood or get abortion legalized in this country by only rocking cradles. Dorothy Height (National Council of Negro Women), Jewell Jackson McCabe (National Coalition of 100 Black Women), Faye Wattleton (Planned Parenthood), Marian Wright Edelman (Children's Defense Fund) and Barbara C. Jordan (professor and former Texas congresswoman) have not contributed to the improvement of hundreds of thousands of lives by rocking cradles. They rock the boat.

To be all that we can be—even if we join the Army—we must control the timing and circumstances of motherhood. Since telling people to abstain from something as necessary, basic and pleasurable as sex doesn't seem to work, that means using contraception in the first place and abortion as a last resort. I'm not saying that every young mother lives a blighted life. I just want to maximize the odds in favor of girls, women and children. That's the name of this tune.

In 1965, Daniel Patrick Moynihan authored The Negro Family: The Case for National Action. *In the controversial report, Moynihan attributed dramatic rises in black female-headed homes, drug-addiction, crime, out-of-wedlock births and welfare dependency to the "matriarchal" structure of the black family. Moynihan's unflattering depiction of the black community prompted scathing criticism that for years discouraged others from evaluating important socioeconomic changes in black America.*

In the following excerpt from her book Families in Peril: An Agenda for Social Change, *Children's Defense Fund founder and president Marian Wright Edelman provides a comprehensive analysis of developments in the black family during the past four decades. Focusing on changes in marriage and birth rates, a shifting economy that has increased joblessness among black males, and decreasing educational opportunities for black youth, Wright clearly illustrates that the major obstacles black families face today are rooted not in racial pathology, but rather in an increasingly complex urban sociology.*

It is impossible to adequately assess the state of black women's health without looking at the condition of the black family. For they are inextricably connected.

The Black Family in America
Marian Wright Edelman

There is only one sure basis of social reform and that is Truth—a careful detailed knowledge of the essential facts of each social problem. Without this there is no logical starting place for reform and uplift.

> —W.E. Burghardt Du Bois
> and Augustus Granville Dill,
> *The Negro Artisan*

After a period of not-so-benign neglect, the black family is back in the public eye. The spiraling percentage of black female-headed households and the problems associated with teenage pregnancies have been graphically chronicled by Bill Moyers on CBS Reports' "Vanishing Family," in *Ebony*, *Time* and the *New Republic* cover stories, and in a spate of front-page series in the *Washington Post* and numerous local and national papers.

The attention of the media is a welcome development. Unless, as so often happens, the glare of the spotlight leads us to despair or to look for quick fixes and simplistic answers to complex family problems that require long-term attention and multiple remedies. Or unless proposed solutions are twisted into general attacks on supposed failures in social programs or are transformed into a new cycle of blaming the victim and greater race and class polarization.

A 1985 Children's Defense Fund (CDF) study, *Black and White Children in America: Key Facts,* found that black children have been sliding backward. Black children today are more likely to be born into poverty, lack early prenatal care, have a single mother or unemployed parent, be unemployed as teenagers, and not go to college after high school graduation than they were in 1980.

Compared to white children, we found that black children are:

twice as likely to

- die in the first year of life
- be born prematurely
- suffer low birthweight
- have mothers who received late or no prenatal care
- see a parent die
- live in substandard housing
- be suspended from school or suffer corporal punishment
- be unemployed as teenagers
- have no parent employed
- live in institutions;

three times as likely to

- be poor
- have mothers die in childbirth
- live with a parent who has separated
- live in a female-headed family
- be placed in an educable mentally retarded class
- be murdered between five and nine years of age
- be in foster care
- die of child abuse;

four times as likely to

- live with neither parent and be supervised by a child welfare agency
- be murdered before one year of age or as a teenager

- be incarcerated between 15 and 19 years of age;

five times as likely to

- be dependent on welfare; and

twelve times as likely to

- live with a parent who never married.

We also found that:

- Only four out of every ten black children, compared to eight out of every ten white children live in two-parent families.

- Births to unmarried teenagers occur five times more often among blacks than whites, although birth rates for black teens, married and unmarried, have been *declining*, while the birth rate among white unmarried teens has been *increasing* in recent years.

- In 1983, fifty-eight percent of all births to black women were out of wedlock. Among black women under the age of twenty, the proportion was over eighty-six percent. For thirty years these out-of-wedlock ratios have increased inexorably. They have now reached levels that essentially guarantee the poverty of many black children for the foreseeable future.

Whether black or white, young women under the age of twenty-five who head families with children are very likely to be poor. The poverty rates in 1983 were 85.2 percent for young black female-headed families and 72.1 percent for young white female-headed families. But black female-headed families are much more likely to stay poor. In female-headed families with older mothers, aged twenty-five to forty-four, there is a twenty-percentage-point gap between black and white poverty rates.

Today black children in young female-headed households are the poorest in the nation. While a black child born in the United States has a one in two chance of being born poor, a black child in a female-headed household has a two in three chance of being poor. If that household is headed by a mother under twenty-five years of age, that baby has a four in five chance of being poor.

We all know that family income is usually lower if there is only one parent or if the parents are black. We often overlook the increasing importance of the parents' age in determining the family's income. For example, as the accompanying table shows, among female-headed families, those with young women as household heads are far more likely to be poor. The poverty rate among all families with heads under twenty-five (including those with two parents) is 29.4 percent, almost three times the national average; nearly as high as among all female-headed families (34.5 percent); and higher than among those families headed by a woman over forty-five.

Correlation between poverty rate and age of female heads of family.

	Poverty rate (percent)		
Age	White	Black	Total
Under 25	73.8	84.8	77.9
25–44	38.7	58.8	45.5
45–64	27.5	51.2	36.2

Black teens are having fewer rather than more babies: 172,000 births in 1970; 137,000 in 1983. The proportion of black women under twenty who have given birth has been falling steadily since the early 1970s and will probably reach the 1940s level before the end of the decade. However, the percentage of those births that were to unmarried teens soared fifty percent—from thirty-six percent in 1950 to eighty-six percent by 1981. Among black women reaching their twentieth birthday between 1945 and 1949, forty percent had given birth. Among black women reaching their twentieth birthday between 1975 and 1979, forty-four percent had given birth—an increase of only four percent. From 1947 to 1977, however, the marriage rate for pregnant black fifteen- to seventeen-year-olds dropped about eighty percent; and for black eighteen- and nineteen-year-olds the marriage rate is down sixty percent.

Today's young white population also is less likely to let pregnancy lead to marriage, but the decline is nowhere near as great. Seven percent of white teen births were out of wedlock in 1960, seventeen percent in 1970, and thirty-nine percent in 1983. Among pregnant white fifteen- to seventeen-year-olds, the proportion marrying before birth fell from sixty-two to forty-three percent during the same thirty-year period (1947 to 1977), while the proportion of pregnant eighteen- and nineteen-year-olds who married fell from fifty-two to fifty percent. The current white prenatal marriage rates are still much higher than the corresponding black rates were even back in 1950. Such changes in marriage rates have a dramatic effect on determining the proportion of all births that are to unmarried mothers. Every prenatal marriage in effect counts twice: by removing a birth to an unmarried mother, and by adding a birth to a married one.

It is important to identify why the proportion of out-of-wedlock teen births is rising. The cause among black teenagers is a drop in marriage rates, not an increase in birth rates. Among white teens the cause is more babies coupled with a decrease in marriage among those who become pregnant.

In 1970 teens accounted for half of all out-of-wedlock births. In 1983 almost two-thirds of the babies born to unmarried women were to women twenty and over. This is true for whites and blacks (63.4 percent white; 63.0 percent black). Again, while the share of out-of-wedlock births for adult women has been going up for both blacks and whites, the reasons for the increase are different. Birth rates for white unmarried women (aged sixteen to forty-four) have been going up (19.3 per 1,000 in 1983) because more unmarried white adult women are having babies. Birth rates for unmarried black women have been going down (95.5 per 1,000 in 1970; 77.7 in 1983), but fewer young black women are getting married, and married black women are having fewer babies. (In 1984 there were 89.1 births per 1,000 white married women aged eighteen to forty-four; there were 79.3 births per 1,000 black married women. In 1984, sixty-five percent of all white women but only forty-three percent of all black women were married.)

In 1980 pregnant *married* black women were two and one-half times as likely to have an abortion as pregnant married white women.[1] Having a child can mean a substantial loss of family income to a married black woman. Among two-parent families with incomes over $25,000, eighty-three percent of black women work, compared to sixty-two percent of white women.[2] And the black woman's salary contributes a bigger share of total family income than does the white woman's. For many married black women, an additional child may tip the scales back toward economic insecurity.

The crux of the problem facing the black family today is that young black women who become pregnant do not marry nearly as often as they used to. Nor as often as young pregnant white women do. Why young black marriages do not form is thus central to our concern about the proportion of black children in female-headed families. That is especially true since the *whole* of the increase in the proportion of black children in female-headed families over the last decade is accounted for by the increase in those who live with un-married mothers, and not by the increase in the proportion who live with divorced or separated mothers.

In 1981, among the infants born to fifteen- to seventeen-year-olds, forty-eight percent of those born to white teenagers were out of wedlock, compared to ninety-four percent of those born to black teenagers. CDF research staff used data to determine what would happen if black teen girls had behaved as white teen girls had. In general the white young women were less likely to be sexually active, more likely to abort if they did become pregnant, and more likely to marry before birth if they decided to carry the child to term. We can project what would have happened if young black women had matched each white rate.

If black teens had been no more sexually active than white teens, the proportion of births to black unmarried mothers would only have fallen from ninety-four to ninety-three percent. Similarly negligible results held for applying white contraceptive efficiency or white abortion rates. But if the black young women had adopted white prenatal marriage rates, the out-of-wedlock ratio would have fallen to only fifty-six percent, not very far above the actual white rate of forty-eight percent.

Some Scholarly Perspectives on the Black Family

Before analyzing the complex economic and social factors that have led to fifty-eight percent of black babies today being born to single mothers, it is important to remind ourselves that the stereotype is just that—a stereotype—true in too many cases but not others: millions of black families are not on welfare, have children who stay in school, stay out of trouble, and do not get pregnant, and, if they fall on hard times, find a way to overcome. Many single mothers are doing a valiant job which we should affirm and learn from. Until recently, two-parent families have been the black family norm, despite great publicity given to black female-headed families. It is only in the 1980s that the majority of black infants have been born to unmarried mothers—the culmination of a trend that began in the 1950s. However, since black families began to be studied from the turn of the twentieth century, black and white scholars alike have been concerned with out-of-wedlock births and single-parenting.

In their concern over the effects of slavery, urbanization, and unemployment on black families, a number of scholars have identified female-headed households or matriarchy as the characteristic and pathological element making and keeping black families "inferior" to white families. Until the 1960s many analysts assumed that there was something wrong with the black family, which was described at best as non-functional and disorganized.

In the last twenty years other researchers have begun to look at black families a bit differently and to emphasize their strengths: to try to distinguish between myths, stereotypes, and facts; to identify African retentions that may make black families different from but equally functional as white families; and to look at the effects of social and economic inequalities and discrimination. These more recent scholars insist that past research suffered from stereotypical historical and sociological judgments and poor empirical methodology. Slavery was assumed to have left American blacks with little culture and no behavioral norms; thus, acculturation to white norms was shoddy and slow. Early researchers blamed black poverty and disorganization on the failure to establish strong marital bonds.

Researchers have used various terms to categorize the differing perspectives on the black family. Those perspectives fall essentially into three groups, according to the way scholars thought black families functioned and the cause(s). I will call the dominant early perspective the *cultural deficiency* view. Black families were seen as different from and unequal to white families, especially white middle-class families, which were the norm used. Most black families were characterized by instability, suffering not only from economic troubles and discrimination but also from promiscuity and matriarchy. Some critics went as far as to suggest pathology in black family functioning. The causes for all this were slavery (the splitting up of families, emasculation of the black male, lack of cultural tradition) and urbanization (the lack of community and behavioral norms, splitting up of families, unemployment). Proponents of this viewpoint, however, did not all agree on how blacks could be helped and whether black families could become more like white ones. They did all tend to see black families as homogeneous and in trouble.[3]

The next perspective, the *cultural variance* view, developed as a response to the first. The scholars holding it considered black and white culture as different but equal and therefore felt that the black family had to be judged according to its own culture and values. These differences had developed because black Americans did retain African mores and behavioral norms; therefore a distinct Afro-American subculture has emerged. According to this perspective, blacks, because of our history in the United States, have had to adapt differently and develop different family structures from whites. However, these structures are as functional for blacks as white structures are for whites. Instead of making judgments about inferiority and pathology, society needs to recognize that blacks function under a different value system and socialization process.[4]

Some researchers who might fit into this category assert that African retentions have contributed significantly to black American culture and that we need to look at ways that black families have functioned positively and have survived over the years (without necessarily comparing them to white families). Yet these researchers may not agree that blacks function under a totally separate value system from the rest of society. Another group concentrates more on similarities between black and white families than on differences. We might add a subcategory for them, calling it *cultural equivalency*. It accounts for those scholars—mostly historians—who find that, throughout history, black Americans have formed two-parent families, have maintained intact families, and have family structures and functioning similar if not identical to whites. Thus, they reject talk about a separate or inferior culture and different black family functioning.[5]

Another major outlook on black families can be called the *social class* view, which assumes that if blacks were not so poor and did not suffer from racism and discrimination, their families would be much like white families. The problem is that economic inequities have left the majority of the black population in the lower income class. Poverty and lack of opportunities have destabilized and handicapped black families. They are not, however, inherently different or inferior to white families. Given equal opportunities and compensation for past inequities, black families would be no different from white ones.[6]

The 1980s found more scholars attempting to take a new look at black families, to reconcile the conflicting views and research, to develop a new methodology based on a cultural understanding of black families and accurate empirical information, to leave behind the stereotypes and misunderstandings of the past, and to look at black families as heterogeneous and functional, as resulting from both African and American traditions, and as exemplary of both weaknesses and strengths.[7]

I am not going to spend time arguing about differing scholarly views. Nor am I able to resolve whether it is the change in black family structure which causes its desperate economic condition, or family destabilizing changes in the economy which have led to black family changes. I believe that poor female-headed households, male joblessness, and poverty are all parts of the same conundrum which we must act to pierce now, rather than just continuing to debate whether the chicken or the egg came first.

Certainly, we need to understand as much as we can, and thoughtful academic research and exchange on cause and effect are needed. But we cannot afford to wait for a precise disaggregation before we act to save another generation of black young.

Where Are the Black Fathers?

Since the main reason that black children live with only a mother is that most unmarried pregnant black women do not marry before giving birth, what has become of the fathers? They remain single. The pattern is quite clear.

According to U.S. Census reports, 27.3 percent of white males aged twenty to twenty-four have married; only 11.9 percent of black males of the same age have married. Among white males aged twenty-five to twenty-nine, 64.9 percent have married; among black males of the same age, only 44.3 percent have married.[8]

If black marital rates for males in their twenties equaled those of white males in that age group, there would be an additional 450,000 married black males. That should be compared to about 750,000 black female-headed families with children where the female head is also under thirty years of age.

If marriage rates were the same, not every one of these men would marry one of these unmarried mothers. Yet any reasonable set of assumptions will show that an increase in the marital rate among young black men to the white level would reduce the proportion of fatherless young black families by between one-half and two-thirds. Thus, the failure of first marriages to form among young blacks is the largest single cause of the very high proportion of all young black families that are fatherless.

It is not the only cause, so I will mention other less important, but real causes.

First, historically young black males have always been institutionalized—primarily imprisoned—at rates much higher than those of white males. In 1980, five percent of black men versus one percent of white men in their twenties were institutionalized. But this excess incarceration rate would, if eliminated, supply at most about 40,000 newly married men (even assuming that they were all single, heterosexual, and that they all married at white rates.) That is less than one-tenth the number to be found if the non-institutionalized young black men were as likely as whites to marry.

Second, young black men are more than twice as likely to be in the military and living in barracks as are young white men. However, this disparity could supply fewer than 20,000 additional fathers. And increasingly, in light of what I will discuss later, the racial difference in marital status disappears for young men in the military. Obviously young men in military service are less likely to be married than civilians of the same age for all races; but almost eighteen percent of white, and over twenty percent of the black males in the military are married.

Third, black males are far more likely to marry nonblack females than black females are to marry nonblack males. But the numbers are small in either case.

Fourth, black males die at nearly twice the white rates. Among males in their twenties this is primarily because of the excess of deaths by homicide among black males. Among twenty-year-old men, 3.3 percent of black males and 1.8 percent of white males will die before reaching the age of thirty. It is urgent that this disparity be reduced quickly in order to recover these wasted lives. Even so, we will not thereby regain more than a percent or so of the missing young black fathers.

The last factor we must take into account is the most difficult to document: those young black males who are missing from the census. The extent of the undercount of young black males is necessarily speculative. A few black males can be shown to be missing among the eighteen- and nineteen-year-olds. But among those twenty and over, the numbers are substantial by even the most conservative count. The CDF estimates that a minimum of 8.1 percent, or about 210,000 black men in their twenties are missing from the census.

These young black men are those who are most often pointed to as members of the underground economy, or as "hidden" within households headed by black women who receive public aid. The reality is more complex. In one simple sense, we know that they are in an underground economy. They don't die, so they must eat. That need not imply a criminal source of support. Men who hide from creditors, including collectors of child-support payments, do so primarily because they have aboveground income they seek to retain. Still, let us suppose them criminals concealing their incomes and themselves from the census-taker. Are they currently adequate, although undetected, fathers for black children? I think not. Criminal earnings average very little and incur great risk when pursued over any substantial number of years; and it takes almost twenty years to raise a child.

Moreover, black males who are criminals do not do well. White-collar crimes are the profitable ones. The data suggest that the missing black males are often even less well-educated than those we record and so are poorly placed to work the richest and safest criminal fields. The remaining violent and heinous crimes—robbery, burglary, drug-dealing and pimping—are not a strong basis for a parent to provide adequately for a child.

The other alternative is that the missing young black males are hidden among the recipients of public assistance. Surely there are some. In almost half our states, an unemployed father must leave the home before the children are eligible for Aid to Families with Dependent Children (AFDC), no matter how low the family's income.

No doubt, not all impoverished fathers strictly abide by such welfare policies. A small minority probably survive in part off the AFDC benefits of their wives or girlfriends. However, if this failure of design in our AFDC program is the cause of a substantial number of the "missing" young black males, especially in states that do not provide assistance to intact families, it will be removed as soon as the program mandates coverage of intact families with unemployed workers.

The proportion of young black families with fathers fell drastically from 1970 to 1980. If the "missing black males" from the U.S. Census are centrally connected to this phenomenon of single-parent-family growth, then the proportion of all young black males who are missing ought to have increased equally drastically between the census of 1970 and that of 1980.[9] Instead, that proportion has been constant. There is no reason to believe that they are the driving force behind the failure of new black two-parent families to form.

What does explain the 200,000 or so young black males who do not appear in national counts? Because of the variety of human existence, there are going to be a few men who fit every description I have mentioned. But I believe the majority are unemployable, disheartened, and derive little if any criminal income. As a matter of public policy, the nation has much to gain by reducing the number of black males who are of little value to the economy, even the criminal economy. The United Negro College Fund slogan is right: "A mind is a terrible thing to waste." How much greater is the loss when we discard the whole person of 200,000 black males.

Let us go back to the 450,000 black males who would be married if black marriage rates equaled white rates for men in their twenties.

Because the real explanation lies not in finding the 200,000 missing men, but understanding the single status of this larger group. One crucial question is: When did the rate of marriage formation drop among young black males? In the 1970s it paralleled the decline of employment prospects of young black males, which resulted in only 29.8 percent of black teens and sixty-one percent of black twenty- to twenty-four-year-old men being employed by 1978.

From 1978 to 1985 things got a bit worse for both black teens and males in their twenties. The year 1986 was the first year in the history of the United States when the average number of black women who are employed exceeded the average number of black men who are employed. In 1985 there were only 39,000 more black male than black female workers. But there were over twelve million more white male than white female workers.

The black teen employment collapse during the 1960s and the employment collapse for blacks in their early twenties during the 1970s portend, distressingly, a currently occurring but not yet clearly quantified collapse in the employment situation of black males in their late twenties and thirties. The way this disaster has rolled up the age spectrum in the black community suggests that we must focus more of our efforts (though certainly not all) on teens—through education, job training, health care, and other services—and even on young children to prevent the repetition of this damage. (I frankly don't know how to get Bill Moyers' thirty-year-old Timothy into the mainstream job market at this point, although we must try. I do believe we must focus more resources on helping to prevent boys of twelve, thirteen, and fifteen, and their younger siblings, from becoming twenty-five- or thirty-year-old dependent men.)

There is more than a correlation between declining black male employment and declining marriage rates among young blacks. There is cause and effect. When a pregnant single woman is resolved to bear the child, marriage is most likely under active consideration. If the father of the child, presumably a few years older than herself, is potentially a good provider, marriage may well result. But if the proportion of young males who are potentially good providers falls, we would expect to see the prenatal marriage rate decline. We have. Indeed, we would expect two substantial changes in young women's behavior to follow a decline in the "marriageability" of young males. First, fewer single women would become pregnant with a child that they had planned to bear. Second, fewer pregnant single women, intent on bearing their child, would marry before giving birth. Those are exactly the two patterns we do find among young black women today.

My basic conclusion is that the key to bolstering black families, alleviating the growth in female-headed households, and reducing black child poverty lies in improved education, training, and employment opportunities for black males and females. (This must be coupled with a community support and value system that prepares young people for work that decent public policies must undergird. A strong community work ethic in the absence of work and training opportunities adds up to frustration and hopelessness.) This view is shared by many analysts of black family and civil rights organizations. William Wilson of the Department of Sociology at the University of Chicago says: "Both the black delay in marriage and the lower rate of remarriage, each of which is associated with high percentages of out-of-wedlock births and female-headed households, can be directly tied to the labor market status of black males. . . . We were able to document empirically that black women, especially young black women, are facing a shrinking pool of marriageable (that is, employed, economically stable) men."[10] The problem of black joblessness, Wilson argues, should once again be placed as a top priority item in public policy agendas designed to enhance the status of families.

Why did this economic disaster for black men occur? It is difficult to say precisely, but I think that the other factors which contributed included the softening of the labor market generally in the 1970s, poor education, continuing discrimination and a reciprocal sense of defeatism among some inner-city and rural men. There is no question that the number of Americans who wanted to work and could not find jobs was larger in 1980 than it had been in 1970. The economy absorbed unprecedented numbers of baby-boomers, women, and immigrants; in the process it left behind the same people who have always been at the end of the American line.

Why? Schooling for inner-city blacks did not improve appreciably. Urban employers, remembering Watts and Newark and Detroit, tended not to trust (and therefore not to hire) ghetto blacks. We saw decline in older, unionized industries that previously provided jobs for black males and an increase in the service industries where black female employment grew.

Some black males, it must be admitted, balked at accepting entry-level jobs that probably would not lead to better things. As more immigrant groups passed blacks by, the message being received by too many black youths was that poor blacks were not going to make it, even if they tried. Overnight, it seemed, jobs in restaurants, hotels and office buildings—jobs not good in themselves, but that might lead to a way out and up for newcomers—became the property of new, often illegal immigrants. Did young black men experience real exclusion or were they the ones who turned away for lack of opportunity or perceived lack of opportunity to move ahead?

There is no doubt that when there is greater unemployment and underemployment those with the poorest education, the greater proclivity to experience discrimination, and the poorest personal and work skills have the worst time. If their own attitude compounds their problems, should we be surprised?

We must continue to try to understand why this accelerated deterioration of black male joblessness in the 1970s and 1980s occurred. To the degree that it arises out of lack of jobs and from job discrimination, government and the private sector must take immediate steps to remedy it. To the degree that it results from a ghetto lifestyle, lack of individual initiative, and poor work habits, a concerted effort by black families, community leaders and agencies to resurrect strong work and family values is imperative. And that latter effort is occurring. But the loss of black community cohesion, through increasing urbanization and desegregation and the drifting away of many black middle-class family and work role models and leaders from the poor black community, has made a sense of hope more remote from the poor blacks left behind.

What Is Being Done by the Black Community?

Because the importance and limitations of self-help permeate all I will say, I want briefly to anticipate the leadership issue here as more white politicians call for shifting the focus of the debate away from outside government and private sector policies to black self-help. I hope we can avoid the useless either/or debate in responding to black family concerns; clearly both elements are required if adequate remedies are to be mounted.

The black community understands the urgent need for self-help and appropriate leadership; it is addressing the growing crisis among its children and families. The subject of children having children was on the cover of *Ebony* a year before *Time* magazine discovered it. During recent years almost every major black organization has made preventing teenage pregnancy and strengthening black families major priorities, as has CDF.

The National Council of Negro Women, the National Coalition of 100 Black Women, and the black Catholic women of the Knights of Peter Claver are coordinating most of the sixty-four Adolescent Pregnancy Child Watch projects in thirty states in conjunction with a broader CDF teen pregnancy prevention campaign. The Links are reaching out to poor teens in Nashville housing projects, and the Concerned Black Men of Washington, D.C. are teaching black teen males the personal and social skills their parents often cannot provide. The National Urban League is working in cities around the country. Byllye Avery's National Black Women's Health Project, headquartered in Atlanta, has developed a national forum and supportive atmosphere for poor black women to come together and define and respond to their own health needs. Avery's self-help network and Daphne Busby's Sisterhood of Black Single Mothers in Brooklyn, New York, are tapping and affirming the enormous strengths of poor black women and communities and helping them organize to ensure their own individual and family well-being; to protect themselves and their children against the physical and emotional abuse of their internal and external worlds; and to protect their families and children against teen pregnancy and other self-limiting activities. The Shiloh Baptist Church in the inner-city of Washington, D.C.—my church—has reinforced its deep-rooted commitment to strong family values by building, without outside help, a five-million-dollar Family Life Center. Scholarships, counseling, and tutoring for young people, day care, family recreation, and a range of other family-centered services and activities are as important a part of its ministry as Sunday-morning services. Numerous black churches are conducting similar education, day care and senior-citizen activities.

This kind of individual, community, and religious group outreach and direct service self-help is being complemented by and hooked up with another kind of black leadership that is emerging from thoughtful black professionals who have committed themselves to strengthening disadvantaged children and families. Dr. Robert Johnson, director of Adolescent Medicine at the University of Medicine and Dentistry, in Newark, is working effectively with poor black adolescents to help them delay too-early sexual activity and pregnancy. Dr. Aaron Shirly has started three comprehensive school-based clinics in Jackson and other Mississippi communities. Dr. Bailus Walker, Massachusetts Health Commissioner, has systematically developed and implemented policies to lower infant mortality and improve the health status of poor children, black and white. They, in turn, are connecting up with the growing number of black social-services, welfare, child-welfare, and child-care officials and advocates around the country for the needed interdisciplinary and comprehensive approach to complex family problems. Collaboration and comprehensiveness are becoming the cornerstones of emerging teen pregnancy prevention and family strengthening efforts, as is an emphasis on building self-sufficiency. More people are recognizing that the traditional fragmented policy and service approach cannot solve social problems that are cumulative and complex. They also recognize that government effort without community awareness and support will not be enough.

These professionals are reaching out to work with the growing network of black elected officials like Jesse Oliver, a Texas state legislator, who, in 1985, skillfully shepherded through his legislature a two-hundred-million-dollar indigent health care package. When fully implemented, it will benefit over 300,000 poor Texas mothers and children. Oliver is one of a growing group of state and local black political leaders mobilizing to use the political process to help black and white children and families in a tough-minded and effective manner.

Effective change strategies today involve the dull, technical details of policy and budget development. The absence of a single overriding national symbol like Dr. Martin Luther King, Jr. must not obscure the valiant and multiple efforts we are finding in black communities across the country that are beginning to rally together to recapture our youth and families.

This surge of black community energy and commitment is essential because we will have to reach many of our vulnerable children, teens, and parents on a one-to-one basis. It is also essential because the black community knows far better than anyone else—knows in its bones and in the hard school of experience—that without its own strong leadership now, as in the past, too little can be expected from government or other institutions. No one is more aware of the folly of relying solely on government to solve black community problems than the black community. The black American journey is one of making a way out of no way because we often had no one, save God, to lend us a hand. For most of our American sojourn, government has been opponent and victimizer rather than ally. Slavery and legally sanctioned segregation left to us the major burden of seeking our own freedom, protecting our own families, creating our own churches in which to worship, forming our own benevolent societies to bury our dead, developing our own home health remedies and hospitals to care for our sick, and opening up homes and churches to teach our own children.

Federal affirmative-action strategies, under so much attack in the Reagan-Bush era, are a blip, like the singular precedent of Reconstruction in a long American history of affirmative action *against* blacks of indescribably greater magnitude. Increasingly we hear political "leaders" and read columnists who state or imply that the black community is asking government in the 1990s to assume responsibility for problems the black community brought upon itself and could and should solve itself, or that blacks are asking government for help different from or greater than that historically and currently provided other groups in the society.

Such politicians and journalists need to be reminded that we seek no more or less than what government has been willing, often eager, to do for others. They need to be reminded that the black community has always and will always do its utmost to solve its problems.

• Harriet Tubman did not wait for government to free the slaves. She made repeated journeys on her underground railroad into the Deep South to spirit out hundreds of slaves to freedom in the North.[11]

• Nat Turner and Denmark Vesey revolted against slavery and paid with their lives.

• Sojourner Truth and Frederick Douglass used their eloquence to speak out against and resist slavery, despite beatings and threats.

• Prince Hall founded one of the oldest social organizations among Negroes in American when, on March 6, 1775, he and fourteen other Negroes chartered a Lodge of Freemasons at Boston Harbor, which mushroomed into the hundreds of Masonic lodges throughout the United States today. As early as 1776 he urged the Massachusetts legislature to support emancipation and in 1797 prodded the city of Boston to provide schools for free Negro children. Before they eventually agreed to do so, he ran a school for black children in his own house, as did many other blacks.[12]

• The unwelcoming attitudes of white churches led Thomas Peel to organize independent Baptist churches, including congregations of Free Negroes in Boston and Philadelphia, and Richard Allen to found the African Methodist Episcopal Church.[13]

• Black journalists excluded from white newspapers started their own, for example, Monroe Trotter's *Boston Guardian*.[14]

• Ida Wells was one of many blacks who led the crusade against lynching.[15]

• A. Phillip Randolph organized the Brotherhood of Sleeping Car Porters in 1925 and fought racial discrimination within the labor unions all his life. He organized the celebrated March on Washington Movement during World War II—a precursor to the famous 1963 March—to prod the U.S. government into halting discrimination in industries having government contracts, the standards and enforcement of which we are still fighting for today.[16]

• Mary McLeod Bethune started Bethune Cookman College on a dump heap, with a ton of faith and a five-dollar down payment on a two-hundred-and-fifty-dollar note she and students worked to pay off.[17] She also founded the National Council of Negro Women, which Dorothy Height now heads and which is a leader in the struggle to strengthen black families today.

• Charles Houston, a black Harvard law school graduate, conceptualized and implemented the legal strategy that undermined legal segregation in the United States. He and a small band of lawyers, which included Thurgood Marshall and James Nabrit, and handfuls of brave black parents, knew they could not depend on the government to ensure fair treatment for black Americans when it was government that segregated them.[18]

• W.E.B. Du Bois spent a lifetime documenting, publicizing, and fighting discrimination against black Americans. Few, if any, ever approached his leadership in helping America become a more just society.

• And no American since Lincoln has aroused the conscience of the nation more than Martin Luther King, Jr.

But as important as black self-help is, and must continue to be, it is not enough. Teenage pregnancy and parenthood and the growth of female-headed households are intimately intertwined with poverty and lack of economic opportunity, which flow from governmental policies or abdication of responsibility for some of its citizens. Changes in the economy have, over the past thirty years, undermined the capacity of black men to marry and support viable families. Short-lived or underfunded efforts to help poor families and children achieve self-sufficiency coupled with government policies that encouraged family breakup have hampered solutions to family problems. These lie at the heart of the black family crisis today.

A few cautions are in order because we are confronting a black and white family crisis that we must not lose and must not mess up by careless rhetoric, political posturing, or media-seeking. Preventing teen pregnancy and black family instability will require the greatest care, effort, and sensitivity on everyone's part, black and white, public and private. Who says what and how it is said will make an enormous difference in whether we see positive solutions or a polarized atmosphere. These complex problems will not be solved just by media or by speeches. They can be derailed by the media or by speeches if we are not all careful in weighing what we say and how we say it, and if the media and political leaders cannot take the time and make the effort to learn about and present complex problems in more thorough ways.

It is critically important that we maintain an appropriately balanced view about who are the poor, both in our definition of the problem and in our consideration of proposed remedies. These remedies must go far beyond needed welfare reform. They must be more than mere moralizing.

In 1967, in *Where Do We Go From Here: Chaos or Community?* Martin Luther King, Jr., reflected on the renewed focus on the black family and cautioned: "As public awareness of the predicament of the Negro family increases, there will be danger and opportunity. The opportunity will be to deal fully rather than haphazardly with the problem of a whole—to see it as a social catastrophe... brought on by long years of brutality and oppression—and to meet it as other disasters are met, with an adequacy of resources. The danger will be that the problems will be attributed to innate Negro weaknesses and used to justify further neglect and to rationalize continued oppression."[19] Today, as the debate about the black family crisis is renewed, Dr. King's caution of more than two decades ago has tremendous vitality.

For God's sake and our children's future, let us seize the opportunities and avoid the dangers that we know are lurking. Let us focus on what unites us, on the poverty that we can do something about now, and on preventing another generation of black babies from becoming the poor black mothers and fathers that we so begrudgingly try to help today through our social policies.

. . .

Footnotes

1. National Center for Health Statistics, "Induced Terminations of Pregnancy: Reporting States, 1981: Final Data," Monthly Vital Statistics Report, vol. 34, no. 4, supplement (2), United States Public Health Service, Washington, D.C., July 30, 1985, table D, page 4, and calculations by Children's Defense Fund. Unmarried black women who are pregnant are less likely to have abortions than unmarried white women who are pregnant, although the rates among unmarried teenagers are converging. Rates are customarily given per 1,000 women rather than per 1,000 pregnant women, and must be adjusted for the higher pregnancy rates among unmarried black women of all ages.

2. U.S. Bureau of Labor Statistics, unpublished tabulations from the March 1984 Current Population Survey, based on 1983 calendar year income; calculations by CDF.

3. E. Franklin Frazier, *The Negro Family in the United States* (Chicago: University of Chicago Press, 1939, rev. 1969); W.E.B. Du Bois, *The Negro American Family* (Atlanta: Atlanta University Press, 1908; Cambridge, Mass., MIT Press, 1970); Daniel Patrick Moynihan, *The Negro Family: The Case for National Action* (Washington, D.C.: U.S. Dept. of Labor, Office of Policy Planning and Research, 1965).

4. Andrew Billingsley, *Black Families in White America* (Englewood Cliffs, N.J.: Prentice-Hall, 1968); Robert B. Hill, *Strengths of Black Families* (New York: Emerson Hall, 1972). See also Robert B. Hill, *Economic Policies and Black Progress: Myths and Realities* (Washington, D.C.: National Urban League, 1981).

5. Herbert G. Gutman, *The Black Family in Slavery and Freedom, 1750–1925* (New York: Random House, 1976); John W. Blassingame, *The Slave Community* (New York: Oxford University Press, 1979); Eugene Genovese, *Roll Jordan Roll: The World the Slaves Made* (New York: Pantheon, 1974).

6. Jessie Shirley Bernard, *Marriage and Family among Negroes* (Englewood Cliffs, N.J.: Prentice-Hall, 1966). See also Joyce A. Ladner, *Tomorrow's Tomorrow* (Garden City, N.Y.: Doubleday, 1971); Robert Staples, ed., *The Black Family: Essays and Studies* (Belmont, Calif.: Wadsworth, 1978); Walter R. Allen, "The Search for Applicable Theories on Black Family Life," *Journal of Marriage and the Family*, 40 (February 1978): 117–129; Robert Staples, "Toward a Sociology of the Black Family: A Decade of Theory and Research," *Journal of Marriage and the Family*, 33 (February 1971): 19–38; William G. Harris, "Research on the Black Family: Mainstream and Dissenting Perspectives," *Journal of Ethnic Studies*, 6 (Winter 1979): 45–64.

7. Harriette Pipes McAdoo, *Black Families* (Beverly Hills, Calif.: Sage, 1981); Eleanor Engram, *Science, Myth, Reality: The Black Family in One-Half Century of Research* (Westport, Conn.: Greenwood, 1982). See also John Reid, *Black America in the 1980s*, Population Reference Bureau, Population Bulletin, 37, no. 4 (December 1982).

8. U.S. Bureau of the Census, Current Population Reports, series P-20, no. 399, "Marital Status and Living Arrangements, March 1984" (Washington, D.C.: Government Printing Office, 1985), and previous annual editions. Since 1950 the Census Bureau also has published a subject report, "Marital Status," as part of volume 2 of each decennial census. Because the current population survey begins in the late 1960s, longer-term comparisons are taken from the decennial census subject reports.

9. The undercount of the population is a matter that has been long investigated by the Bureau of the Census. It is established by comparing the counts taken during the Census with many alternative sources: vital statistics, administrative records, special intensive campaigns to locate persons missed, and smaller random surveys that employ better methods and more skilled interviewers than are used in the full census.

The most reliable alternative is the vital statistics system. Birth and death reporting in the United States is essentially complete. The sex ratio at birth is almost exactly equal; a tiny excess of male over female births is reduced by a slightly greater death rate among male infants in the first year of life.

Deaths are accurately reported and, given the higher rates of male deaths over female deaths, available by five-year age groups for each sex within each race. One can then compare the theoretical sex ratio among twenty- to twenty-five-year-old blacks to that actually found in the Census reports, and observe how that comparison has changed over the decades. The conclusion—that there was no increase in the young black male undercount to explain the decline in young black family formation during the 1970s—is consistent with the Census Bureau's own internal studies. The most recent published review is: U.S. Bureau of the Census, Current Population Reports, series P-23, no. 115, "Coverage of the National Population in the 1980 Census, By Age, Sex, and Race: Preliminary Estimates by Demographic Analysis" (Washington, D.C.: Government Printing Office, 1982).

10. William J. Wilson, remarks at Children's Defense Fund National Conference, February 1986, as a panelist in a session entitled "Teen Pregnancy and Welfare: Part of the Problem or Part of the Solution"; see also William J. Wilson, "Poverty and Family Structure: The Widening Gap Between Evidence and Public Policy Issues" (unpublished paper, February 1985).

11. Sarah Bradford, *Harriet Tubman: The Moses of Her People* (New York: Corinth Books, 1961, reprint 1986); and Gerda Lerner, *Black Women in White America: A Documentary History* (New York: Vintage, 1973).

12. Russell L. Adams, *Great Negroes, Past and Present* (Chicago: Afro-Am Publishing, 1984), p. 26; Rayford W. Logan and Michael R. Winston, eds., *Dictionary of American Negro Biography* (New York and London: W.W. Norton, 1982), pp. 278–280.

13. Logan and Winston, eds., *Dictionary of American Negro Biography*, pp. 12–13.

14. Ibid., pp. 602–603.

15. Adams, *Great Negroes, Past and Present*, p. 109.

16. Ibid., p. 121.

17. Lerner, *Black Women in White America*, pp. 134–143.

18. Genna Rae McNeil, *Groundwork: Charles Hamilton Houston and the Struggle for Civil Rights* (Philadelphia: University of Pennsylvania Press, 1983).

19. Martin Luther King, Jr., *Where Do We Go From Here: Chaos or Community?* (Boston: Beacon, 1968), p. 109.

THREE: CLIMBING HIGHER MOUNTAINS

Hypertension, or high blood pressure, afflicts one out of three blacks—making it one of the major medical problems affecting African-Americans today. Not only is high blood pressure more prevalent in blacks, but it begins earlier in life, is often more severe and results in a higher death rate at a younger age. Blacks have a sixty-percent greater risk of death and disability from stroke and coronary disease than whites because of high blood pressure, according to the American Heart Association. If you have high blood pressure, it can't be cured. But you can control it and live a normal, healthy life.

A nutritious diet, limited alcohol, regular exercise, paying attention to family medical history and quitting smoking are some of the preventative measures you can take to minimize your chances of developing hypertension.

Controlling Hypertension
Pamela Sherrod

When I turned thirty, I was looking forward to entering a new age of maturity, a period in which I could comb my well-earned graying strands of hair proudly to the front. I looked and felt great. I'd held my five-foot-four-inch frame at a steady weight of 108 pounds for most of my adult years. A non-smoker, I'd never used drugs, had avoided junk food and never added salt to my meals. I thought I was doing all the right things to ensure my health and longevity. So it was hard for me to believe that I had high blood pressure. But like my mother who has struggled with it since her early thirties, and her mother who died of it at age forty, I had inherited the family tendency toward this disease, which is a frequent killer of Black Americans.

Before starting a new job, I was required to undergo a routine physical examination. When the nurse took my blood pressure, the reading was 170/100, well above the normal rate of 120/80 and even above the high normal rate of 140/90. Startled by the result, she tested me several times and advised that I see my regular doctor. But like many Black Americans with this "silent killer," I delayed going to the doctor because I felt fine. About a month later I decided, out of curiosity, to have my blood pressure checked again. This time the reading was 160/100. I was reminded of all the years while I was growing up that my mother's blood pressure stayed near 190/100 and how short of breath she would get just by walking up the six steps to our front porch, all the time insisting she was fine.

At this point I checked with my doctor, who monitored my pressure for one month. The readings consistently hovered around 150/90. He advised that I get more exercise, cut back on my usual twelve-hour workday and eliminate salt-laden processed foods from my diet. Then he gave me a prescription for Dyazide, an antihypertensive diuretic.

Determined not to be sentenced to taking drugs the rest of my life, I maintained a low-sodium diet, adding fresh produce, fish and poultry to my grocery list. I also worked aerobic activities such as weekly exercise classes and swimming into my schedule.

It took three years before my doctor was able to reduce the dosage of my medication, then finally to put me on a trial run without any drugs, using only diet and exercise to control my blood pressure. But the plan worked. Now my pressure ranges between 125/75 and 130/80, which is considered normal for me. I monitor my blood pressure regularly and do my best to stick to my diet and exercise schedule. If I can't take a weekly exercise class, I walk the length of Chicago's "Magnificent Mile" (actually about three quarters of a mile), instead of taking a taxi, or climb the four flights of stairs at work to get to my office. Although I'm not perfect in adhering to my routine, I know that my low-sodium diet and exercise have made a difference.

My experience with hypertension is not unique. According to the American Heart Association, about thirty-nine percent of all adult Black females and thirty-eight percent of all adult Black males suffer from high blood pressure. Hypertension is found almost twice as often in Blacks as it is in whites, and some physicians are now treating Black children as well for this disease.

The symptoms of high blood pressure usually build internally and do not surface until irreparable damage has already been done. Results can be kidney failure, heart attack or stroke. In rare instances there are warning signals such as swollen feet, ringing in the ears, nosebleeds, shortness of breath, chest pain and dizziness. These symptoms usually occur five to ten years earlier in hypertensive blacks than in whites with high blood pressure.

Hypertension is not caused by any one factor. While a diet high in sodium is a major contributor, so is family history, as in my case. Stress in the home and work environment is also a cause. Dr. Bambi Nickleberry, who specializes in family medicine and sees a variety of women in her Los Angeles practice, says, "A growing number of Black women in their thirties and forties are experiencing problems with high blood pressure. I'm seeing it among women who are homemakers, those who have their own businesses and those in upper-management positions. The aggressive, supermotivated, compulsive woman with a family history of hypertension is a prime candidate for this disease."

"But it's not only professional career women," says Dr. James H. Carter, professor of family medicine and director of the Morehouse Medical Clinic in Atlanta. "The poor, the unemployed and those in low-paying jobs also have high blood pressure." Dr. George Rowell, a psychiatrist in Los Angeles, agrees, adding that hypertension can be compounded by outside factors. "Elevated blood pressure can be related to changing conditions on the job, such as stress due to shift changes, extreme work overload or racial tension."

The stress of daily living is not the only culprit. Smoking, alcohol, some antihistamines, birth control pills with high estrogen levels and street drugs such as cocaine can also increase blood pressure.

To manage hypertension, first have your blood pressure checked regularly, either by a health care professional or by using a home blood pressure machine. Though the range may vary slightly, doctors generally consider blood pressure to be high if it consistently measures about 140/90. The top number, the systolic pressure, is the force exerted when the heart is beating. The bottom number, the diastolic pressure, is the force exerted when the heart is at rest. The top figure, the systolic, is the one most people use to describe their blood pressure. However, both measurements are important.

High blood pressure can be controlled in a number of ways, such as restricting salt intake, losing excess weight, limiting alcohol, decreasing cholesterol and fat, quitting smoking, exercising regularly, controlling stress and taking medication as prescribed. A health care provider can help you determine which treatment plan is the best for you.

There are several drugs used to treat hypertension. They generally fall into one of the following groups:

Diuretics—drugs that promote salt and water loss in order to decrease the amount of fluid that the heart has to pump.

Beta-blockers—drugs that reduce the force and rate of the heart's contractions.

Calcium channel-blockers—drugs that relax the muscular walls of the arteries, reducing the resistance to the heart's pumping action.

Angiotensin converting enzyme (ACE) inhibitors—drugs that prevent the formation of angiotensin-II, a hormone that constricts the blood vessels.

Many community groups and organizations are creating hypertension-screening and awareness programs to help reduce the incidence of high blood pressure in the black community. HealthPITCH —People Involved to Control High Blood Pressure—is one such coalition that offers one-day screening clinics, medical referrals and educational information in major cities around the country. "Too often victims of hypertension suspect or even know that they have high blood pressure, but aren't sufficiently motivated to commit themselves to treatment," says Dorothy Height, president of the National Council of Negro Women, a participant in the HealthPITCH campaign. "Through this program, we aim to convey a sense of urgency about this terrible killer and share current information about the effectiveness of modern treatment."

High blood pressure does not have to be debilitating or lead to premature deaths for Black Americans. As I learned, it does mean taking control and responsibility for your health by changing your lifestyle. Here are some ways to do it:

• If there is a family history of hypertension, make sure you check your blood pressure regularly—as often as once a month.

• Make the necessary eating and behavioral changes to improve overall health and well-being while lowering blood pressure and reducing the risk of complications, by maintaining ideal weight, exercising, limiting alcohol and quitting smoking.

• Use meditation, prayer or other relaxation techniques to help relieve stress. You may not be able to control the stress you're under, but you can control how you respond to it.

• Take your medication as prescribed by your doctor. If you have side effects or complications from the medication, see your physician immediately. Don't stop taking your medicine until you have been so advised. The type, as well as the dosage, can be adjusted. Discuss improvements in your blood pressure with your doctor. If you can lower your pressure through lifestyle changes, your doctor may reduce or eliminate your medication.

Sickle cell anemia is an inherited disease, affecting mainly people of African or Mediterranean descent. About one in 600 African-Americans has sickle cell anemia, which results when a person inherits defective genes from both parents for the hemoglobin protein found in red blood cells.

Most people with sickle cell anemia live normal lives. However, the disease can prompt periodic "crises" which can cause fevers, great physical pain, severe weakness and sometimes even death.

Because of her struggles with the disease, the author of the following article fell behind in school and did not learn how to adequately read or write until her mid-twenties. She is now actively involved in literacy work in New York City.

Sickle Cell Anemia and Me
Forrestine A. Bragg

At age seven, I sat in my first-grade class in Brooklyn as my teacher asked, "Who can spell the word 'want'?" "Ooo oo me, I can spell it," I said excitedly. Looking around the room to see if any of my classmates had their hands up, I wiggled out of my seat. "Ooo me, I can spell that word." As I stood to spell the word, my teacher looked at me quizzically and asked, "Are you all right? You don't look too well." "Oh, I'm fine," I replied. "Maybe you should see the nurse," she said.

After visiting the nurse, I was sent home because I had a high fever. When I got home, my mother looked at me worriedly and asked, "Are you having one of your attacks?" "Just a little pain in my arms and legs." "Then go to bed right now and get some rest," my mother told me.

Poking out my lip, I trotted off to bed. At three a.m. I woke everyone in the house with my crying and screaming. My mother came rushing to my bedroom and found me with a fever of 106 degrees. My hands and feet were swollen like balloons. Later that morning my mother took me to see our family physician, Dr. Patrick. After he examined me, the doctor told my mother that he suspected I had sickle cell anemia.

I was hospitalized immediately. I awakened several hours later in an oxygen tent. I was freezing and crying. My mother tried to soothe me. While she was trying to calm me down, Dr. Patrick came in to confirm that I had sickle cell anemia, a disease that causes red blood cells to fold in on themselves. The cells form sickle-like shapes which diminish their ability to carry oxygen, causing excruciating pain. The disease can prompt other complications such as joint problems, leg ulcers, pneumonia, strokes, gallstones and jaundice.

After a few days, I was discharged from the hospital and went back to school. But as time passed, I found myself spending more time in hospital beds than in school rooms. This was very frightening for me.

A few years later, on a cold wintry Saturday morning, I went Christmas shopping with my family. As we were going through the revolving doors at the store, my brother Tyrone noticed a familiar look on my face. "Are you in pain?" he asked. "Just a little."

Two seconds later, I had passed out cold. When I came to, I was in the hospital again. When I tried to get out of bed, I discovered that my right leg and arm had lost their feeling. "I can't feel them," I said in a panic.

The doctor arrived and informed me and my mother that I had had a stroke and needed to be in the hospital for at least a week or two, or maybe a couple of months. This was too much for a ten-year-old girl to handle.

Because of the stroke, I became paralyzed on my right side. I had to learn how to walk and talk all over again. There was a physical therapist in the hospital who helped me. But most of the work I did on my own, with the help of my mother.

By the time I reached fourth grade, I had missed a lot of school because of my illness. I would feel okay and then I would get an excruciating attack and wouldn't be able to breathe. But unless I was having a really bad crisis, I stayed at home instead of going to the hospital because it was too expensive. "These medical bills are so high, I don't know what to do," my mother would say nervously. She missed quite a bit of work and almost lost her job with the Internal Revenue Service because she had to stay home and take care of me.

Because their parents didn't understand anything about sickle cell anemia, the kids in my neighborhood teased me a lot. "You're contagious, we can't play with you," a little girl said to me one day as I was sitting on the front stoop. I felt sad and depressed because other children were afraid of me. I wish their parents had been able to educate them better and teach them that sickle cell anemia is not a contagious disease.

With my own education, I was slipping further and further behind. I repeated several years to try to catch up, but it didn't help. I had mostly white teachers and I kept asking them to help me, but I never got their attention or concern. Instead of helping me, they said that I would never learn to read or write and put me in special education classes. They just passed me from one grade to the other so I went straight through school without learning a thing.

When I finally graduated from high school, I was twenty-three years old. And just as the teachers had predicted, I didn't know how to read or write.

Because the teachers were unwilling to understand how sickle cell anemia had made it difficult for me to keep up in school, they simply gave up on me. They treated me like I was retarded instead of helping me overcome my struggles with the disease.

After finishing high school, I tried to get clerical jobs in insurance or medical offices, but I couldn't because I didn't know how to fill out a job application. "Maybe you should go back and take basic education classes," my mother said. But the classroom setting was very discouraging to me and I eventually dropped out. I thought maybe I could pass the General Equivalency Degree, or GED, test on my own. I tried and failed about ten times.

I became so depressed that I started getting sick again. Before I would have a crisis maybe twice a year; now it seemed that I was sick every other week. "I'm afraid to speak. I'm afraid to go through my life not knowing how to read or write," I would think in despair. Finally I decided I would have to do something to change my life.

Someone told me about a literacy program and I went to find out what it was about. I got an individual tutor and then I moved into a group with two other students who also were learning how to read and write. At first, it was hard and I wanted to give up. During those times I would remember how hard I had fought against the pain of sickle cell anemia and to keep breathing when I had a crisis. And just as surely as I had always gotten my breath back, I began to slowly understand the words I was trying to learn. For the first time in my life I was able to skim through a book and understand what the writer was saying or figure out a headline without struggling. A whole world that had been closed to me began to magically open up.

Today I am a student advocate with the Literacy Volunteers of

New York City. I am so grateful for how much the program helped me that I want to help others.

I think that black women with sickle cell anemia should get in a support group so they can communicate with other people who have the disease. I found one through a local hospital and it has been very helpful to me. It is also important not to over-exert yourself, to eat healthy foods and to drink lots of fluids. Most of all, you have to think positively and tell yourself that you can hang in there no matter how much pain you're in. Like me, you can get a crisis under control, pick up the pieces and go on with your life.

Systemic lupus erythematosus, or lupus, as it is more commonly referred to, is an illness that disproportionately affects black women. The symptoms of this disease vary from person to person. What exactly is lupus? This article describes the illness and provides an understanding of its social and psychological ramifications.

Lupus and Black Women: Managing a Complex Chronic Disability
Vida Labrie Jones

Lupus, a Latin word which means *wolf*, is a chronic inflammatory disease of unknown cause that can affect almost any part of the body. It is no longer considered a rare disease, but rather a chronic illness that can be managed over time. Research conducted in major cities throughout the United States indicates that black females are three times more likely to develop lupus than the general population. Women of childbearing age also comprise a disproportionate number of newly diagnosed cases. Thus, being young, black and female poses an increased risk of developing lupus.

New patients with lupus generally develop distinct abnormalities of the immune system: that is, in addition to making antibodies (special substances that help destroy foreign material entering the body) against bacteria and viruses, lupus patients produce antinuclear antibodies, which mysteriously attack healthy cells. A diagnosis of lupus is likely to follow the discovery of these antinuclear antibodies, especially antibodies to DNA (deoxyribonucleic acid), the substance that governs heredity.[1]

Lupus produces changes in the structure and processes of the skin, joints and internal organs. Unfortunately, the number and variety of symptoms of lupus are great. The disease may begin in a single organ or system and/or progress to any combination of several organs or systems. For instance, in some ninety-five percent of the cases, the lining of the joints becomes inflamed, resulting in arthritis. In still others, the lungs or the lining around the lungs and heart may become inflamed, causing pleurisy and fever. In most cases, lupus is a mild non-progressive disease. Episodes of active disease may be short-lived or arrested by therapy, and the patient remains completely well for long periods. However, if kidney or neurological systems are affected, the disease can have severe and sometimes fatal consequences.

Medical crises, commonly referred to as "flare-ups," are often totally unpredictable for lupus patients. This makes the management of the disease particularly difficult because a life-threatening flare-up may be triggered by any number of things, ranging from the flu and too much sun to emotional upsets. For example, a case is cited in which a woman had lupus for thirty-eight years and was in her sixties before she had a severe flare-up resulting in kidney failure. In another case, a patient who was diagnosed with lupus at age sixteen, died at twenty-eight from a stroke that was caused by the disease. Many doctors believe that lupus patients should have periodic check-ups which can help in predicting potential flare-ups.

One of the most striking aspects of lupus is that it appears as individual as each person who has it. Although the symptoms may overlap, no two persons with lupus can "compare" their disease or the path it may take.[2]

Among the many indicators of lupus are a distinctive "butterfly" rash on the face, fatigue, loss of hair and inflammation of the blood vessels. Because blood travels throughout the entire body, the inflammation will affect the particular organ where the blood has lodged. Therefore, if the inflammation is of the blood vessels to the skin, one will develop a skin rash; to the kidney, kidney trouble; to the heart, heart problems, etc. The inflammation can be episodic, but when it occurs, it presents problems particular to lupus patients. Some cases of lupus are drug-induced. Stop the medication, and you stop the lupus. In other cases, spontaneous lupus can disappear, unaided. This happens about ten to fifteen percent of the time. Overall, individual symptoms have to be diagnosed and the whole person must be examined to come up with a therapy suitable to control the disease.

There is no present cure for lupus. Degrees of treatment may range from no medication to aspirin to corticosteroids, anti-inflammatory agents and immunosuppressants. Aspirin and corticosteroids are "anti-inflammatory" agents and decrease the swelling that causes so many problems for lupus patients. Other medications such as anti-malarials are used when steroid therapy is not adequate. Caution in the administration of medications is particularly important, and patients must be kept keenly aware of the ramifications of their drug therapy and possible complications that may result.

Because lupus can vary so markedly in its manifestations, it is difficult for investigators to establish the frequency of the illness in the population. Very little comprehensive or systematic effort has been invested in the epidemiology of lupus and it is clear that more research needs to be done.

In general, scientists and medical experts believe that the illness develops in individuals predisposed to it, and that a viral infection or similiar stress can alter the delicate balance between normal immunity to foreign substances and reactions to one's own cells. It is known that the single factor most dramatically increasing risk of lupus is family history of the disease. If an identical twin has lupus, the unaffected twin has a seventy percent chance of getting the disease. More than ten percent of lupus patients have at least one affected relative.[3]

Because lupus is such an ambiguous, sometimes vague and difficult to diagnose illness, it is important for black women to be aware of some of the symptoms. Unfortunately, many women have gone years suffering with lupus and having family members question the veracity of their complaints because medical professionals have been unable to diagnose the illness. If you become aware of the biophysical properties and the key symptoms of lupus, you can be an active patient and demand that your doctor consider lupus as a possible cause for your health problems.

The following list of symptoms is used by the Bay Area Lupus Foundation (San Jose, California) in its various screening programs. Patients who answer yes to at least three of these symptoms are tested for the illness. However, if you respond strongly to any of these symptoms, it is advised that you discuss lupus with your physician. If your doctor is uninformed about appropriate diagnostic tests, seek out a good rheumatologist, or go to a university medical center where physicians are more accustomed to seeing a wide variety of illnesses. Review carefully this list of symptoms, keeping in mind that it is very important not to self-diagnose and that it does not mean you have lupus if you answer yes to one or more questions.

1. Have you ever had arthritis or rheumatism for more than three months?

2. Do your fingers become pale, numb, or uncomfortable in the cold?

3. Have you had any sores in your mouth for more than two weeks?

4. Have you been told that you have low blood counts (anemia, low white cell count, or low platelet count)?

5. Have you ever had a prominent rash on your cheeks for more than a month?

6. Does your skin break out after you have been in the sun (not sunburn)?

7. Has it ever been painful to take a deep breath for more than a few days?

8. Have you been told that you have protein in your urine?

9. Have you ever had a rapid loss of hair?

10. Have you ever had a seizure?

The most important tool to help you deal with lupus is awareness. It is extremely important to be familiar with up-to-date information. If you do not have a local organization like the Bay Area Lupus Foundation, contact the Lupus Foundation of America in Washington, D.C. (see *Resources* at the back of this book). It provides information on lupus and recommendations on where to seek appropriate medical care.

The lack of knowledge about lupus causes many lupus patients the additional agony of coping with misinformation. It should be clear from the preceding discussion that lupus is NOT:

1. Contagious—you cannot catch it from anyone.

2. Like AIDS—while the immune system is involved in lupus, it is not an illness that is infectious or primarily fatal. It can be a managed illness.

3. A sexually transmitted disease—while a false positive test for syphilis is sometimes a part of the diagnostic process, lupus is definitely not syphilis nor related to any other sexually transmitted disease.

4. Psychosomatic—many women in the long, arduous diagnostic process are frequently thought of as hysterical hypochondriacs or chronic complainers by family, friends, co-workers and medical professionals.

Lupus is a complex, unpredictable, and, at times, life-threatening chronic illness. But it is an illness that is manageable, and many patients cope with it for many years while living productive lives. It is much easier for them to cope with lupus if their peers have an accurate understanding of the disease. Friends and family members can help by acknowledging that lupus, at times, is difficult to manage; that lupus patients can feel awful while looking healthy; that careful monitoring of symptoms is essential to preventing serious life-threatening flare-ups; and that avoidance of stress aids in abating serious episodes of the illness.

The following information was collected from black female lupus patients in the San Francisco Bay Area. The purpose of the research was to tell the "lupus story" from women who knew it first-hand.

It is common for women to have difficulty in receiving a definitive diagnosis for lupus. Some of the reasons have been explained in the discussion of the biophysical properties of the illness. Others can be attributed to a lack of knowledge about the illness and to race and gender bias; that is, the way many white male physicians view medical complaints of black women. Like Donna, many women said they had difficulty in getting someone to actually believe they were ill:

"One problem was being told I was a hypochondriac and that I should see a psychiatrist. Even though I was genuinely ill and I was hospitalized, no one could tell me why I was sick. I had pericarditis and other life-threatening episodes, but no one could explain why these medical problems were happening to me. I felt that since they could not explain what was wrong, the doctors somehow blamed me for 'inventing' the problems."

Because many people are unfamiliar with lupus, their ignorance often creates a multitude of problems for lupus patients like Pam:

"The startling and difficult thing about lupus is so many people don't have the slightest idea what having this disease means. I have had people ask 'Can I catch it?' from simply being in the same room with me, or 'Should I eat out of utensils that you have eaten out of?' This is ridiculous; lupus is not contagious."

Or Saundra:

"My mother and father, as well as sisters and brothers, do not believe there is anything wrong with me. They think I'm just looking for excuses to avoid taking care of my children. Because lupus changes, sometimes from day to day in the way it affects you and because the medication affects my moods, they all think I am strung out on cocaine and alcohol. The times when I am o.k. and "up" they associate my behavior with cocaine, and the times when I am down, they feel alcohol is the cause. They simply feel the only chronic condition I am suffering from is that of being a chronic complainer."

Discussing the lack of information about lupus, Joanne said:

"I do not blame my doctor for not providing me with an appropriate diagnosis. I blame him for not entering into a positive struggle with me to search for such a diagnosis. . . . Even my husband thought my vague complaints were the products of my imagination, and what else could he think? The medical profession had proven there was nothing wrong with me."

Stress also has a great impact on lupus. Many lupus patients who deal with stress effectively are often successful in managing their illness. As Renee said:

"I haven't had an attack or had to go to the hospital since I separated from my husband. We were arguing all the time. So I finally told him to leave. My friends tell me that I should have gotten rid of him a long time ago since I feel so much better now that he is gone."

Many lupus patients find full-time work a hardship and make career changes that, at times, are more rewarding. For example, Barbara is a young black female newscaster who was working in the highly competitive and stressful television industry. When her lupus was diagnosed she switched to a job in radio:

"I am happy now with more time for my son, reading and creative writing. A lot of people think I have taken a step down, but what they don't realize is that television is a cruel business. Every moment you're aware that your job is on the line, every second. I am relieved to be free of that stress."

Thus, the redesigning of work habits and lifestyles can help make lupus more manageable.

Because of the complexity and variability of lupus it is important for patients to be aware of their individual symptoms and to work interactively with physicians, not passively. Remember to trust your own knowledge of your body and to be a partner in managing and controlling your illness.

There are women all over the world who are fulfilling their dreams and making enormous contributions while living with lupus. Once identified and treated, the illness does not usually severely restrict a woman's life. If you have lupus, there are individuals and information available to help you. There is no reason for the illness, or anything else, to hold you back. Reach out and you'll find help.

Footnotes

1. Henrietta Aladjem, *Understanding Lupus* (New York: Charles Scribner and Sons, 1985).

2. Peter Schur (ed.), *The Clinical Management of Systemic Lupus Erythematosus* (Orlando, Florida: Grune and Stratton, 1983).

3. Bay Area Lupus Foundation, *Information on Lupus*, San Jose, CA.

*There is much exciting and promising new research on potential causes
and cures for diabetes. There are new drugs being developed and even the
prospect of inoculation against juvenile-onset diabetes, according to the
American Diabetes Association. In the meantime, medical supervision and
general good health practices can help black women successfully manage
this disease.*

*Many doctors believe that regular exercise, a proper diet and vitamin
supplements can help prevent or minimize the effects of diabetes. They say
that reducing stress and stopping smoking will also help to avert the disease.*

*In the following piece, a Berkeley journalist with an interest in health
care issues tells the story of a black woman with diabetes who has adjusted
to her illness and is living life to the full.*

The Best Foot Forward:
A Black Woman Deals with Diabetes
K. Malaika Williams

A month ago, Juanita Bryant's doctor gave her a clean bill of health
and said she wouldn't have to return for three months. Juanita was
elated.

"After what my body has been through, for her to tell me I'll see
you in three months was like saying 'congratulations,'" Juanita
said.

Juanita, a fifty-six-year-old grandmother and San Francisco preschool teacher, became a diabetic a year and a half ago. Though she
has followed her doctor's orders and adjusted her diet to maintain
her health, she has still seen her body go through changes. Her eyesight changed, her skin became softer, and for a time her blood
sugar level was fluctuating beyond her control. Now it is stable, and
Juanita leads a basically normal life.

Juanita's symptoms began in late December, 1987. She was thir-
sty all the time and drank a lot of water to quench her thirst. She was
also losing a lot of weight.

"I drank so much I couldn't go thirty minutes without using the bathroom," she said.

When Juanita called her doctor early in January 1988, she was told to make an appointment immediately. After the examination, her doctor diagnosed Juanita as a "borderline" diabetic, gave her detailed instructions on how to care for herself and referred Juanita to a dietitian. Her condition quickly developed into diabetes type-II, or non-insulin-dependent diabetes, which can be controlled by diet and exercise.

Diabetes is a disease that hinders the way the body uses food, thereby causing high blood sugar levels. Normally, the body changes sugars and starches into a sugar called glucose. Glucose is carried through the body in the blood with the help of the hormone insulin, which is produced in the pancreas. People with diabetes have problems with the production of insulin. In diabetes type-I or insulin-dependent diabetes, the pancreas does not generate any insulin. This form of diabetes (also known as juvenile onset) usually begins fairly early in life. In type-II diabetes, the pancreas does not produce enough insulin and/or has difficulty using the insulin produced. These conditions are cause for concern because without sufficient insulin, energy cannot be produced in the cells and glucose levels build up in the bloodstream.

Juanita's symptoms—excessive thirst, frequent urination and dramatic weight loss—are three of the major indicators of diabetes. Other signs of the disease include extreme hunger, irritability, fatigue, blurred vision, nausea, vomiting, drowsiness, itching, tingling or numbness in the extremities, slow-to-heal skin abrasions and a family history of diabetes.

While cancer and AIDS have perhaps become the most feared diseases in America today, diabetes is the fastest growing of all the major health hazards. Trailing cardiovascular disease and cancer, diabetes is the third leading cause of death for African-Americans, with black women showing a particular vulnerability to the disease. For instance, while black men are nine percent more likely to develop diabetes than white men, black women are nearly fifty percent more likely to become diabetic than white women.

Researchers do not know what triggers the pancreas malfunction that causes diabetes, but there are a number of theories about why black women are prone to develop the disease. For example, research shows that overweight people tend to have problems using insulin in food digestion and that sixty to eighty percent of diabetics were overweight when first diagnosed with the disease. This is telling, because black women are more likely to be overweight than white women.

There also is some evidence that black Americans are less physically adaptable to the contemporary American diet, which is high in sugar and fat. Historically, Africans have had a high-carbohydrate diet, which takes longer to break down into glucose in the bloodstream. Consequently, such a diet does not require the body to produce as much insulin at one time.

Although her mother and one of her sisters were diabetic, Juanita never suspected she was likely to develop the disease. No one ever told her that diabetes might be hereditary or that overweight black women more than forty years old are at particular risk. However, once she discovered she had the disease, Juanita was willing to fight.

Juanita's doctor gave her all the armor she needed: literature, precautionary instructions, and diet tips to stabilize her blood sugar level and to help her avoid some of the problems associated with diabetes such as blindness, kidney disease, amputations of legs and feet, heart disease and strokes.

Juanita also had to learn to test her own blood. Using a kit available at drug stores, she pricks her finger with a supplied needle and places the blood on a strip of litmus paper. After a few minutes, she compares the color of the strip to a chart to find out if her blood sugar level is satisfactory.

When she first started, Juanita tested her blood three times a day: "I would go from one extreme to the other. I'd either have it extremely low or extremely high. I was totally frustrated."

Her doctor told her the variations are common at the onset of diabetes. Her pancreas was spitting out various levels of insulin, making it difficult for Juanita to control the levels.

After a year of careful maintenance Juanita is able to keep her blood sugar stable, and only needs to test her blood twice a week.

Diet and proper nutrition are the key to controlling diabetes, so to do so Juanita became an amateur nutritionist. She revamped her eating habits to include more fresh vegetables and foods high in fiber and less red meat, fatty foods and sugar. For example, Juanita starts her day with oatmeal and coffee. Once at work, she might have another cup of coffee, a piece of toast and sometimes fresh fruit. For lunch and dinner, she'll eat a starch, such as noodles or rice, lean meat or chicken and a fresh vegetable. Occasionally she'll have a piece of cake with no frosting or "lite" ice cream for dessert. And as a snack when she comes home from work, she'll sometimes drink a large glass of water and eat popcorn.

Juanita wore glasses before she became a diabetic as she was nearsighted. But when diabetes set in, she became farsighted and had to get a new pair of glasses. Diabetics are often at risk for eye problems that prompt gradual loss of vision, and even blindness. As a preventative measure, Juanita has her eyes checked every six months to make sure her sight is not deteriorating.

Because injuries to the extremities of diabetics often do not heal properly, diabetes is a contributing factor in about forty-five percent of the leg and foot amputations in the United States, according to health officials.

Wiggling the toes of her small feet as they rested on a foot stool, Juanita said, "If they cut off anything of mine, I won't be able to handle it. I know that."

So she takes very good care of her feet. To keep her feet clean she has twelve to fourteen pairs of shoes so she never has to wear the same pair two days in a row, and she wears clean stockings every day. She oils and lotions her feet every night and makes sure to keep her toenails even.

Soon after the diabetes started, Juanita was in a grocery store. A little boy was playing with a shopping cart, coming dangerously close to bumping it into other customers. Juanita recalls being terrified that the boy would hit her and injure her legs or toes.

Now she is less fearful because her doctor told her that as long as her blood sugar level is stable, injuries to her feet and legs will have a better chance to heal. But she still avoids walking barefoot in her apartment after her grandchildren have visited. She does not want to be nicked by any sharp objects they might have accidentally left on the rug.

One of the other ways Juanita takes care of herself is to stay fit. She walks for exercise and her job with preschool children keeps her active and limber. As an added precaution, she always carries a bottle of micronase pills with her. The medication is frequently prescribed for diabetics because it helps balance blood sugar levels.

During the first few months of her diabetes, Juanita was very frustrated and credits her oldest and youngest daughters with being supportive. Her doctor also made things easier by explaining everything and taking her step-by-step through the changes she would need to make in her life. However, she said she wishes she could have found a support group of black women going through the same thing she was going through. Unfortunately, the other diabetic black women she knows are not handling their condition well.

"Black women with diabetes need to take better care of themselves. They don't realize how important it is," Juanita said.

Despite the precautions she must take and the changes diabetes has brought about, Juanita's resolve is strong.

"I love me. I never get tired of doing anything for Juanita. Anything in the world that I could do for me, if it's in my power or in my price range, I'll do it for me," she said. "The only problem I have is my diabetes. And that is under control."

Beverly Smith has been a dedicated crusader for people of color, women and gays since the 1960s civil rights era. A respected lecturer, consultant and organizer, Smith has been on the cutting edge of progressive causes ranging from anti-apartheid efforts to reproductive rights to AIDS activism. As Program Coordinator of Black Women's Health at the Massachusetts Department of Public Health in Boston, she has a comprehensive view of the myriad health issues confronting black women.

The following interview was conducted by Andrea Lewis, a black feminist writer from the San Francisco Bay Area.

Looking at the Total Picture: A Conversation with Health Activist Beverly Smith
Andrea Lewis

Andrea: What kind of situation did you grow up in?

Beverly: My family was part of the large migration of Black people who came from the South to the North during the period from about 1915 to 1940. My sister Barbara (publisher of Kitchen Table: Women of Color Press) and I were raised in Cleveland, Ohio, but my family was originally from Georgia.

Andrea: Were there particular events that politicized you in your earlier days?

Beverly: (Laughs.) Everything! When I was entering primary school Truman was still president. Although I was brought up in the North, there was still a tremendous amount of racism and discrimination. For example, public accommodations were still segregated, and that was true in Cleveland, let me assure you. I knew early on that Black people were oppressed, but awareness came long before activism. It's hard to figure it out, but I know that I was very aware and very observant of race and racial differences from a very young age. It may have been the family. I think that the fact that issues of race were at least talked about in my family had a lot to do with shaping our political values. I grew up in a family of women. My mother worked and my grandmother took care of us. I never had any contact with my father or his side of the family. In fact, I had very little contact with my mother because she was working most of the time.

Many of the experiences in my family led directly to my becoming involved in women's health, beginning with the long illness and death of my mother. She died of rheumatic fever when I was almost ten years old. The hypothesis was that she had probably had rheumatic fever as a child and it went untreated—which was typical for someone growing up in poverty in rural Georgia in the 1920s and 30s. So when she got it again, her heart was already very damaged. Then during my first year of college, one of my great aunts who had lived with us and who had always had lots of health problems, began having blackouts and fainting spells and things like that. The symptoms began to manifest themselves as mental illness, though I don't really think that was the origin. She was in a private mental hospital for a few weeks, but when the cost became too much she had to go to a state mental hospital. Then my grandmother got very senile and would wander away from home. She was very confused and had to go into a nursing home, and of course there were limits to what we could afford. The whole thing of getting her into the nursing home was very traumatic and it was very depressing to go down there.

The coup de grace was about two years after I graduated from college when my mother's sister died very suddenly from a stroke and my grandmother died about three years after that. So that's my family. It's ugly, and telling you about it is very upsetting to me. I have to deal with the realities of it everyday because I don't have relatives around. I'm very aware of how it has affected my life and my family's.

I came to public health rather precipitously. As I look back on it now, I realize that it may not have been such a singularly considered decision, but I can see the process. I remember saying to my aunt when we were trying to get my grandmother into the nursing home, "I don't care what I have to do, but I'm going to do something so that people don't have to go through this."

Andrea: Was there a time when you became specifically aware of feminist politics?

Beverly: There were memorable incidents there also. I remember reading something about the battle of the sexes and thinking, "What is this all about?" In college I did have exposure to a lot of activism including the women's movement, but I can remember going to one of the first Women's Liberation organizing meetings in Chicago and thinking, "What are these women talking about?" I just didn't get it. I can't tell you how much racism was right in front of my eyes during college years. We're talking about the transition from the civil rights period to the Black Power, Black Nationalist movements, so maybe I couldn't see much of anything else.

Andrea: The women's meetings that you did attend, were they very white and middle-class?

Beverly: Oh, absolutely.

Andrea: So what did you see yourself doing? You had this degree in history and an interest in health issues.

Beverly: I had no idea. In college I didn't really have any interest in health as a career. I really didn't know that one could do something in health and not be a doctor or nurse. So I didn't know what I was going to do. But a few years after doing some graduate work in American Studies and History, all of a sudden I thought, "Well, I could go into public health." It was just like that. I started checking into classes and public health schools, and I took an excellent course in community health at the The New School for Social Research in New York City. Then I applied to public health school, went to Yale and pretty much simultaneously got involved in feminism. I had been to some N.O.W. (National Organization for Women) meetings in New York during the early 1970s, but what really made a great difference was in the fall of 1973 when there was a National Black Feminist Organization Eastern Regional Conference. That was the first time I was able to be in contact with a lot of Black feminists and that made a tremendous difference. One of the workshops I attended there was on Black women's health, so my involvement in both feminism and health came at about the same time.

Andrea: Let's talk in general about Black women's health. Why do you think we don't have it, and what do you think we can do to get it?

Beverly: There is no question that Black women have some of the worst health problems of any group. Two words came to mind immediately when you asked me that question and those words are *freedom* and *safety*. Those are the things that are most needed for us to have good health. We're supposed to have freedom but not one Black in this country does and particularly as women we do not have safety. The reason that Black women don't have good health in this country is because we are so oppressed. It's just that simple. It's about social conditions. That's really what poor health status is for most people in this country.

Andrea: Do you think that most Black women in this country are aware of this? Are they conscious of the problems? Do they think, "Hey, the reason that health is a problematic issue for me is because I'm Black and oppressed?"

Beverly: No, because having the time to think about one's health in that way is really a luxury. For most Black women who live from crisis to crisis—and not only health crises—you think of health when it becomes a crisis for you. You think of health when your child gets sick. So things get handled in episodic fashion. One of the things that you find in poor cultures is that people define illness as being nigh on to death. You have to be terribly sick in a lot of cultures to be considered socially sick.

Many years ago the World Health Organization made a somewhat holistic definition of what health is and they talked about how it's not merely the absence of disease, but it is also the presence of well-being—physical, emotional, mental and social. Well-being is definitely something different than the absence of disease. When you look at Black women's health status, and this is true for Black men as well, you find tremendous discrepancies between Blacks and whites; the lack of longevity, incidence of certain killer diseases, infant mortality—and I think that the incredibly awful infant mortality rate in this country indicates the poor health of Black women and of the entire Black community.

Andrea: When you talk about freedom and safety are you also referring to freedom of access to health care?

Beverly: Yes. Access is a very important issue, but the reason that freedom came to mind is that, to me, freedom means control over your own life and how you live your life. I have been haunted by a story that I heard on National Public Radio a few weeks ago about women who were mostly Black and definitely poor, who were working in a chicken factory. There's an occupational disease called repetitive strain injury that people get from doing the same physical motion over and over again too fast and too often. These women were cutting up four chickens a minute and suffering from this disease. Their health was tremendously compromised by what they were doing, but they didn't have control over how they were going to earn a living, or over their work lives. It's not like they decided, "Well, I'll clean toilets even though I could be a corporate lawyer" or "I'll go cut up chickens though I could go and be a college professor." Those people don't have freedom of choice. That's what I mean by freedom: control over your life and the choices that you have in the context of a just society.

Andrea: And what about safety? Can you expand on that?

Beverly: By safety I mean a lot of things. Specifically protection from and the absence of violence, whether that be racial violence, or sexual violence, or racial/sexual violence. Like when a Black woman is raped by a white man, how do you tell exactly what is going on there? Is it racism? Is it sexism? It's undoubtedly a combination of both. I also mean safety from emotional violence as well—everything from the personal abusiveness that can occur in an individual relationship to the violence that is done to our psyches as Black women because we are so devalued.

Andrea: Things have really changed for the better in some ways. When I was a kid terms like domestic violence, child abuse, emotional abuse were just not used.

Beverly: It might be that emotional child abuse is the last to be uncovered and it's true that it's good to know about it, but I feel like this society is an abusive society and knowing about the existence of rape doesn't necessarily change anything. There was a time that battering had not been conceptualized and yet the amount of battering hasn't diminished just because of it being named and services being there. A big factor now in the minds of battered women is homelessness. I mean, if you leave this man you may very well end up on the streets.

Andrea: It often seems that the inequities of our society are completely out of control and I wonder what can happen that will shake people enough to realize it. How are Black women ever going to be able to achieve the amount of freedom and safety that they need for better health? And even if you did have a legitimate plan of action to solve the problems, would it be heard?

Beverly: I ask myself the questions you've just asked me night and day. I am engaged at the Department of Public Health in trying to work toward creating that kind of world. And I ask myself, it seems, hundreds of times a week, "Well, is it making any difference? Is it worth it?" I feel that even if it's not making much of a difference, it's very important for me to be fighting for these things and to resist oppression. It's the difference between being a compliant slave or being a resistant slave. I think your orientation or your posture to your oppressor is important. To me, the potential is in how much and how far the oppressed can push against and resist oppression. If every woman who has the potential to become politicized around her own health and her own well-being was in fact engaged in doing so and empowered to do so and organized to do so, how much farther could we get? The people who I despair over are the ones who could be doing something but for whatever reason are not. Someone might criticize me for saying that and they might say, "Well, don't you understand that the very nature of oppression is to keep people immobilized and not doing things to fight against it?" Yet I know that if I'm able to do it, then other people can too.

Andrea: Yes. I think that the fixation with self-gratification is a problem in our culture. It's hard for people to get beyond it. So many people seem to only be interested in getting as much personal pleasure out of life as they can. Do you feel that health issues are pretty far down on the list of priorities for Blacks?

Beverly: Health doesn't exist in a vacuum, so I think that working to guarantee, for instance, good housing for Black women is a measure that would impact Black women's health. A lot of people don't understand that the availability of medical care is not the primary thing that impacts health status. Economic and social forces such as good nutrition, good housing, a clean water supply, adequate clothing, and sanitation influence health care the most. Having adequate access to those things is going to go much farther to enhance your health status than lots of medical care. Let's say you have a clinic set up in a poor neighborhood or in a Third World country, where you provide all the things needed to deliver fairly decent primary care. If the people you want to treat are drinking contaminated water, living exposed to the elements or not getting proper nutrition, then the health center really isn't going to help them that much. This is important for people to consider when they're thinking about health care. So even though health may not be high up specifically on the agenda of Black women, I think that implicitly it is in some ways. The things that poor Black women are struggling for would go some distance in improving their quality of health.

Andrea: One of the things that I personally find troublesome is society's attitude toward weight issues. One of the most inspiring things I've ever read was at the beginning of Alice Walker's book *In Search of Our Mother's Gardens* where Bernice Reagon [Black activist and founder of the vocal group Sweet Honey in the Rock] talks about the Black community being a place where having hips is okay. She says that it's the nature of our culture and many of the images we are fed about how we should look come from the white community. What are your feelings about it? It's certainly a medical issue, but is it also a social standard that has been put on us by white society?

Beverly: I think that it's complicated. Clearly there are imposed patriarchal standards about what women should look like. So how do you find a pro-health position on obesity that validates some of the things Bernice Reagon says, which I think are true? African-American women do not tend to be sylph-like in their natural form, though we don't know what that natural form is exactly. The long, thin anorexic look that is so favored is really probably not natural for white women either. I do believe that there is such a thing as obesity —of weighing so much that it impairs your health and/or the quality of your life.

Black women are more likely to be obese than any group in this country. We are more overweight than others and that includes Black men. I think that's very significant. Some of the destructive eating may have to do with some of the pain we experience in other parts of our lives. I think that the emotional well-being of Black women is pretty much ignored. The condition of our psyches, the inner lives, thoughts and feelings of Black women are not paid much attention to. One of the lines in Sojourner Truth's speech "Ain't I a Woman?" that I think is heart-rending is when she talks about her children being sold into slavery. She says, "I cried out in my mother's grief and none but Jesus heard me." That's what can be said about the emotional devastation that Black women have experienced.

Andrea: I know that you do a lot of work around women with AIDS. Why do you think that so little attention is being paid to the subject?

Beverly: More than fifty percent of the women with AIDS are Black and that group is followed closely by Latina women. I think this is because these are women who are forgotten and are some of the most reviled people in society. They have everything going against them. They're often intravenous drug users, or they are partners of IV drug users. It's also a group that is in the least position to be able to do anything about it. For women whose major concern is not that they may be HIV-positive or in a high-risk group, it's difficult. They may be concerned about getting food on the table and having a place to even put the table because homelessness is such a tremendous issue. Food, shelter and violence of various kinds are probably much more important to them, and they are not in much of a position to organize around the myriad issues which impact their lives.

Andrea: It also seems that despite all of the media attention that has been given AIDS, people still feel very removed from what is happening.

Beverly: We as Black women and Black people really need to get over that because I feel that the way AIDS is developing in our community, the consequences are going to be tragic. I think it could lead to a diminishing of the Black population, a quite sizeable decrease, because that's how the epidemic is running. We have to do whatever it takes to get over our sense of separateness. The class and anti-drug issues are tremendous. One of the things that gets me is how narrow self-interest can be. One's response to AIDS can't always be based on how likely one is to be at high risk. That's crazy.

Andrea: Let's talk a little about abortion. How do you feel about the Supreme Court decision that may lead to an overturning of *Roe v. Wade* and the anti-abortion groups like Operation Rescue which have stolen their demonstration tactics from the left? Things seem to have turned so upside down.

Beverly: I think what has happened since *Roe v. Wade* has really affected the reproductive rights of Black women. Access for Black women to abortion has been seriously compromised in the past several years. I heard an excellent speaker at a conference I attended recently. She said that it's a luxury to be able to focus on a single political issue because so often one's life is about surviving a host of different oppressions and then dealing with all of the problems and struggles at once.

Andrea: In an article [*Gay Community News*, February 19–25, 1989], you discussed abortion in terms of genocide of the Black race.

Beverly: I think that being the target of racial oppression both as individuals and as a community can in some ways distort your views of reality. I have always marveled at the fact that some Black people consider abortion and birth control as genocidal, when to me, they are the precise things that might enable a Black woman to take control of her life. I think that genocide comes up in relation to birth control and abortion in part because of the generalized distrust that we as Black people have toward a system that has never meant us any good and which has behaved in a genocidal fashion toward us. I think that genocide for Blacks in this country is systemic. We are systematically deprived of things that make it possible to live decently—everything from a decent education, jobs and health care. The whole combination is what I would describe as genocide against Black people.

Andrea: What can you say to Black women about taking control of their lives and their health?

Beverly: We need more people. We need more people who are willing to get out there and do the kinds of things that need to be done on a host of issues, not just Black women's health. But I think that it's very hard for people to be creative. It's hard to start things from scratch and to keep things going. That's one of the things that is particularly challenging in AIDS work because much of the stuff that is happening in AIDS is really new. In the work that I'm doing, I think the biggest challenge is building coalitions among Black women and dealing with and acknowledging the differences that we have. There are always conflicts between Black women—the problems we have dealing with each other.

Andrea: Around issues of sexuality for example?

Beverly: That's one of the places where it can be played out. But there are others. Audre Lorde talks about how we can be very, very reluctant to connect in positive and real ways with other Black women because it's real hard when you are a member of a group that is so despised. When you look at another Black woman you see all of this reviled stuff—you see all of the stuff that you embody and have been told is bad about you. It's intense.

Andrea: Do you think that many gains have been made in Black women's health in the past decade?

Beverly: I think that it's helpful that people are talking about Black women's health and that organizations like the National Black Women's Health Project have been formed. So I think there has been some progress in terms of consciousness-raising. But the overall status of Black women's health has not improved measurably; in fact, if you look at all the indicators, our health is worse, primarily because of the Reagan and Bush administrations and what has gone on economically in this country. So on the one hand, I think there is more awareness of Black women's health and more of a desire to do something. But on the other hand, we are working in an environment that is more hostile than it was ten years ago. I think that the more hopeful things that are going on are happening at a local grass-roots level rather than at the national governmental level.

Besides the dreadful statistics and the specific health problems, I think we need to be talking about Black women's health because our position and condition is unique. Our history, culture and present situation in this country all have impact on our health. So it isn't just about the diseases we get or our terrible infant mortality rates. It's much more complex than that. It's about how difficult it is to be who we are. When I talk about health, as I said before, I think of it in a very holistic sense which takes into account women's emotional, social and spiritual well-being as well as their physical bodies. Again, what does focusing on Black women's health mean? For me, it means services that are consciously constructed to take into account the whole life situation of Black women. There are hundreds of thousands of places and people in this country in neighborhood clinics and elsewhere who are providing medical care for Black women. But that is not the same as *practicing* Black women's health. What makes the work we do Black women's health work is that we really try to look at women's life circumstances and value the meaning of those lives. At the very least, we acknowledge the importance of language and culture and the experience of immigration and war and sexual assault—all of the things that happen to women. We look at the total picture. That's what you need to do if your mission is to heal Black women.

AIDS is claiming black lives at a rate three times faster than that for whites. During the past two years, forty-one percent of reported cases of AIDS have occurred among people of color, according to Louis Sullivan, U.S. Secretary of Health and Human Services.

For black women with AIDS, the disease is not a singular issue. For many of them, it is just another piece in the mosaic of joblessness, poverty, drug abuse, teen pregnancy and illiteracy that is rampant in inner-city neighborhoods.

In the following piece, the author analyzes AIDS and its impact from the perspective of black women and calls for advocacy efforts that address the disenfranchisement of ethnic minorities.

AIDS: In Living Color
Beth Richie

As the most serious health crisis to affect black women in recent history, AIDS is a vivid symbol of the havoc that has been wreaked on women's quality of life in contemporary American society. In addition to presenting major life-threatening conditions, the AIDS epidemic represents a widespread social, political and cultural backlash. With racism and sexism on the rise in our society, AIDS has given leeway for individuals and social institutions to ignore or further exploit black women.

Once thought to be a disease that only affects white gay men, in recent years the epidemiology of the AIDS epidemic has dramatically shifted. According to the Centers for Disease Control in Atlanta, Georgia, today twenty-five percent of all people with AIDS are black. Fifty-two percent of all women with AIDS-related illnesses or positive HIV status are black. And fifty-nine to eighty percent of all children afflicted with the virus are black. AIDS has become the leading cause of death for black women between the ages of twenty-four and thirty-six. Moreover, black women who contract AIDS do not live as long or die as well as their white or male counterparts.

The problems commonly associated with AIDS, such as poor nutrition, drug use, incarceration, lack of preventative health services and inadequate housing are not new problems for the black community. Nor is denial of the existence of a black gay and bisexual community or competition with other oppressed groups for scarce resources. Premature death is not a new trend among African-Americans. AIDS, in many ways, is like every other health, social and economic crisis tthat black people have faced for generations. What is alarmingly different about AIDS is the severity of the infection and the particularly repressive political timing of the emergence of the disease. The combined effect of all these elements leaves the black community in an extremely vulnerable position. AIDS has the potential to cripple black people in a way that few other health or social forces have since slavery.

One of the most significant tolls that AIDS has had on our society is to seriously overtax the already strained health care system. Federal, state and local reductions in health care budgets, lack of health planning and punitive health policies have resulted in a dangerously poor quality of health care in most metropolitan areas. In particular, the staffing shortages among nurses and health technicians have become a critical factor contributing to the health service crisis.

Black women comprise a large percentage of the low-level nursing population that provides most of the daily care for people with AIDS. Black female nurses aides, home attendants and medical technicians have been caught in the middle of an inadequate health system, irresponsible government policies and a tremendous increase in patients who require intensive care, usually as they die. Although extensive research has proven that health care workers do not constitute a high risk category for contracting the HIV virus, it is reasonable to assume that there are mental health consequences from working under the stressful conditions that the AIDS epidemic has created. This is especially true for black women in the health care industry who are routinely underpaid, required to work long hours without adequate compensation or support, not given equal access to the necessary training or supervision, and who are otherwise exploited by the health organizations that employ them. This problem is exacerbated by the multitudes of health agencies that hire undocumented black women and do not provide basic health insurance or job protection for them. Such agencies further abuse immigrant black women (primarily from the Caribbean) by threatening deportation to ensure compliance. In the AIDS crisis, the health system is exploiting black women workers just as other industries have done for more than a century.

The culturally dictated gender role of most women in black families requires that they be responsible for the health and well-being of their children, husband or sexual partner. This means when family members become sick, black women care for them, usually alone. The nature of AIDS-related illnesses creates a high level of fear, and requires constant health surveillance, repeated medical appointments and hospitalizations. It is exhausting and expensive, and black women usually carry the burden by themselves.

While the white gay male community has banded together to share resources in the AIDS crisis, the extended family support system which is characteristic of most black communities has been drained. The pattern of the illness is such that many black women are simultaneously caring for children, sex partners and friends dying of AIDS-related illnesses. And of course, many black women are themselves sick.

Institutionalized racism is another critical factor that compounds the situation for black families. Black men are often absent from their families because of poor job opportunities in urban areas, biased criminal justice systems that lead to higher incarceration rates for black men, or the internalization of despair that can result in drug or alcohol abuse. Again, black women are left to devise systems of survival for themselves.

Statistics indicate that the most frequent mode of transmission of the HIV virus to black women is through sexual contact with black men who are intravenous drug users and/or gay/bisexual. This means that to fully understand the impact of AIDS on black women, attention must be given to the politically charged issue of sexuality.

There have always been gay men and women in the black community. However, because of homophobia, their identities and activities have rarely been acknowledged. The AIDS epidemic has forced the black community to address the religious and cultural intolerance that has prompted many black men to live dual existences in both the heterosexual and homosexual worlds.

The prevailing societal view of black women's sexuality is that they are promiscuous, irresponsible and involved in illicit sexual activity such as prostitution. This misrepresentation has serious consequences in that it contributes to sexual harassment, rape and a general lack of sensitivity to the range of sexual expressions black women choose. In the face of these damning images of black women's sexuality, the community has become defensive and hesitant to openly discuss any issue related to sexuality. This silence has, in turn, left black women particularly vulnerable to HIV infection because of a lack of opportunities to discuss sexual behavior or AIDS risks.

This problem is manifested most seriously in the health education campaigns designed for women about condom use and other safe sex practices. These advertisements are not generally culturally sensitive. The result is that the black community (usually the male leadership) rejects the safe sex efforts because they are viewed as either sexually suggestive or culturally inappropriate.

Safe sex campaigns designed for women also must be examined from another angle. On the one hand, all women need information and strategies to protect themselves and their unborn children. On the other hand, many of the safe sex campaigns aimed at women reinforce the premise that women must be responsible for men. The result, unfortunately, is that women are blamed if they become pregnant, contract the HIV virus or another sexually transmitted disease from an infected male partner. For black women, this situation is complicated by the racial stereotypes of black heterosexual couples: the man being highly irresponsible (and consequently excused for his behavior in intimate relationships) and the woman being dominant and controlling.

As previously mentioned, black women are enormously overrepresented in the population of people with AIDS. The lack of AIDS prevention programs in communities of color, the lack of primary health care and the virtual absence of social and emotional support for black women with AIDS have exacerbated the problem. A black woman's health needs are likely to be considered secondary to the needs of her children, her partner, her community or the convenience of the health care system. That is, she is treated as a risk to others rather than in need of assistance herself.

The threat of sterilization abuse has re-emerged as a risky complication of AIDS. When black women are infected by the HIV virus, they may be overtly or covertly pressured to delay pregnancy or to undergo a sterilization operation or abortion. This risk has raised the politically volatile issue of genocide for black people, especially those who are poor, drug-users or sick. Given the repressive social climate and the increase in racial intolerance, it is expected that this risk will become even more profound in the near future.

For black women who are HIV-positive and pregnant, the situation becomes considerably more complicated. There are few prenatal care providers who are trained or willing to help pregnant women who may have contracted AIDS through the use of intravenous drugs, and those that do usually require drug detoxification as a condition of service. Because of a waning commitment to human services during the Reagan-Bush era, most drug detoxification programs have long waiting lists. This means that a growing number of drug-addicted pregnant women who are HIV-positive are completely underserved, and if current trends continue, they may be criminally penalized for giving birth, even though there are few service systems to protect or assist them.

For sure, black women with AIDS who give birth are extremely vulnerable within the child welfare system. There is a great risk that their children will be taken away should their health status be revealed.

The well-being of black women is seriously threatened by the AIDS epidemic and the complexity of its related problems. Yet black women have historically endured in the face of overwhelming odds. Lots of people have wanted us dead before now and thought they had us dying long ago. The challenge we face as individuals and community activists is to develop creative strategies for survival— one more time. As we've done since slavery, we must define issues for ourselves and establish strong and empowering sources of support to combat AIDS. Organizations such as the National Black Women's Health Project, the California Prostitutes Education Project and Kitchen Table: Women of Color Press are in the forefront of this effort. Reassessing our roles as health care workers, family and community caretakers and sexual beings will also bring insight for solutions. Certainly the AIDS epidemic calls for us to challenge the system to reverse trends that oppress groups based on their race, gender, sexuality and economic status.

After a long silence, black people are beginning to realize just how serious this epidemic is and to address the emergency it has created for our community. As AIDS sufferers and strategists, black women have a lot to gain by battling this new menace with the tenacity with which we have always confronted the obstacles put in our path.

Imani Harrington is an HIV-positive black woman who was a victim of sexual assault and is recovering from drug addiction. She states:

"In the five years in which I have been abstinent from self-abuse, I have come to realize that we all must look to that mirror and face who we are and tear down those false layers covering our true spirit and begin to build new ones. Living in a country that fosters the destruction of women, I echo these words to all sistahs who have been left to die in grave silence on isolated corners that meet dead-end streets. If we must die we shall die speaking our truths."

Aid of AMERICA
Imani Harrington

Small bones crushed by the foot of racism
will be placed in an archaeologist's grave
precious red wet eyes run deep
with blood dripping staining our bodies
onto canvasses to be hung in a dying gallery
blending colors of pain-o-sorrow-o-grief
into the heart open lonely space of a mother's mouth
crying for the loss of her child
the rich sweet acrid taste of a mother's love
has been lost in this war

I am/we are/they are
you are now it a veteran in AMERICA
with the aids of AMERICA
crossing life's war
combatting a disease infiltrated
with the aid of AMERICA

When you make your living at night under the red light
girl you will be charged
with the aids of AMERICA
hissing chimes the men throw dimes to slide
on your wet body your blood line is a crime
you are a black woman in AMERICA without a face or a voice
stop the denying lesbians do die
with the aids of AMERICA
until you are dead and gone every thing you do
will be wrong
with the aids of AMERICA

How can we forget what it means to lay down
on a pissy homeless bed with cardboard hanging
over cold black heads lynching fear
Bein' a black woman in this country is to look
at the racist virus that's got you, us and me
like the black blood that dripped off southern trees

Little children will suffer from a never
to be gotten disease
with the aids of AMERICA
again the old red/white and blue stands true
for who's got who
with the aid of AMERICA
with the aids of AMERICA

Contrary to early predictions that prostitutes are "walking AIDS time bombs," there is scant evidence that sex workers are major transmitters of HIV infection. In fact, because of their rigorous safe sex practices, prostitutes can be excellent resources for AIDS education and prevention programs.

The author of the following piece is one of the nation's most prominent leaders in the movement for sex workers' rights. After working as a prostitute for nearly two decades, she is today director of the California Prostitutes Education Project and co-director of COYOTE. Both organizations advocate on behalf of prostitutes and are based in San Francisco.

Black Prostitutes and AIDS
Gloria Lockett

Prostitutes have been blamed for the heterosexual transmission of AIDS in this country since it was first recognized that the disease was sexually transmitted. Despite the large number of sexual contacts that prostitutes have, sex work does not appear to be a major risk factor for HIV infection. Most of the prostitutes who have become infected with the AIDS virus have either been intravenous drug users or lovers of IV drug users.

Prostitutes have been practicing safe sex with their clients for several years and have developed ways of eroticizing the use of condoms. As a former prostitute, I know we can be excellent AIDS prevention educators and vital resources to the black community as it struggles with the AIDS epidemic.

There have been a number of studies to determine the prevalence of HIV infection among prostitutes in this country. The studies have found that the rate of infection among prostitutes varies greatly from city to city in direct proportion to the rate of infection among IV drug users in the respective locale. The rate of infection also varies according to the category of prostitutes evaluated (i.e., street prostitutes, escort service workers, brothel workers) and according to the specific site of the study (i.e., jail, methadone maintenance program, medical clinic, brothel). In all instances, there is a direct correlation between prostitutes with HIV and the prevalence of IV drug use.

The rate of infection ranges from nearly nonexistent among prostitutes in Las Vegas to about fifty percent in New Jersey, according to the Centers for Disease Control in Atlanta.

The results of these studies and others suggest that HIV infection among prostitutes is virtually always related to a personal history of IV drug use or sexual involvement with a partner who uses IV drugs. In a San Francisco study, only one prostitute who tested positive was not an IV drug user.

One common misconception about prostitutes is that they all work on the street. In truth, about ten prostitutes work off the street (in massage parlors, bars, brothels and escort services) for every prostitute who pounds the pavement. People who work as prostitutes come from all racial, ethnic and class backgrounds and have all levels of education and work experience. The impetus for beginning work as a prostitute is virtually always money—money to get out of debt, money to pay medical bills, money for college tuition. A second common trigger is a history of childhood sexual abuse. Nearly fifty percent of adult female prostitutes were victims of childhood sexual abuse compared to about twenty-eight percent in the general female population. Among juvenile prostitutes, the prevalence of sexual abuse, especially incest, hovers at around eighty percent. Many of the juvenile prostitutes are runaways who left "the comfort of their homes" because of ongoing sexual assault.

COYOTE has estimated that about one percent of American women have worked as prostitutes at one point in their lives, with the average stay in the occupation being four years. COYOTE reports that over a sixty-five- to seventy-year life span, some ten percent of women have worked as prostitutes. However, the group reports that up to twenty percent of black women have turned to prostitution to pay the bills—about double the rate of the general population.

Black women are disproportionately represented among street prostitutes and consequently at greater risk for arrest. The job discrimination that plagues black women in legitimate employment also operates in the sex industry. For instance, escort services, massage parlors and brothels tend to hire mostly white women, although some black women are hired to offer customers "variety."

Because of the economic realities facing black men and women in this society, many blacks know women who have worked as prostitutes and are therefore less likely to carry cultural stereotypes about prostitutes as bad, immoral, dirty or diseased. They are able to empathize with the black female sex worker and distinguish sex on the job from sex in the context of relationships.

Because black prostitutes have often had more money than their neighbors and have frequently been benefactors to other black people, they have earned the respect of their communities. Admittedly, the respect is often tinged with religious disapproval, or lurid fascination.

Although their knowledge is kept from the public, stigmatized, and even punished, prostitutes are nonetheless experts on sexual matters. We believe that if more prostitutes were utilized as AIDS prevention educators in the black community they could convey information about safe sex that people would really take to heart and begin to practice.

For instance, prostitutes know that for sex to be safe, it must prevent the direct contact between one person's mucous membranes and the other's bodily fluids, particularly semen, blood and vaginal secretions. Latex condoms have been found to effectively block the transmission of the AIDS virus, provided they do not break. Studies have also found that the spermicide nonoxynol-9 kills the AIDS virus in the laboratory. Thus latex condoms fortified with nonoxynol-9 have proven to be wise safe sex choices.

COYOTE recommends that latex condoms be used for all fellatio (oral sex), vaginal and anal intercourse. For fellatio, it is best to use a plain, unlubricated condom because the lubricated ones, as well as those coated with nonoxynol-9, often taste extremely bitter. The spermicide can also sometimes leave the mouth numb. For vaginal and anal intercourse, COYOTE recommends nonoxynol-9-prepped condoms with an extra dab of spermicidal jelly or foam as a lubricant. For those who are sensitive to nonoxynol-9, "double-bagging," or the use of two plain condoms with a touch of nonoxynol-9 spermicide between them, is recommended. The friction of the two condoms rubbing against each other increases the pleasure of the man wearing them. This added erotic sensation should help to reduce the resistance to the idea of double-bagging.

For many black women, the issue is how to get their black male partners to wear condoms. Many prostitutes have had success with Blackies, which are made of black latex, and with Rough Riders, made of textured latex to increase the friction. They have also learned to make the condom part of the erotic experience. An old prostitute's trick is to put the condom on her partner with her mouth—without him realizing it. It is not very difficult to do, and can easily be practiced on a banana, zucchini, dildo, or even one's own fingers. The trick is to get the condom facing the right way in your mouth so that it can be rolled down over the penis. You can use your fingers to help it along, but it is the oral cavity that makes it erotic, especially if accompanied by sounds of pleasure. The object is to make the experience pleasurable so that the man does not object.

AIDS is not going to go away and, unfortunately, the black community will suffer many deaths before this epidemic is over. Black prostitutes should not be made scapegoats for the transmission of this disease. They have been practicing safe sex with their clients for years and are struggling, like other women, to enforce safe sex with their lovers. The black community has much to gain by engaging the help of black prostitutes in the battle against AIDS. The risk is too great to exclude them from this struggle.

. . .

The author thanks COYOTE co-director Priscilla Alexander for her contributions to this piece.

In assessing black women's health, it is important not to overlook black women who are serving time in correctional facilities. Far from being hardened or heinous criminals, most of these women are incarcerated because of relatively minor crimes committed to make ends meet, such as check forgery or petty theft, reports the National Institute of Justice.

Because of racism in the criminal justice system, black women are likely to be sentenced more severely for similar crimes than white women. Black females represent 1,251, or forty-three percent, of the 2,907 women in our nation's federal prisons, according to the NIJ, an alarming number, given that blacks comprise twelve percent of the nation's total population.

In the following piece, the author looks at the health status of black women inmates and offers support for a segment of the black community that is too often ignored or forgotten.

Bar None: The Health of Incarcerated Black Women
Sean Reynolds

In July 1987 I began working as a health educator for women in jail. Although I had previously worked as a volunteer AIDS outreach worker with various community organizations in San Francisco (most of them gay and/or lesbian), I was particularly interested in improving the health of people of color, especially black women. My job in the city jails provides me with an opportunity to do this, though I had no idea what kind of lessons I would learn when I first started the job three years ago.

I tried to prepare myself for working in the jail by recalling some past experiences. I had been to jail myself in the late sixties for engaging in civil rights and anti-war demonstrations, so I presumed to know what being behind bars would be like. I had also visited friends in the County Jail in Chicago (then known as the Bridewell) and, again, assumed that I would be met by similar people—relatively savvy and sophisticated, just down on their luck. Victims of the system. People caught in the trap. Unwilling accomplices to uncontrollable forces which many of us, because of our privilege and/or consciousness, had managed to avoid.

The first day on the job all of my attitudes, opinions and beliefs were challenged. I knew that people of color were disproportionately represented in jails all over the country; however, I was still surprised to find that in San Francisco, where black people comprise less than fifteen percent of the total population, people of color comprise eighty-five percent of the inmates. Upon entering the jail dayroom (the area where most of the women spend most of their time), I felt as though I were in a fun house hall of mirrors, seeing my own distorted reflection staring back at me from everywhere I turned. That day I counted sixty-two women, four of whom were white, three Hispanic. The rest were black like me. Most were in a state of both physical and emotional disrepair. Some appeared to be catatonic and one woman shuffled back and forth, logging several miles going no place in no big hurry.

Although basic consciousness-raising had not been defined as part of my job description, it was clear from the jump that issues such as racism, domestic violence, sexuality, class, feminism, neglect, disenfranchisement and most of all *self-esteem* would have to become an integral part of my health education efforts with the inmates. I realized immediately that for me to do my job effectively, I would have to rethink my approach and concentrate primarily on attempting to change many of the behavior patterns prevalent among incarcerated black women.

With this plan in mind, I began to evaluate the services for incarcerated black women and how they are utilized. I noted that inmates receive relatively good health care while in the San Francisco County Jail system. There are doctors, nurses and a dentist in the facility who provide care. From what I've seen, there are not that many differences between the health status of black women in jail and that of black women in the general population. In fact, unlike the thousands of black women who do not have adequate access to health care, incarcerated black women can take advantage of jail health services.

Unfortunately, however, these services are basically stop-gap measures. Jail medicine is not geared towards prevention, but rather is designed primarily to remedy the immediate health problems of inmates. For example, the consumption of the typical jail diet, combined with many hours of inactivity, causes many inmates to suffer from digestive and eliminatory problems, which are then treated by jail medical staff.

For pregnant black women who are incarcerated, the period in jail is frequently the only time they receive prenatal care. Black women who are arrested while under the influence of alcohol or other narcotics are detoxed and closely monitored while in custody. Though involuntary, the experience may be their first step toward recovery from substance abuse. Inmates who were on methodone maintenance programs before they were arrested can continue receiving the drug while behind bars. Epilepsy and other seizure-causing illnesses are routinely treated. AZT (which stems the progression of AIDS in some patients) is often provided free of charge to inmates who elect to take it.

In sum, jail doctors become the primary physicians for many black women who serve time. When they are released from custody, the emergency room at a nearby hospital then becomes the primary health care provider. This is a practice that is common in the black community because of the high cost of routine and regular medical care.

There are some physical, mental and social problems that are more pronounced among black women in custody. I have observed more drug and alcohol dependency, unemployment, illiteracy, homelessness and isolation among incarcerated black women than in the general population. After working with more than three thousand incarcerated black women, it is clear to me that most suffer from a debilitating inner sense of defeat. When I put all the bravado and toughness of jailed black women aside, I find that the majority of them have poor self-esteem and a heartbreaking lack of purpose in life. This sense of hopelessness is compounded by the racism and sexism in society and often leads incarcerated black women to a vicious cycle of substance abuse, criminal behavior, jail time and compromised health. It is a pattern I've seen in my incarcerated sisters more times than I care to count.

Especially troubling these days is the high rate of sexually transmitted disease among incarcerated black women. Dr. German Maisonette, a physician at Vacaville State Prison in Vacaville, California, has done extensive research on venereal disease in the black community. He reports that AIDS, syphilis, gonorrhea and chlamydia are skyrocketing among black female inmates. Many of the women contract these diseases as a result of swapping sex for drugs, particularly crack cocaine.

Although the San Francisco Jail Medical Services Department has a comprehensive AIDS education program, many inmates still ask if they can contract AIDS through kissing or sharing cigarettes. This problem exists because many of the women are unable to read or retain the health information that are provided for them. Consequently, they fall prey to the rumors and misinformation that are circulated among their peers. Improved literacy programs would empower incarcerated black women and help them better understand the dangerous connections between substance abuse and sexually transmitted disease.

Despite the many obstacles they face, there are black women with criminal histories who manage to rise up and create healthy and productive lives. The following interview highlights one such woman.

Stephanie Henderson is a black, thirty-six-year-old native San Franciscan who has been arrested more than ten times for possession and sale of heroin. She has also served time for prostitution. The mother of two children, ages nineteen and six, Stephanie told me she began using drugs and alcohol in her teens to mask her feelings about her parents' divorce and an abortion she had undergone. She said that her substance abuse provided an escape mechanism that covered up her sense of abandonment and loss and helped her to feel better about herself.

After being arrested and released numerous times for drug-related offenses, Stephanie was finally sentenced to six months in jail for prostitution. After serving her time, she got caught up in the "mix" (street life) again.

She recalls: "It was two weeks to the day that I was re-arrested for the same fucking charge—prostitution. I felt humiliated and ashamed and that's when I actually started thinking about my life. I had my daughter and I just wanted more. When I first started going to jail, my family would tell my daughter that I was in the hospital. Since I've been clean and sober I've talked with my children about my 'hospital' stays and now they know the truth."

It took eight years from her last incarceration for Stephanie to straighten out her life. She had slips and backslides but she kept her resolve to stay clean and out of jail. She credits the support she received from Narcotics Anonymous with helping her get back on her feet. Today she provides AIDS outreach to youths as a Juvenile Field Supervisor for the California Prostitutes Education Project. She is also a published poet who is frequently invited to read at black and feminist gatherings.

"You see, I've always had a lot of ego and I was determined to make a decent way for me and my kids, and somehow we made it," Stephanie says. "It wasn't easy, but being a junkie wasn't easy either. I'm a big believer in change and moving in more positive directions by doing one thing different at a time. I started with the alcohol, then the drugs, then the crime."

Stephanie Henderson is just one example of a black woman with crime in her past, who has reclaimed her health, her sense of purpose and her self-esteem. As I walk through jail each day and see the multitudes of black women behind bars, I am mindful of Stephanie's uplifting words:

"Love yourself. Believe that you are worth something and know that you've got to do most of the work. The government is not going to do it for you. Welfare is as big a trap as drugs. Both keep you powerless and out of control. But first and foremost, you've got to love yourself and believe that you have a right to live. That's the only way to stop yourself from self-destructing."

Without the license to give breath to all our dimensions, it is impossible for black women to achieve true health. For black lesbians, anti-gay sentiments compound the racism and sexism that circumscribe all black female lives. In the following piece, two black lesbian writers discuss the debilitating toll homophobia takes on black gays. Furthermore, they challenge blacks to address and relinquish *the oppressive religious traditions that have historically made homosexuality taboo in our community.*

Jewelle L. Gomez is author of several volumes of feminist prose and poetry. Barbara Smith is co-founder and publisher of Kitchen Table: Women of Color Press. Like their thousands of black lesbian foremothers, the authors have uplifted the black community through their dedicated art and politics.

Taking the Home Out of Homophobia: Black Lesbian Health

Jewelle L. Gomez and Barbara Smith

Barbara: One of the things we've been asked to talk about is how homophobia affects Black women's mental health. I think that in addition to affecting lesbians' emotional health, homophobia also affects the mental health of heterosexual people. In other words, being homophobic is not a healthy state for people to be in.

Jewelle: I'd like to hear more about that.

Barbara: Well, it's just like being a racist. I don't think that most Blacks or other people of color would vouch for the mental health of somebody who is a rabid and snarling racist. Because that's like dismissing a part of the human family. Particularly within the African-American community, when we are so embattled, it's just baloney to dismiss or say that a certain segment is expendable because of their sexual orientation. Anyone who would do that hasn't grown up, they're just not mature.

Jewelle: I think it's even more dangerous for people of color to embrace homophobia than it is for whites to embrace racism, simply because we're embattled psychologically and economically as an ethnic group. We leave ourselves in a very weakened position if we allow the system to pit us against each other. I also think it renders Black people politically smug. That's the thing about homophobia, racism, anti-Semitism, any of the "isms"—once you embrace those you tend to become smug.

And once you take a position of smugness you lose your fighting edge. I think Afro-Americans who've taken the position of "we are the major victim" in this society and nobody else has suffered like we've suffered, lose their edge. They don't have the perspective that will allow us to fight through all the issues.

Barbara: Right. From the time we get here, we are steeped in the knowledge that we are the victims of a really bigoted and racist society. But we also have to acknowledge that there are ways that we can be oppressive to other groups whose identities we don't share. So I think that one of the challenges we face in trying to raise the issue of lesbian and gay identity within the Black community is to try to get our people to understand that they can indeed oppress someone after having spent a life of being oppressed. That's a very hard transition to make, but it's one we have to make if we want our whole community to be liberated.

Jewelle: At this point, it seems almost impossible because the issue of sexism has become such a major stumbling block for the Black community. I think we saw the beginning of it in the 1970s with Ntozake Shange's play, *For Colored Girls Who Have Considered Suicide/ When the Rainbow Is Enuf*. The play really prompted Black women to embrace the idea of independent thinking; to begin looking to each other for sustenance and to start appreciating and celebrating each other in ways that we've always done naturally. I think that the Black male community was so horrified to discover that they were not at the center of Black women's thoughts, that they could only perceive the play as a negative attack upon them. I think that for the first time, that play made the Black community look at its sexism. And many people rejected Ntozake Shange and things having to do with feminism in a very cruel way. So years later, when we got the Central Park incident with the white woman being beaten and raped by a group of young Black males, all people could talk about was the role racism played in the attack.

Barbara: I happened to be at a writers retreat in April 1989 when that incident occurred. It was a radicalized retreat run by a group of old lefties, so everybody there had to have a certain level of political consciousness. There was one woman there who had been involved in progressive politics for decades and she and I were discussing the Central Park rape. Her sole concern was whether these young Black and Latino men were going to get a fair trial. I couldn't believe what I was hearing. And I thought, this is why a Black feminist analysis is so important. It's important because my concern was that there was a woman lying up in the hospital almost dead. A woman who if she ever recovers physically, is likely to be profoundly psychologically damaged for the rest of her life. Black feminism is important because we can look at these issues from a holistic and principled perspective as opposed to a reductive one.

There was an article in the *Village Voice* in which some Black women were asked what they thought about the Central Park rape and most of them came down very hard on sexual violence and sexism in the Black community. They indeed cited sexism as a cause of the rape. This incident is not a mysterious fluke. It is part and parcel of what African-American women face on the streets and in their homes every day. There was a Black woman standing in a supermarket line right here in New York City and they were talking about the rape. There was a Black man behind her and he was apparently wondering why they had to beat the white woman, why they had to do her like that. And then he said, "Why didn't they just rape her?" As if that would have been okay. So you see, we have a lot to contend with.

Jewelle: I think that the sexism continues to go unacknowledged and even praised as part of the Black community's survival technique. The subsequent acceptance of homophobia that falls naturally with that kind of thinking will be the thing that cripples the Black community. During the civil rights movement, it was a single focus on desegregation that gave us an impetus to move and hold onto our vision. But it is that same single focus that has left us with these half-assed solutions to our problems today. I mean a movement toward the middle-class is not a solution to the problems in the Black community. And I think it's just pathetic that the narrowness of vision in the Afro-American community has left us with that. Therefore, it's not surprising that homophobia is part of the fall-out. Nor should people be surprised about the anti-Semitism in the Black community. It's just one more of the "isms" that xenophobic oppressed groups justify themselves in taking on simply because they are oppressed groups.

Barbara: Right.

Jewelle: It's been said that people to whom evil has been done, will do evil in return.

Barbara: Who said that?

Jewelle: W.H. Auden. So I don't think we should be surprised about homophobia. It sneaks up in a very subtle and destructive way, even though homosexuality has always been an intrinsic part of the Black community.

Barbara: Absolutely.

Jewelle: When I was growing up, everyone always knew who was gay. When the guys came to my father's bar, I knew which ones were gay, it was clear as day. For instance, there was Miss Kay who was a big queen and Maurice. These were people that everybody knew. They came and went in my father's bar just like everybody else. This was a so-called lower-class community—the working poor in Boston. It was a community in which people did not talk about who was gay, but I knew who the lesbians were. It was always unspoken and I think that there's something about leaving it unspoken that leaves us unprepared.

Barbara: That's the breakpoint for this part of the twentieth century as far as I'm concerned. There've been lesbian and gay men, Black ones, as long as there've been African people. So that's not even a question. You know how they say that the human race was supposed to have been started by a Black woman. Well, since she had so many children, some of them were undoubtedly queer. (Laughter.) Writer Ann Allen Shockley has a wonderful line about that which I use often. "Play it, but don't say it." That's the sentiment that capsulizes the general stance of the Black community on sexual identity and orientation. If you're a lesbian, you can have as many women as you want. If you're a gay man, you can have all the men you want. But just don't say anything about it or make it political. The difference today is that the lesbian and gay movement prides itself on being out, verbalizing one's identity and organizing around our oppression. With the advent of this movement, the African-American community has really been confronted with some stuff that they've never had to deal with before.

I grew up in Cleveland in a community very similiar to the one you described. Today the issue is not whether gay people have been here since forever. It's that we are telling our community that it has to deal with us differently than before. That's what contemporary Black gay and lesbian activists are doing.

Jewelle: I was thinking, as you were saying that, that if one embraces the principles of liberation, gay liberation and feminism, then you have to assault the sexual stereotype that young Black girls have been forced to live out in the African-American community. The stereotype that mandates that you develop into the well-groomed girl who pursues a profession and a husband.

Barbara: High achiever.

Jewelle: Or the snappy baby machine. You tend to go one way or the other. You're either fast or you're well-groomed. I think that for so many young Black women, the idea of finding their place in society has been defined by having a man or a baby. So if you begin to espouse a proud lesbian growth, you find yourself going against the grain. That makes embracing your lesbianism doubly frightening, because you then have to discard the mythology that's been developed around what it means to be a young Black woman.

Barbara: And that you gotta have a man. The urgency of which probably can't even be conveyed on the printed page. (Laughter.) I was just going to talk about when I was younger and meeting people who would want to know about me. Not so much about my sexual orientation, because they weren't even dealing with the fact that somebody could be a lesbian. But I always noticed they were more surprised to find out I didn't have children than that I wasn't married. Marriage was not the operative thing. It was like, "Why don't you have any children?" That really made them curious.

Jewelle: Right. They had no understanding at all that you could reach a certain age and not have any children.

Barbara: And not having children doesn't mean we're selfish. It means we're self-referenced. Many Black lesbians and gay men have children. Those of us who don't may not have had the opportunity. Or we may have made the conscious choice not to have children.

One of the things about being a Black lesbian is that we're very conscious. At least those of us who are politicized about what we will and will not have in our lives. Coming out is such a conscious choice that the process manifests itself in other areas of our lives.

Jewelle: Yes, it's healthy. Having grown up with a lot of Black women who had children at an early age, I've noticed a contradictory element in that that's the way many of them come into their own. I have younger cousins who have two, three, four children and are not married and will probably never be married. It seems that the moment they have the baby is when they come into their own and their identity after that becomes the "long-suffering Black mother." I think it recreates a cycle of victimization because a lot of these young women carry the burden of being on a road that wasn't really a conscious choice. On the other hand, when I look at Black lesbian mothers, I see that yes, many of them are struggling with their children. But there is also a sense of real choice because they've made a conscious decision to be out and have children. They are not long-suffering victims. They are not women who have been abandoned by their men. They are lesbian mothers who have made a place in the world that is not a victim's place. Now that doesn't necessarily mean that things are any easier or simpler for them. But there is a psychological difference because most Black lesbian mothers have made a choice and have a community they can look to for support.

Barbara: In talking about choice, another thing we've been asked to address is why do people become lesbians, or why did we become lesbians, or why do we think there is such a thing as lesbianism?

Jewelle: It was all those vegetables. Eating too much spinach. (Laughter.)

Barbara: Well, I was a notorious non-vegetable eater all my life. Maybe it was the candy bars in my case. Seriously, I don't know why people are lesbians. All I want to say is that I think the reason women become lesbians is because they are deeply attracted—sexually—to other women. To me, that's the bottom line. There was a notion during the early women's movement, in which I was involved, that you could choose to be a lesbian. But I think the important point is whether you choose to be out, or to act on your lesbian feelings. Those of us who were coming out before there was a women's or lesbian and gay movement, understand this a little bit better. I teach students who are in their early twenties and they really perceive their coming out as say, a political choice because they are doing it in such a supportive context. Those of us who were coming out just before Stonewall[1] knew that we had feelings, passion and lust for other women. We didn't necessarily have a place for our feelings that felt safe. But we knew intuitively—not because we read it a book somewhere—that gay was good. Today people have women's studies courses, out lesbian teachers, all kinds of stuff that we didn't have. So they can indeed perceive their coming out as following in the footsteps of a role model.

Jewelle: I grew up in a bar community and I knew I was a lesbian when I was quite young. But the only available role models weren't anything like who I thought I was going to be when I grew up. I knew I wasn't going to be sitting up in a bar all day, or hustling on the streets. So what was I going to be? There were no other role models.

Barbara: That was the complete terror. Talking about how being a lesbian and homophobia affect one's mental health—I lived my adolescence and young adulthood in terror. I knew I was a lesbian, too. But likewise, I saw no way to act on it and stay on the path. This was a path that I had not necessarily chosen for myself, but that my family had worked very hard to give me the option of choosing. I'd think, How the hell can I excel in school, go to college, graduate school—and then become low-life by sleeping with women? I mean it just didn't jibe. Some people think that when I came out during the women's movement it was an easy thing. But I'd just like to say right here for the record, that from puberty on, I had screaming nightmares because I was having dreams of being sexual with women. I would wake up and my grandmother would be standing looking over me and I thought she knew what I was dreaming. She knew that I was disturbed about something, even though I never revealed to her what it was. So, I was really terrified.

I think that conscious lesbianism lived in the context of community is a positive thing. It can be a really affirming choice for women. The connection to sexism is deep, though. Homophobia is a logical extension of sexual oppression because sexual oppression is about roles—one gender does this, the other does that. One's on top, the other is on the bottom.

Jewelle: I think the interconnection of racism and sexism has been so profound that we don't even know how the homophobia is going to be difficult for us as Black women. I've just recently begun to separate them out. I didn't really come out through the women's movement. For me, my sexuality didn't have a political context until later. I always had a sexual identity that I tried to sift out, but I was most concerned about how I was going to fit it in with being a Black Catholic, which was very difficult. Once I realized that one of them had to go—sexuality or Catholicism—it took me about five or ten minutes to drop Catholicism. (Laughter.) Then I focused on racism, to the exclusion of homophobia and everything else. That left me unprepared. I had a woman lover very early. Then I slept with men until my mid-twenties. They were kind of like the entertainment until I found another girlfriend and got my bearings. I didn't have the political context to deal with what it meant to want to sleep with both men and women. I skipped past the feminism until much later. So homophobia came as a total shock to me because I had never experienced it. Nobody seemed to be homophobic in my community, because no one ever talked about it. I hadn't experienced it because I wasn't out. I didn't know that I wasn't out. But I wasn't.

Barbara: Because you weren't out, you weren't really experiencing homophobia consciously.

Jewelle: Right. I thought it was an aberration. I didn't quite understand what it meant. It reminded me of the first time I heard about child abuse. That happened when I was a teenager and I thought child abuse could only have happened once or twice in the history of the world because it was so appalling to me and beyond my comprehension. And of course as I read more and realized it was . . .

Barbara: Pandemic.

Jewelle: Yes. I had to withdraw for a little bit to figure it out. It seemed as if someone had just stabbed me in my heart. I think I felt the same way when I understood there was such a thing as homophobia. A couple of years ago, I had an eye-opening experience while looking for an apartment in Jersey City. Now, I had experienced racism in Manhattan. In fact, someone had told me that when I called for an apartment not to reveal my last name because Manhattan landlords would think I was Puerto Rican.

Barbara: This is America.

Jewelle: So I'd just say that my name was Jewelle and show up at the apartment. This was in the early 1970s and it seemed that back then, being Black was a little bit more acceptable than being Puerto Rican, so they would rent to me. And also because I worked for television at that time, the landlords somehow took that to mean that I was okay, that I was better than just the average "Joe Blackperson" off the streets.

But looking for an apartment in Jersey City with my then lover, who was Black, was very different. Frequently, we'd be dealing with people who had two-family homes and were looking to rent one of the units. I remember we called this one place, and I was in stark terror. In my mind, I was thinking about a white couple looking at us and seeing two Black people that they were going to potentially bring into their home. It terrified me because I could see them insulting us or even possibly slamming the door in our face. And then just as we were about to get out of the car, it occurred to me that this white couple would also look at us and see two lesbians. (Laughter.) I was literally shaking. I had been so focused on them seeing two Black women, that it hadn't occurred to me that they would also see two lesbians. They'd see the quintessential butch-femme couple, both of us going into our forties.

Barbara: Yes. Well beyond the college roommate stage.

Jewelle: It terrified me. But as it turns out, they would have rented to us if we had decided to take the place, which we didn't. But the anxiety I suffered during those minutes before we rang the doorbell was devastating and definitely scarred me internally.

Barbara: Of course. It's deep. This is one of the permutations of how homophobia and heterosexism overshadow our lives. One of the things that I'm very happy about now is that I live in Albany, New York. And they did allow me to buy a house there. I don't know how many Chase Manhattans I would have had to rob down here in New York City in order to get enough money to buy a house. (Laughter.) My house is in the heart of Albany's Black community. And one of the really nice things about it is that I know that nobody can put me out of my house because of what I have on my walls, who I bring in there, or whatever. That's very refreshing. Of course, it's the first time I've ever felt that way. What I'd always done before, because of homophobia and racism, was to be pretty low-key wherever I lived. I just felt that around my house, I had to try to be very cautious, even though I'm known to be a very out lesbian, both politically and in print. I didn't want anybody following me into my house who thought that bulldaggers shouldn't be allowed to live.

Jewelle: I know. When the plumber is coming to my Brooklyn apartment to fix something, all of my lesbian things get put away.

Barbara: Because he knows where you live and may even have a key to the apartment.

Jewelle: Yes. I have no desire to wake up and discover the plumber and his helper standing over me.

Barbara: That's right. That's real. This gets into an area that is very important for all people, especially Black people in this country to understand. And that is that we pay a heavy toll for being who we are and living with integrity. Being out means you are doing what your grandmother told you to do, which is not to lie. Black lesbians and gays who are out are not lying. But we pay high prices for our integrity. People really need to understand that there is entrenched violence against lesbians and gay men that is much like and parallel to the racial violence that has characterized Black people's lives since we've been in this country. When we then say that we are concerned about fighting homophobia, and heterosexism, and changing attitudes, we're not talking about people being pleasant to us. We're talking about ensuring that the plumber and his assistant aren't standing over our beds with their damn wrenches or knives. Everyone should have safety and freedom of choice. We have the right not to be intimidated in our homes or on the streets because we're Black, or on welfare, or gay.

Jewelle: Right. My lover and I went camping in New Mexico recently. One day we camped on the Rio Grande in a fairly isolated area. We put up our tent and went away for while. When we returned, there were these guys fishing nearby and it made us really nervous. In fact, we had a long, serious discussion about our mutual terror of being a lesbian couple in an isolated area with these men nearby. I was especially conscious of us being an interracial couple and how much that might enrage some people.

Barbara: Oh yes, absolutely. Speaking from experience, I think it's easier for two Black women who are lovers to be together publicly than it is for a mixed couple. To me, that's a dead give-away because this is such a completely segregated society. Whenever I had a lover of a different race, I felt that it was like having a sign or a billboard over my head that said—"These are dykes. Right here." Because you don't usually see people of different races together in this country, it was almost by definition telling the world that we were lesbians. I think the same is true for interracial gay male couples. So, you see, the terror you were feeling was based on fact. Just recently a lesbian was murdered while she and her lover were on the Appalachian trail in Pennsylvania. This is what colors and affects our lives in addition to Howard Beach and Bernhard Goetz.[2]

Jewelle: The guy who murdered the lesbian on the Appalachian trail claimed his defense was that he had been enraged by seeing their blatant lesbianism. He believed he had a right to shoot them because he had been disturbed by their behavior.

Barbara: What is that defense called? The homophobic panic?

Jewelle: To me, it's equivalent to the Twinkie defense.[3]

Barbara: Yes. There's a term of defense they try to trot out that suggests that the mere existence of gay people is so enraging to some that they are then justified in committing homicide.

Jewelle: It's sort of like saying that because you are scared of the color black you are justified in running over Black people in Howard Beach.

Barbara: Right. We as a race of people would generally find that kind of thinking ludicrous. Yet there are Black people who would say that those murdered lesbians got what they deserved. I think that some Black men abhor Black lesbians because we are, by definition, women they are never going to control. I think something snaps in their psyche when they realize that Black lesbians are saying, "No way. I'm with women and that's that."

Jewelle: I think it's a psychological thing. Black women are perceived as property and they are the means by which Black men define themselves. It's another way they are like white men. They use female flesh to define themselves. They try to consume us to prove themselves as men because they're afraid to look inside of themselves. The final note about our terror in New Mexico was that it was both a positive and negative thing. It was positive because we refused to give up ground. We decided to stay where we were because we liked the spot. Of course, it meant that I slept with a large rock in my hands and she with her knife open. But I'll tell you, I slept very well and she did too.

Barbara: I'm glad you said that about not giving up ground because as out Black lesbians we have to live and do live with an incredible amount of courage. I've always felt that if anybody tried to physically violate me, that I would do my best to kill them. That's just fact. I'm taller than average. I'm as tall as most men and I don't slouch. When they're looking for people to harass, I feel like they skip me. (Laughs.)

Jewelle: I've frequently felt that way too because I'm big. But I think that one of the things that's happening now with the homophobic backlash is that our size and presence enrage them too.

Barbara: That's why self-defense is so important. As people of color, as lesbians and gay men, we live with potential or actual danger.

Back to the point about courage, I attended a conference several years ago for women organizing around poverty and economic issues in the deep South. The Black women who came to the conference were wonderful and they treated me gloriously. As usual, I was out as a lesbian at this conference. Homophobia was the one issue they had not considered as a barrier to women's leadership. Funny thing, they skipped that. (Laughter.) But there was a little quorum of white and Black lesbians and we raised the issue. We got up on the stage and read a statement about homophobia. Then we invited other lesbians and people in solidarity with us to stand up. Almost everybody in the room stood up. Later we were talking about the incident in our small groups and a woman said something I'll never forget. She said that what we'd done had taken a lot of courage. And I have never forgotten those words because they came from a woman who was in a position to know the meaning of courage. She knew what it meant because she had been hounded by white bigots all her life. For her to recognize our being out as courage meant a lot to me.

Jewelle: That's a very important point. I think that for those of us in Manhattan, Brooklyn, Albany, we have a certain leeway in being out. We have a diverse women's community that supports us in our efforts to be honest about being lesbians. I find it sad that there is a larger proportion of Black lesbians in small, rural communities who won't and can't come out because they don't have this suppport. I think they suffer an isolation and even a kind of perversion of their own desires. That's one of the things that Ann Allen Shockley writes about so well—the Black lesbian who is isolated and psychically destroyed because she doesn't have a positive reflection of herself. These are the stories that aren't often told. Such Black lesbians don't get many opportunities to share what is going on for them.

Barbara: Yes. Class is a factor, too.

Jewelle: Certainly. Your whole view about what it means to be lesbian is colored by whether you were able to get an education—to read different things about the experience.

Barbara: Another point I want to make is that the people who are not out and have the privilege of good education and jobs need to be more accountable. It really bothers me that there are closeted people who are perceived as leaders within the Black community. This is something I find very annoying, because I think they are skating. If they were out on the job or in the community, they would automatically bring together issues that have been counterposed to each other for too long.

Jewelle: Yes. They are skating on our efforts and devotion. It happens all the time. Another thing we need to talk about is religion in the Black community and how it has been such a sustainer in our lives. I find it despicable and a desecration that our spiritual beliefs are perverted and used against Black gay people. Anyone who understands what the spirit of Christianity is supposed to be would never use it against gays.

Barbara: Love thy neighbor as thyself.

Jewelle: Right. Christianity does not say pick and choose which neighbors you're going to love. And any of those biblical quotes that are used against Black gays need to be looked at in the context that that self-same Bible has been used to depict Blacks as inhuman. Racists use Christianity against Black people and then Black people turn around and use Christianity against gays. It doesn't make any sense to me.

Barbara: We also need to discuss some of the young Black men who are so prominent today in the Hollywood movie and television industry. People like Arsenio Hall, Eddie Murphy, etc. I think they are homophobic to their hearts.

Jewelle: And sexist. I think it's telling that Spike Lee, the most popular Black filmmaker in the country today, includes the rape of a Black woman in his films. Sexism is so pervasive in our community that we don't even think of this as awful. Imagine what it feels like to sit in a movie theater watching his film *School Daze* in which a Black woman is raped. The so-called Black brothers in the movie are saying, "Yeah, bone her. Bone her." And the Black women in the audience are giggling.

Barbara: They were probably giggling because they knew they had to go back home with those kinds of guys. This gets back to the Central Park rape that obsessed and terrorized me so much. The question I was raising at that time is: Do men understand that they can kill a woman by raping her? Do they understand that rape is torture and terror for us?

Jewelle: I think that as Black lesbians, in some ways, we are very fortunate. This is because we are in a community that supports us in growing past racism, sexism and homophobia. But as you've said, our heterosexual sisters have to go home with these guys.

Barbara: We have to acknowledge that there are heterosexual Black females who are not putting up with that stuff. There are definitely Black heterosexual feminists who are saying—"No way. I'm not taking that kind of abuse, negation or suppression." And as more Black women become feminists, the men are going to have to change. My impression is that there used to be more cooperation between Black men and Black women. Back when lynching was a daily American pastime and the crazed white man was our common enemy, we were not as inclined to lash out against each other as we are today.

For instance, there was an article recently in *Publishers Weekly* about Black writers. The thrust of the piece was that Black male writers are suffering because Black women writers are getting lots of attention. This kind of thinking is based on the scarcity model that says there is only so much approval for Black writers within the mainstream white publishing industry. And that may be true. But there should be infinite approval within a Black context. Everybody who wants to write should write so we can all keep moving on up a little higher.

Jewelle: Can you believe we've had this whole discussion without mentioning *The Color Purple?* To me, the criticism of the book and the film was very much like what happened to Ntozake Shange. People couldn't handle seeing Black women bond, even if it was only on celluloid. So it prompted unbelievable scenarios like grown men sitting at conferences debating whether Alice Walker should have been *allowed* to write *The Color Purple.*

Barbara: What does that say about where we are? And as I've said at exactly those kinds of discussions—if people think *The Color Purple* is an exaggeration of Black women's lives, they should go to any emergency room, battered women's shelter or rape crisis center in this country. If they did that, they would see that *The Color Purple* is mild, bland and minimal compared to what is actually happening to women and children in this society.

Jewelle: I'd like to close by saying that homophobia is particularly dangerous for Black lesbians because it is so insidious. There have always been acceptable places for gay Black men to retreat and escape from the danger, i.e. the "choir queen" or the Black gay man who embraces the white gay male community. But as Black gay women, we haven't been interested in removing ourselves from our families or communities because we understand the importance of that connection. The insidiousness of the homophobia lies in the fact that we've been forced to find ways to balance our contact with the community with our need to continue to grow as Black lesbians. We straddle the fence that says we cannot be the uplifters of the race and lesbians at the same time—that's what makes it so dangerous for our emotional health as Black lesbians. But you know, I think that our ability to see the need to keep the family intact is what is going to be our savior and help preserve the Black community. As lesbians, we have so much to teach the Black community about survival.

Barbara: I'm very glad that you said that about family. One of the myths that's put out about Black lesbians and gay men is that we go into the white gay community and forsake our racial roots. People say that to be lesbian or gay is to be somehow racially denatured. I have real problems with that because that's never been where I was coming from. And that's not the place that the Black lesbians and gays I love, respect and work with are coming from either. We are as Black as anybody ever thought about being. Just because we are committed to passionate and ongoing relationships with members of our own gender, does not mean that we are not Black. In fact, the cultural and political leadership of the Black community has always had a very high percentage of lesbian and gay men. Although closeted in many cases, Black lesbians and gays have been central in building our freedom.

Jewelle: I think the political code has always been that you don't bring people out who don't want to come out—you don't force anyone out of the closet. But I think that's changing.

Barbara: (Laughs.) I'm delighted, very delighted.

Jewelle: With the way the media works now it's almost impossible to stay closeted. And I don't think people who are out feel as morally obligated to protect the ones who stay in the closet.

Barbara: Especially now that there's AIDS. The ideology that you can just sit back and let a part of your community die off because of homophobia is untenable at this time. There won't be anybody here.

Jewelle: Yes. It's very important that all our voices be heard. Everyone asks why do we have to talk about homophobia? Why can't we be quiet about it? The fact that we have to talk about it means that a lot of people don't want to hear it. And as soon as there's something they don't want to hear, it's very important that we say it. I learned that as a Black person.

Barbara: I'd like to challenge all the non-lesbians to think about what they can do to improve the chances that we'll all be free and sisters.

Footnotes

1. In response to repeated police harassment, a group of gays rioted at the Stonewall Inn bar in New York in June 1969. The rebellion is heralded as the start of gay liberation.

2. In December 1984, Bernhard Goetz gunned down four Black youths on a Manhattan subway after alleging they had tried to rob him. In 1987, a gang of white New York teenagers attacked several Black men who had stopped in their Howard Beach neighborhood for pizza. One Black youth was killed by a car as he fled.

3. A defense used by San Francisco Supervisor Dan White in his 1979 trial for the slaying of the city's mayor and a politically powerful and openly gay city supervisor. White's attorney argued that his client's consumption of junk food contributed to his state of diminished capacity.

A Tribute to a Sister: Pat Parker, 1944–1989
Evelyn C. White

When I think of Pat Parker, I usually picture her reading from her poetry collection, *Jonestown and Other Madness.* I can hear her husky voice chanting: "Black folks do not, black folks do not, black folks do not commit suicide." I can see her, dark and majestic, vindicating the souls of those who perished in Guyana with her refrain.

Most people knew Parker as a dynamic and visionary lesbian poet who spoke the unspoken and loved the unloved issues and individuals of the black and gay communities. When Parker strode on stage in her colorful garb, with that mischievous glint in her eye, we knew she was going to rock the house with her passionate poetry and presence. In a poem about her friendship with a gay black man, Parker wrote: "We Be—Something Else." As always, she hit the nail right on the head.

Fewer people are aware of Parker's work as a health activist. From 1978 to 1987 she served as a board member and medical coordinator at the Oakland Feminist Women's Health Center. A strong advocate for the self-care movement, Parker believed that women should take an active role in their health. Under her direction, the agency offered a variety of women-centered services including family planning, pregnancy screening, alternative insemination, prenatal care, home births, abortions and general medical treatment. She believed that *all* women deserved competent, comprehensive and affordable health services. Through her work at the Center, she transformed her belief into a reality.

In early 1987, Parker left the Center to concentrate full-time on her writing. She was eager to work on her craft, to hone her already considerable talents. In a bitter twist of fate, Parker was diagnosed with breast cancer within the year. A year and a half later on June 17, 1989, she died with friends and family members by her side.

In October 1989, I went to Parker's home with her literary executor, Laura Brown, in search of a piece to include in this book. In a quiet, wood-paneled studio with book-filled shelves, I journeyed through volumes of Parker's prose and poetry. And though I felt loss, I also felt an enormous sense of appreciation for the gifts that Parker gave us. The sister did not labor in vain.

I chose the poem that follows because I believe it is important for us to see our heroines in all their dimensions. Parker was indeed a powerhouse, but she was also a vulnerable black woman. She shed tears and she suffered great pain.

In Parker's studio, there is a picture of Zora Neale Hurston with a caption that reads: "Ms. Parker—Would Zora Be Proud Of Your Work Today?" In her life and in her work, Pat Parker strove to lift up and inspire black women to grab every inch of life. I'm sure that Hurston is proud of her, and we are, too.

Massage (for Margaret)
Pat Parker

In the days following my mastectomy,
my body was covered in bandages—
mountains of tape
hid the space where
my breast had been piled so high.

My body was numb—
hard like my mother's body
in her casket.
And I mourned.
I mourned for the passion gone
and I numbed my mind.

No one had seen my body
except my lover and my surgeon.
I protected my friends with robes
and gym mates with towels.
Protected myself from looks of
horror, disgust or pity.
Let the numbness be still.

I brought my numb self to you
turned my body into bread
for your hands to knead and mold,
to stroke the tension
away-away-away—

And like fine bread I rose
my body feeling loose and
smooth and passionate
and I wanted to sing of my
re-wakening
wanted to kiss you
with gratitude.
Instead I said
thank you and went home.

FOUR: ROCKA MY SOUL

There is an enormous amount of grief and sorrow in the black community. Because of high infant mortality rates, high homicide rates and low life-expectancy rates for blacks, many black women have suffered premature loss. Medical and mental health experts report that unresolved grief can contribute to hypertension, stress, depression, anxiety and drug and alcohol abuse.

Realizing that it is healthy to release emotional pain, growing numbers of black women are turning to counselors, friends family members and the church to help them deal with their sorrows.

In the following piece, the author writes of her personal grieving process.

Speaking of Grief:
Today I Feel Real Low, I Hope You Understand
Bridgett M. Davis

I don't go to cemeteries. In a cemetery barely one mile from the family home lie my father, my eldest sister and my only brother. In another, a few miles away, lie my middle sister and her toddler son. I am twenty-nine years old and don't go to cemeteries.

I don't even want to pass by one, as I had to do every day, twice a day, when I was a newspaper reporter in Philadelphia. A tiny piece of me would die each time that I rode to and from work. Days and days of getting slowed by a funeral procession—little flags waving off car antennas and headlights glaring in the daylight. After two years of that agony, I escaped.

What led to my escape was the build-up of emotion that accumulated over that eight-year span from 1978 to 1986 when my family buried five of our loved ones. Five. During those years, I mourned and I cried and I suffered a lot. But I did so against my will. I never really took the time to grieve. Finally, the grief overtook me and I knew I had to stop everything and just get away.

I have slowly, slowly begun to heal. What I am now trying to do is make sense of that grieving process. I don't know that I can.

Loss is painful no matter what. But when the loss comes so fast and furious, and in succession as it has in my life, the pain reaches a piercing height, has a menacing spin to it. So little time exists for growing a protective crust over the open wounds caused by one death before another one happens. A deep survival instinct led me, I think, to grow numb after a while. Or as numb and unfeeling as I could be.

Every day of my life, I am reminded of either my sisters, my brother, my nephew or my father. Or all of them. Or some combination. That means a Motown song on the radio, a white car on the road, a familiar smirk on a stranger's face or a bowl of oatmeal at breakfast can force my thoughts backwards, force me to experience the hurt anew. It's as if I'm compelled to visit my pain periodically throughout the day, checking on it as you would a sleeping child through the night. Those daily digressions have worn on me over the years, robbing me of the luxury of resting my brain, of walking down a street with nothing on my mind. I can never think about nothing.

Sights, smells, sounds and even tastes bring them—and their deaths—back to me with relentless frequency. Lately, I'm haunted by young black men who remind me of my brother. Sometimes it's a hairstyle, a body build, a nose, a smile. Sometimes it's just knowing a stranger is probably the same age my brother was when he was murdered. They are everywhere, these men. On street corners, in subways, at construction sites, in the laughter of my brother's son, in the face of a man I fell in love with.

I pray that in time, my memories of those who've died will be poignant and welcomed. But for now, they are still catalysts that trigger vivid and horrid images. When I think of my sister Deborah, I see her stretched out on a hospital floor, nurses flying about yelling "Code Blue" over her head. I see my brother Anthony bleeding, dying on his porch steps with the house keys still gripped in his hand. I see my sister Selena raising her hand over her heart by reflex just before her husband's shotgun blasts into her chest. And I can see my Daddy, lying in a hospital bed, tubes everywhere, trying desperately to say his last words, words that I cannot understand.

Yet the pain of memory, however difficult, is bearable. Because it comes in flashes, like sharp chest pains that grip you for a few seconds, then pass. I've learned to live with it and to mask it. Beyond a pensive expression on my face or a sudden quietness, I like to believe I don't draw attention to myself when the images attack.

What has been harder to manage is the sorrow, the overwhelming sadness that permeates my life. Sometimes I get used to the feeling and forget that it's there, but like a dull toothache, it remains. I have no answer for how a person learns to overcome the sorrow. I think it lingers long after the grief has gone, long after the mourning is over. For me, death's presence has become a fact of life. Every laugh, every happy feeling, every good time is laced with a faint melancholy. And at those moments, a voice whispers to me, asking how can I be having fun when those I've loved are gone forever?

In the early days, I fought myself not to break down. I wouldn't cry. I wouldn't talk about it. I wouldn't give in. I was afraid. Afraid that if I let go, all hell would break loose and they'd be taking me to a mental hospital that same day. I didn't want to lose control. My primary incentive was to spare my mother the heartbreak—my mother, who has had to bury three of her children. I had to bury my siblings and a father, but that is different from looking down on a person you brought into the world. She has been so strong throughout these tragedies, even though I know she feels a deep pain that those of us around her can't comprehend or save her from. To break down and give my mother someone else to worry about was a selfish indulgence I didn't think I deserved.

Looking back, I realize I also managed to "hold it together" because a nervous breakdown was never an option for me. It seemed a given that I would go back to work because I had to. I would get on with my life because I had to. I would live my life because nothing I did short of that would bring my loved ones back to me.

Also, it seemed a betrayal of faith, of a belief in God to totally surrender myself to grief. And I felt this even at a time when I was angry at God for what had happened. I tried to tell myself it was indifference, but it was anger. I felt cheated and betrayed. I also felt guilty. I kept thinking: If prayer changes things, then if I'd prayed longer and harder, could I have saved their lives?

It was a thin little book written by a rabbi that helped me reestablish my faith. *When Bad Things Happen to Good People* offers a simple but revolutionary premise: God can help bring good into our lives, but he cannot prevent the bad. He can simply be there afterward to help us through the pain. So now I pray for strength—strength to make it through whatever it is that will happen.

Finally, I didn't know *how* to grieve. It does not get easier with practice. Do I visit gravesites? Do I try to force myself to cry? Do I check myself into a hospital? Do I close myself off from others?

I ran from my grief by looking for solace in my work and in people. I tried to figure out which job or person would help me feel better. I never considered just allowing myself to feel bad for a while and saying to people, "Today I feel real low. I hope you understand."

I did try, just after my brother was killed, to seek help. I went to a white psychoanalyst whom a professor had recommended. It was a disaster for me. Maybe it was the cozy comfort of her Manhattan office and the sense I had that she couldn't understand the context of my life experience. When I told her of all the deaths in my family, she looked appalled. Her face screwed up, turning into a mixture of pity and what looked to me like disgust. I think she was trying to be sympathetic, but she seemed shocked instead. And that made me feel abnormal, like a freak. That hurt me because despite what had happened to our family, we were struggling to remain a family—to hold ourselves together and survive. I left her office shaken and feeling violated.

I didn't talk about my pain with other people, except maybe one friend and my sister. And even with both of them, I had my limits on how much to say, how much to admit. I go back and forth between wanting to talk of my loved ones as they were and wanting to talk about how I feel about their deaths. What hurts most is when my sister reveals some new detail about my brother's or sisters' deaths that I hadn't known, that denial had kept me from knowing. I still can't get over how the simple, cold facts hurt as much as they do.

I've found that grief is as private and personal as handwriting. Every person has his or her own style. It may alter according to moods, age and circumstances, but it's always distinct and individual. And imitating somebody else's doesn't make it your own.

This knowledge has helped me realize, three and a half years after the last death in my immediate family, that all the irrational choices and unexplained unhappiness I experienced over those years were a form of grieving. When I refused my mother's invitation to escort me six hundred miles from home to my first day of college, I was grieving. When I plunged into a whirlwind engagement and subsequent break-up, I was grieving. When I ignored my bills for six months and debated whether to drop out of graduate school, I was grieving. When I started a new job in a new city and hated both the place and my work, I was grieving. But I didn't know I was. And even if I had, I didn't know how to ask for help. Instead, I'd lay in my bed night after night and feel I was suffocating, as if the scent of death was everywhere, settling over my life.

Yet, when I decided to quit my job, move to a city I loved, near friends I trusted, to do the kind of writing I craved, I knew I was healing.

Time has been the key to my healing. By switching from daily journalism to a freelance writing career and allowing myself spaces in my day, I've finally given myself permission to grieve. Before, being "too busy" to cry was both a reality and an excuse. I think I was afraid of too many free moments, moments that would be eaten up by the pain of it all. It was all too close and fresh to me. I needed the space that only time provides to take some of the edge off the loss. I needed time to get used to, and to accept, the finality of their deaths.

I also learned to mourn each person's death separately. I realize now that the accumulated losses had overwhelmed me, immobilized me. I couldn't dare get depressed about anything—not a bad day at the office or problems with a man or an argument with a friend—lest I be ready for a chain reaction of bad feelings. I had so much to feel bad about. Now, I take it one day, one memory, one tear at a time.

I think I now know, too, why I was grieving. Not just because the deaths had each been, to my mind, senseless and avoidable. Not just because I would miss my loved ones intensely, knowing I could never share my discoveries, my triumphs, my own life with them again. But because I felt helpless. And because I believed, deep down, that living as a struggling black family in a hardened urban city had more than a little to do with my family's fate. At times, I blame the individuals who pulled the trigger in the case of my sister, my brother and my nephew. At other times, I blame the system—a system that can allow black people to struggle so hard for so little, to work against arbitrary obstacles to acquire the basics that all human beings want, to accept multiple hardship and loss as a given way of life. To bleed inside and think all we deserve is a bandaid and a lecture about working harder. As writer Michelle Cliff has put it: "At times they felt the cause of their losses lay in themselves." That kind of self-blame is suicide.

I believe that on some deeper level, black women are used to tragedy. We expect it. Death is not a stranger to our lives, to our worlds. We've lost our fathers to hypertension and heart attacks, our brothers to frontline battles in American wars, our husbands and lovers to black-on-black crime or police brutality and our sons to drug-laced streets or upstate prisons. All this while grappling with the stress and burden of all that is black life in America: Babies born to babies, dehumanizing ghettos, inferior schools, low wages, on-the-job racism... the slow but steady death of our people. We are just used to pain.

I feel cheated sometimes. Sometimes I want the option of falling apart and I wish I could do that. Let go and just wail. But everything in my genes, in my family's tradition, has coerced me into being strong. Both of my parents come from a line of strong, willful people. That ability to be strong has saved me day-to-day, but I wonder if it has slowed my overall healing process.

I wish, too, that I had been gutsy enough to talk about my losses more openly with more people. But I worried about what "they" would think. I felt others were unwilling to listen to me talk about death. I think often of a line from a poem a friend of mine once wrote: "They say they know how you feel while secretly thanking God they don't."

It's true. The odor of tragedy is often offensive to those who haven't had to smell it in their own lives. They don't want to be around it. Often, I would find myself trying to make others comfortable at the expense of my own gut feelings. But I've come, gradually, to a place where I can acknowledge that I've been through some tragic experiences, that those experiences have helped shape who and what I am, and I see no need to apologize. If someone cares for me, that person will be willing to help fill the spaces left by my losses.

Losing my loved ones and learning to accept their absence in my life has taught me how to need other people—and not be ashamed that I do.

I've also learned to become bolder, to take risks. I think that's because I don't see failure or disaster in the same way most people do. I balance every fear against a simple test: Could the outcome be worse than what I've already gone through? No.

My patience is gone for people who seem overcome by minor, petty problems. I want to say to everyone: "You're alive, aren't you? Then get over it." It's as though I've been forced to see life stripped down to the raw, to its starkest, simplest elements. I concentrate on the biggie: Love. Little else matters to me. Yet, love matters so much that its fierceness frightens me at times. I'm seeing myself love others in a way I never knew I could.

Because mortality is real to me, I rush through life at times. I feel this need, this sense of responsibility to get some things said before it's all over. Each of my deceased siblings died while still in their thirties. I know that I don't have all the time in the world, so I try not to live as though I do.

That is the attitude that I've come to take toward my writing. I can't say why my life has been spared thus far. I can't say, for sure, where I get the strength to carry on. But I do know that I have a mission. That mission is to make my voice heard and to immortalize those I loved who've left me behind. I can do both through writing. And I will.

Confronted with both racism and sexism, black women experience a multitude of psychological pressures. The National Black Women's Health Project reports that more than fifty percent of black women live in emotional distress.

In the following piece, a black feminist psychotherapist speaks about the need for women of color to have culturally sensitive therapy and suggests methods for white feminist therapists to improve their work with black female clients.

Ethnic and Cultural Diversity in Feminist Therapy: Keys to Power
Julia A. Boyd

This article, as it was originally written, was delivered at the 1988 Advanced Feminist Therapy Institute Conference in Seattle, Washington. As a black feminist therapist, I have what I believe to be legitimate concerns about the quality of mental health care available to black women. I feel it is particularly important for white feminist therapists to recognize that the traditional constructs of psychotherapy need to be expanded to include ethnic and cultural diversity and that they themselves must become sensitized to the needs of women of color.

At the end of the article I have listed basic guidelines for black women to help select a therapist who will meet your needs.

. . .

"Difference is that raw and powerful connection from which our personal power is forged."
—Audre Lorde

The black woman's self-image, her confidence (or lack of it), as well as her perceptions of the world around her have evolved out of personal experiences. Many of these experiences are rooted in myths and stereotypes surrounding her ethnic and cultural heritage and gender. The negative attitudes and feelings brought about because of these experiences are not always measurable, but they are generally harmful to the self-esteem of black women. From early adolescence to adulthood, black women are inundated by messages telling them that to be different is societally unacceptable. Anyone who has watched television recently or thumbed through a magazine knows the media present women with flowing hair and strong European features as ideals of Western beauty. Even when black women are used within the commercial context they are chosen to reflect these characteristics—i.e., long straight hair, light coloring, thin lips and noses that often make them indistinguishable from white women. From early childhood, children in our society hear and read stories and fairy tales that are dominated by beautiful blond princesses and heroines who are often being rescued, fought for and cherished. The message that minority children receive is that attractiveness, success and popularity are basically unattainable for females of color.

"Our strategy is how we cope—how we measure and weigh what is to be said and when, what is to be done and how, and to whom ... deciding/ risking who it is we can call an ally, call a friend. We are women without a line." —Cherrie Moraga

How does the black woman know she can trust her feminist therapist to be a friend and ally? Her reality is based on the constant struggle for survival, which demands that she be cautious. Generational teachings regarding trusting others outside the ethnic and cultural community have been strongly enforced by family and respected community members. From early childhood, black women have been taught that personal disclosure outside the community is synonymous with treason. This strong devotion to non-disclosure has for many years silenced black women in personal crisis. In order for the feminist therapist to effectively help a black woman in therapy, the therapist must first understand the ethnic and cultural framework that supports the black woman's world.

In order to illustrate this concept in concrete terms, I have included the following story (which I wrote), as a miniature portrait of what I mean.

The Gospel According to Me

Yesterday during lunch Beth told me that I was her best friend. Now, I'll never understand why it is that this woman always chooses to get relevant when I'm trying to do justice to my stomach. Knowing Beth as well as I do, I knew she was expecting some tactful response on my part. But it's tough being polite when you're hungry, and my stomach had been throwing some large hints to my brain and everybody else's within earshot all day about its empty state of affairs. So as I bit into my grilled cheese sandwich, I told Beth that I'd have to give the matter of her being my best friend a lot of thought, because having a best friend, someone who was really ace, numero uno in your life, deserved some heavy contemplation.

Thinking back on it, I guess I could have given Beth an answer during lunch. But how do you tell a white woman that it's still politically dangerous to have white folks for best friends, even if it is the 1990s. I mean now really! Mama always taught me that a dollar bill was a black person's best friend, and so far as I know, Mama ain't never lied. The gospel according to Mama states that a dollar bill don't give you no lip, it keeps food in your stomach, clothes on your back and a roof over your head. If you treat it right it multiplies and if you don't it disappears. But the bottom line is if you've got a dollar, you've got a friend for life. I know Beth wouldn't understand Mama's logic because we come from two different worlds. It's not that I'm trying to discourage Beth, I really do like her. But having an ace partner means more to me than just sharing office space and having lunch together a couple times a week. I know that Beth made her comment sincerely. She wants me to notice that she's trying to bridge the gap, but what she doesn't understand is that it may take me longer to come over the water, because bridges have a way of not being stable when the winds blow too strong.

As it is, I've already got the neighbors talking because I've invited Beth to my apartment a couple of times. Wilda, my downstairs neighbor, almost broke her neck running up three flights of stairs to my place after Beth's first visit. It's not that Wilda's nosey, you understand, it's just that she was concerned. Wilda knows that white folks driving 280Z's and wearing Calvin Klein jeans don't come around the projects very often and they never come in the building unless they're after something or somebody.

I had one tough job on my hands explaining to Wilda that Beth really was okay and that through Beth's volunteer work at the Women's Center she and I had become friends. Now Wilda, who is a whole lot like Mama in her logical thinking, feels it's her sworn duty to look out for me. And she will generally tell anyone within earshot, including me, that she thinks I'm a little strange but likeable in my own fashion. But the look she gave me out of the corner of her eye let me know that now she really thinks I've lost all my street school'n. But like I said before, Wilda preaches from Mama's gospel and

Mama's Word states that you don't trust nobody two shades lighter than black.

When I think about the pros and cons of my friendship with Beth, both sides of the scale don't always equal out. Seventy-five percent of the time we get along pretty good: we believe in the same political causes even if our personal reasons are miles apart; we share similiar interests in books, movies and music, and we share the belief that going after what you want in life is the name of the game. However, the other twenty-five percent of the time is what divides us. Beth would like to believe that as women and activists, we are equals. She professes confusion when I speak about my blackness being more than just skin color and hairstyle, but a generational lifestyle that is rich in culture and value. Beth wants to form a friendship and bond with my woman-ness, the part of me which she can relate to as a white woman that bears a striking resemblance to her feminist ideals. What she fails to understand is that in only identifying with that part of me she denies my existence as a whole person. I don't know about Beth, but I'm greedy. I want a whole friendship or none at all. Beth has the privilege to forget that she's white and middle-class and I have the right to remember that I'm black, folk ethnic. Our relationship as friends may never equal best, but at least it's a start to something better, and that's the gospel according to me.

This story points out some of the real issues acted out in therapy between black women and white feminist therapists. While it was painful, I understood Beth's concept of me as a black woman/feminist. Her assumptions were based on the limited interactions and information she had with people of color prior to our friendship. I could see the parallels in our shared cause and the contradictions based in our realities of black and white. Beth assumed that our parallel interest, feminism, would be enough to bridge the gap between our worlds. However, my assumptions about Beth as a white woman/feminist were based on my reality (read survival) as a woman of color living in this society. Black feminist health advocate Beverly Smith states, "It is impossible, I think, to be a black person in this country and not be deeply aware of white people. Part of our awareness is knowledge we need to survive." Joining the ranks of feminist leadership did not/could not erase the historical legacies that Beth and I brought to our relationship as friends. All too often, therapists have entered the counseling relationship with women of color in similar ways—unmindful of the intrusion of their excessive, white, middle-class, cultural baggage.

"As women, we have been taught either to ignore our differences or to view them as causes for separation and suspicion, rather than as forces for change."   —Audre Lorde

Fear of being stereotyped and misunderstood appear to be two of the major reasons that women of color give for avoiding psychotherapy. There is a very real fear that the therapist will view ethnic and cultural behaviors as pathologic, as opposed to legitimate survival responses. Women of color are acutely aware that much of the social research involving them has only served to perpetuate myths and stereotypes concerning ethnic groups. A prime example of distorted research that has caused a continuous backlash for black women is the 1965 Moynihan Report in which the black family was viewed as disintegrating because of the "matriarchal" family structure. In her 1981 book, *Ain't I A Woman*, bell hooks eloquently points out that labeling black women as matriarchs is analogous to labeling female children who are playing house and acting out the role of mother as matriarchs. *In both instances, no real effective power exists that allows the females in question to control their destiny.*

Moynihan's report only served to heighten the racist, socially accepted myth that black females are unable to sustain interpersonal relationships. The mythological portrait of the black matriarch is a folk character fashioned by whites from their distorted image about the involuntary social and economic conditions of black women in a system that devalues women of color. Black women are highly aware of the racist labeling that is used to define their person and environment, and they are therefore legitimately cautious in seeking professional therapy. Feminist therapists, unfortunately, are not exempt from bias in their attitudes and beliefs concerning women of color, especially when their professional training has been designed to exclude ethnic and cultural concerns.

Categorizing women of color as neatly packaged groups defined by customs and traditions might be an easy task, if the groups were not made up of individuals. In her book, *Tomorrow's Tomorrow: The Black Woman*, Joyce Ladner points out that there is no monolithic concept of the black woman, but there are many models of black womanhood. Black women are distinct individuals who make choices as to the many ways in which they gain their strength. There are black women who may not always look to their ethnic and cultural traditions for subsistence, but it is very likely that on some level such a woman will periodically seek comfort that only her community or family of origin can provide. This attention to both group and individual needs may sound complex to a white feminist therapist. However, being of one body yet sharing many voices is the daily life and strength of black women.

In order to survive, black women have become masters in the art of being bicultural. In an article in *Aegis Journal*, written in 1983 and entitled "Some Thoughts on Racism," Beverly Smith states, "There is a lot of propaganda in this culture for the normality of the rightness of whiteness." Generations of exposure to the socially accepted norms of whiteness have made it virtually impossible for black women not to adopt specific behaviors such as standards of beauty, language and mannerisms associated with white culture that would allow them to survive. In order to survive, Audre Lorde points out, "those of us for whom oppression is as American as apple pie have always had to be watchers, to become familiar with the language and manners of the oppressor, even sometimes adopting them for some illusion of protection." For black women, learning to comply publicly with white standards has not been as much a choice as a dictate necessary for survival. The following quotes were spoken at a women of color support group meeting I led in Seattle. The subject was racial harassment on the job:

"Sometimes you can hear them thinking in your bones."

"They don't know this is my life they're playing with and I was born knowing the rules."

"Why do they play these silly head trip games, I don't trust any of them."

"I'm afraid of God, dogs and the dark in that order; anybody else I'll fight."

Many of the women at the meeting had been seen individually by a white therapist who had referred them to the group after the women of color had started expressing pent-up feelings of anger and rage at white employers. The continued challenge of being caught in a system that values only one set of standards is a constant burden for women of color. For the woman of color to openly fight back is an invitation to become a target of institutionalized racism designed in the form of rules and regulations to keep one in the proper place.

Feminism that denies freedom of ethnic and cultural differences is not feminism; therapy that covertly denies the validity of a woman's ethnic and cultural experiences is not therapy.

Innocence does not alter the reality for the large number of white feminist therapists who remain in a passive state of denial concerning the therapeutic needs of black women. Many white feminist therapists forget that they were white long before they chose to become feminists or therapists. Being a feminist therapist does not negate the societal privilege that is inherent in being born white. In America, racist oppression runs deep and dies hard. As Elsie Smith says in her 1981 piece in the *Journal of Non-White Concerns*, it is nurtured by generations of "hand me down" hatreds. White feminists who exercise race privilege on a daily basis often lack awareness that they are doing so. Unconscious cultural awareness or race privilege by the white feminist therapist is for the most part accepted and validated as being the norm in a society that promotes difference as being other or alien. Activist Barbara Smith summarizes the common experiences of black women this way: "I have the feeling that no one white understands our daily experiences."

To understand is to obtain knowledge, and for white feminist therapists that understanding/knowledge must begin with the recognition that their personal relationship with the woman of color client is reflective of the larger world in which they both live. As a feminist, the therapist must recognize that the balance of power between herself and her client is unequal. She can begin to equalize the division of power by becoming knowledgeable about her world and the world of women of color. The following example illustrates how I have attempted to go about this process in my own way:

Recently I had the experience of treating a young Southeast Asian woman for depression. She told me that she had been in treatment in the past, only to find that it had not been helpful. She explained that she had little hope that therapy would be helpful this time, but she had promised her physician that she would try once more. During our first interview, I obtained a full family history which included a detailed history of her family life prior to coming to the United States. In taking the history, I encouraged the woman to elaborate, which allowed me to gain some insight regarding her world as she experienced it. After the first interview, I began doing my homework, which was to network with other Southeast Asian women and to research material that would help me to know my client as a bicultural person. During subsequent sessions, as she related information concerning her depression, I was able to shape the therapy into a context that included some of her traditional ethnic values, such as family loyalty, and a circular concept of harmony between self and nature. In listening to this Southeast Asian woman, I was able to glean information regarding her lifestyle, her needs, her wants, and her disappointments; many of which were not the same as mine. However, I was able to recognize that her depression was in some part linked to an ethnic and cultural deprivation she experienced living in the United States. While she may deal with depression again, I feel that I made the right choice by addressing this client's ethnic and cultural needs as well as her emotional ones. I believe that my approach gave her a constructive format in which to deal with her issues.

In doing therapy with women of color, feminist therapists must recognize that they will again become students. The feminist therapist will have to learn about her client's world through her history, networking with agencies and individuals in the client community and through researching relevant ethnic and cultural literature. For to ignore the meaning of the client's identity is to ignore the person. If that occurs, treatment cannot take place. Only through recognizing that the client has a history and an identity that is completely different from one's own, can one take an effective look at the symptoms presented.

"Now is the time for our women to lift up their heads and plant the roots of progress under the hearth-stone."
—Frances E.W. Harper, black abolitionist, 1870

Feminist therapists have become pioneers in establishing previously uncharted courses in therapy. This practice must be continued for black women to receive meaningful treatment. The feminist therapist must be willing to examine her own beliefs regarding black women. In addition, she must be willing to analyze the myths, stereotypes and misinformation that she has received in previous training and look at which of these have been erroneously applied to women of color. She must be willing to examine whether the framework and techniques she is using in therapy encourage ethnic and cultural diversity. As a feminist, the therapist will need to broaden her range of awareness through reading, networking and researching the lifestyles of black women. She must teach other feminists and relearn the art of being a student of ethnic diversity. In this way feminist therapists working with women of color will help their clients to receive effective professional mental health care.

Ideally therapy is the art of self-healing. It enables the client to draw on personal resources to empower and enrich her life. Black women have the right to accurate, safe and effective mental health treatment by feminist professionals who are culturally sensitive. Ethnic and cultural literacy can only be accomplished if the feminist therapist is open to exploring ways in which traditional therapy can become more colorful and diverse.

Information for Black Women for Selecting a Therapist

1. Ask respected friends and acquaintances for recommendations of good therapists. This may sound like a scary thing to do at first, but you would be surprised at the number of people living in the community who actually seek professional help.

2. Interview, either by phone or in person, several therapists before making the choice. Write down beforehand a list of questions you would like to ask. Some examples of things you might want to find out include: the therapist's educational and professional background, including her years of experience and practice; the therapist's knowledge of ethnic and cultural diversity and how the knowledge was obtained—for example, through schooling, living or working in communities of color, or working with people of color; professional fees and availability of a sliding scale for fees; personal references.

Remember that you will be trusting this individual with private, personal information about yourself and that you have a right to know whom you are trusting.

3. Evaluate your satisfaction with the counseling process. Trust your own feelings and comfort level with the therapist—you have the right to terminate therapy at any time if it is not meeting your needs.

Cutbacks in student aid are having a distressing impact on minorities in-
terested in pursuing careers in the health professions. Simply put, more
government dollars are being given to military efforts than to education.
According to the American Dental Association, there are 137,817 practic-
ing dentists in the United States. Of that number only about 1,200, or less
than one percent, are reported to be black females.

As we struggle to make government and academic institutions more
accountable to our health needs, we are fortunate to have role models to
encourage and guide us. In the following piece, a successful black female
dentist writes a personal account of her achievements and also offers basic
dental advice.

One Determination: A Black Female Dentist Speaks

Denise Alexander

I was raised in a central Los Angeles neighborhood where few positive role models existed, particularly for a young black woman wanting to pursue a professional career. When I was about sixteen, however, a visit to the dentist began a process that changed the direction
of my life. I was experiencing discomfort from my wisdom teeth, so I
asked my mother for my Medi-Cal card and made an appointment
with a dentist recommended by a friend. Fortunately for me, the
dentist was black. He was also gentle, had a wonderful sense of humor, and most important, he took the time to talk to me about his
profession. This experience prompted my interest in dentistry as a
career goal.

At the time of the visit I was about a year away from high school
graduation and my grades were poor, to say the least. I decided it
was now time to meet with my high school counselor to tell her that I
wanted to take the preparatory courses for college my dentist had
mentioned. When I met with her to explain that I had decided to go
to college, my words seemed to stun her into silence. When she
regained her ability to speak, she reminded me that my grades were
lousy and my attendance worse. She recommended that I just keep

the courses as already prescribed. She said she would assist me with graduating on time by talking to my teachers about my mother's frequent illnesses, which had interfered with my school work. And last, she suggested that I get a job and then maybe go to trade school later.

I knew she was right about my grades and my attendance, neither of which improved over the next year. I graduated from high school with a grade point average that was equivalent to a D-minus.

I worked full-time for a few years at a local hospital after graduation, but I was still determined to go to college. I tried to attend a local community college part-time while I worked, but I seemed unable to accomplish anything. I felt distracted by my mother's poor health and other family matters, as well as the Southern California party scene. When the opportunity arose, I decided to move to Northern California and enroll at Nairobi College, a black private two-year school in East Palo Alto. I had no relatives or friends in the area, so I was able to immerse myself in my studies. I realized that good grades were important if I wanted my education financed, so I improved my grade point average and won several scholarships.

Because of financial constraints, Nairobi College provided a limited number of natural science courses, which forced me to take some of these courses at other nearby schools. But Nairobi College offered much on black history and black pride. It gave me the tools for success and helped me learn how to move through traditional institutions without losing my identity as a black woman.

After completing my coursework at Nairobi College, I transferred to San Francisco State University and got my bachelor's degree. Then I applied and was admitted to the University of California, San Francisco, School of Dentistry.

Dental school was not an easy challenge. In fact, it was the most intellectually, emotionally and physically stressful situation I had ever encountered. I felt the emotional stresses were related to being both black and female. Both students and instructors would casually imply that blacks were not qualified to be in the school and were only admitted through special programs. If I mentioned the *academic* fellowship I received that paid my tuition, our conversations would end abruptly. It was clear that they didn't want to accept the fact that blacks were as intellectually capable as they were. I often wondered how I was going to continue through four years of school under those circumstances, but I refused to give up, so I struggled on.

There were positive experiences with many of my instructors and their help was gratifying. However, my greatest support came from joining forces with the few other black students in my class. We studied and learned together. We formed a bond with one another and our individual determination became one determination. The result was that I did very well in dental school, and upon graduation I immediately opened a private practice in family dentistry in Berkeley, California.

I built and started my practice from scratch with the help of a very special friend and it has become quite successful in a short time. If I could convey the single most important motivation throughout my struggle, it was my belief that academic achievements and rewards are not just for a select group of people. Black people have always fought systematic exclusion. Educational exclusion is just another of our battles; don't turn away.

If this discussion motivates black people, black women in particular, I will feel I have helped to arm our community with information that will enhance the quality of our lives. As black women, we are in the unique position to be the examples who can instill a sense of health in our communities, and with good health we can and will achieve all that we desire.

Improving Dental Health

Because most blacks do not get adequate dental care or receive compassionate treatment from dentists, I would now like to discuss dental health as it relates to your children's development, and follow with some specific dental information for adults. This information is not intended to replace regular visits to a trained and culturally sensitive dentist. Probably the best way to find a good dentist is to ask for referrals from friends you trust.

Children's teeth begin forming long before the children are born. Once the teeth become visible, usually when the child is age six to ten months, the teeth can develop cavities. To reduce the possibility of cavities, it is very important to begin to clean your child's teeth on a daily basis. Initially this can be accomplished by wiping your baby's teeth with a damp cloth or gauze. Later, as your child's size increases, you may use a child-sized toothbrush and a very small amount of toothpaste. This can be accomplished by having your child lay his or her head on your lap in the backward position. Use one of your hands to hold the lips apart and the other to brush the child's teeth. (In time you will be able to teach your child not to swallow the toothpaste.)

Bottle-related cavities are the most common cavities in baby teeth. They arise from giving a baby a bottle of a sweet, sugary substance at naptime or bedtime. This causes sugar to stay on the teeth for long periods and severe tooth decay can occur. To minimize this possibility, always rinse your child's mouth with clear water after sweets are given and never put your child to sleep with a bottle of sweet liquid. As your children get older it is important to frequently check their teeth for discolorations or brown spots. Such signs could indicate cavities.

When your children are one to three years of age, you should begin to prepare them for their first dental visit. At first, your child may not be completely cooperative, but the dentist should attempt to make the visit a pleasant experience. The following tips can help prepare your child for the first visit:

- Read books to your children about going to the dentist.

- Play tooth counting with your child and switch roles to let your child count your teeth.

- Answer questions about the visit in simple, positive terms your child can understand.

- Make the appointments for early in the morning so your child will be well rested.

- Most of all, remain low-key about the visit. Children are not born with a fear of the dentist. They inherit it from adults. If your children sense that you are afraid of the dentist, they will feel fear, too.

Your children can begin to brush their own teeth at age two to three, but it will still be important for parents to do a thorough back-up brushing and flossing. Later, when your child has mastered brushing and flossing, usually at seven to nine years of age, you should still check to make sure all is going well. Because flossing is so important, parents should teach their children how to do it as soon as their children's teeth have grown close enough together to trap food.

A growing number of adults are facing dental problems because of periodontal or gum disease. Periodontal disease (sometimes referred to as pyorrhea) has four stages:

- *Gingivitis*—This is the beginning stage of the disease. The signs are slightly swollen, inflamed gums that may bleed when brushing and flossing.

- *Early Periodontitis*—If gingivitis is left untreated, this next stage develops. The signs include all of the above plus a loss of gum attachment to the teeth and some loss of underlying bone structure around the teeth.

- *Moderate to Severe Periodontitis*—At this stage destruction of the underlying bone around the teeth advances to a degree that the individual will probably begin to notice the teeth feeling loose in the socket.

- *Advanced Periodontitis*—This is the last stage of the disease. At this point the gum tissue and bone around the teeth have been destroyed, eventually resulting in tooth loss.

Studies show that smokers have a higher incidence of gum disease, as do people who have crooked or malpositioned teeth. The most effective method for controlling the progression of gum disease is daily plaque removal through brushing and flossing. You should also see your dental health professional for routine cleanings. Gum disease develops gradually and can progress slowly with very few signs or symptoms. But with regular dental care, it can be diagnosed early and treated before serious damage is done to your teeth.

During my years of practicing dentistry, I have treated multitudes of people who have avoided routine dental care because they are afraid of the dentist. If fear is preventing you from receiving dental care, I assure you, you are not alone. As a black female dentist who cares deeply about the health of my community, I encourage you to address your dental fears now. Seek a dentist who will be sensitive to your special needs and who has the ability to calm your concerns with gentle, understanding techniques. With good dental care, you'll be the beneficiary of a healthy mouth and a beautiful smile that can last forever. I think you deserve it, don't you?

In the 1850s, Mary Seacole, a black woman of Jamaican descent, nursed along with Florence Nightingale during the Crimean War. For black women, a nursing career has historically represented a way to a better life and a means to serve others. Partially because of recent cutbacks in financial aid, fewer black women are pursuing nursing careers. Health officials estimate that there are about 1,600,000 nurses in the United States. Of this number about 61,000 or 3.7 percent, are black.

In the following piece, the author discusses her multifaceted career as a nurse. She also offers provocative views about changes in the nursing profession and how black women can best respond to improve their lives and the collective well-being of African-Americans.

Service Without Subservience: Reflections of a Registered Nurse
Cheryl M. Killion

No single dramatic event significantly influenced my decision to become a nurse; it was something I just knew at an early age. My career choice was based primarily on what was available at the time for women, African-American women in particular. Of the two prevailing choices, nursing and teaching, I opted for nursing because it seemed to be more noble and more challenging than teaching. My daily interactions with teachers gave me enough exposure to their role; however, I knew very little about the specifics of what nurses did. That they helped the sick, wore crisp uniforms and had a warm, efficient manner was appealing to me. Moreover, I was acutely aware that even though becoming a nurse would be difficult, I would never want for a job.

Economic security was important because I had grown up under modest circumstances in a midwestern industrial town in Illinois. My father was a steelworker and my mother a housewife. Although my brother, two sisters and I always had the essentials, our family regularly bought day-old bread, wore cardboard squares to reinforce the broken soles of our discount-outlet shoes, and ate beans and cornbread to help make ends meet. We lived on the outskirts of town in a basement until I was seven. Then a family friend, with the assistance of my father, built the five-room house that currently stands. It was not until I was in high school that we had a closed sewage system. Every year until then, my father and other neighbor men had to dig out the raw sewage to unclog the cesspool that flowed in open ditches in front of our house. A child growing up in midwest America should not contract typhoid fever, but one of the boys next door did. He nearly died, and I remember his long hospitalization and the painful inoculations other members of his family and our family had to go through to avoid this dreaded disease.

My neighborhood symbolized the marked racial divisions in the town. We lived in a row of houses that was opposite a golf course and an exclusive country club. The hilly landscape, cool, mossy ponds and the carpetlike greens were a beautiful immediate sight from our picture window and provided a prohibited playground in the evening and in the winter, when the golfers were gone. On occasion, it was also the scene of cross burnings to signal to the entire neighborhood that we were not welcome there. Within a five-block radius of our house were five or six frame houses similar to ours, but the majority were pieced-together, dilapidated shacks. Around the corner from us was a family of fourteen, a mother and her thirteen children, who occupied a two-room house; and there were two or three small houses of prostitution, interspersed here and there. Almost directly behind our house, one street over, was a booming night club, from which we could hear the loud music, traffic and scuffles every weekend. Violence and killings were common; however, after years of the community's fight for its demise, the club was finally closed and replaced with a community center. A church and a cemetery were also nearby.

Church was the focus of my family's life. Regular church attendance was mandatory and involvement in related functions actively promoted. My parents were consistently involved and often the leaders in civic, religious and social organizations. This involvement fostered a sense of social responsibility and altruism, and our family was guided by the adage: "A family that prays together, stays together."

In our town of about 40,000, the number of African-American professionals was limited, particularly in the health professions. There was one general practitioner, one surgeon, no dentist and two or three registered nurses. Consequently, most African-Americans sought health care only when they were pregnant, acutely ill or severely injured, or had a persistent problem that could not be managed at home. Going to the doctor's office was either an ordeal or a social event, depending upon the reason for the visit or how sick a person was. Generally, no appointments were given since the physician usually did not have a receptionist (nor an office manager, nor a nurse). People merely trickled in and were seen on a first-come, first-serve basis. Often the waiting line would extend from the waiting room, along a dimly lit corridor, down a steep flight of stairs and out onto the sidewalk. There were complaints, but not loud ones. The procedure was generally accepted by everyone. During the waiting, toddlers played on the floor while mothers swatted flies and fanned. Elderly women swapped stories about their ailments and the self-care remedies they used. Men engaged in small talk or plugged a sporting event or athletic team. Once inside the office, the doctor, who had delivered almost all the babies in the African-American community, dealt with the presenting problem, but afterwards spent as much time catching up on family milestones and community gossip. And this was half the medicine. The general practitioner was liked and respected—and made house calls. Yet, this limited access to health care took its toll on our community and undoubtedly had long-term, pervasive effects.

Since I wanted the "college experience" and a broader education, I attended a four-year university nursing program rather than a three-year-diploma, hospital-based school which was the usual route of education for nurses at the time. I enrolled in physical and behavioral science courses, many of which were taken by pre-med students, and liberal arts courses at a local university for the first two years. During the entire time I was in school, I worked summers and part-time at a number of jobs, including nurses aide and unit secretary in a psychiatric hospital. My last two years constituted the clinical portion of my nursing education. Actual "hands-on" technical skills, which were integrated with concepts from prior courses, were learned and practiced in several hospitals in a large metropolitan area twenty to thirty miles from my home. County/public and private facilities were used, and part of the clinical rotations were in public health/community agencies and in the homes of patients.

Through this clinical component, I was introduced to a full range of problems that were a testimony to the human condition, and I witnessed the extent to which such problems could be assuaged by nursing. One vivid example was a fifteen-year-old quadraplegic, who was cared for at home. She had developed multiple bed sores, some of which were so deep that the bone was visible. Her family had stuffed the exposed areas with newspaper to absorb the fluid that oozed from the wounds, and her bedroom had an unbearable smell. Some of my goals with this patient were to teach the family the proper way to dress the wound, to stress the importance of frequent changes in position, to investigate the type of mattress used, to explore the family's financial sources for obtaining these materials, to assess the impact that this patient had on the family, and to determine whether or not, or to what extent, the patient was being neglected or mistreated.

Another example was a man who had to be re-admitted to the hospital because of a maggot-infested cast. The man had signed out of the facility against medical advice because eviction proceedings had been initiated against him during his hospitalization. After he left the hospital, he had lived in his car. The nurses' immediate problem was to take care of this man's cast. He also needed to be guided to resources that could help him find housing and improve his mental state, since he was very depressed. I was also shaken by my obstetrics/gynecology experience at a county hospital. The stench from the women's clinic seemed to linger in my clothes after I left its small room, where five women would lie side-by-side on examining tables with a half screen to separate them and no curtains to screen their bottoms. Viewing the room crosswise, all that one could see were the exposed genitalia of each of the women as they were propped up in readiness for evaluation. An examiner moved down the row, from vagina to vagina, performing a quick exam, dropping cold, discharge-dripping speculums in a nearby basin as he went. The women got up without assistance or comment, almost in a chorus-line synchrony, then went on their way or moved to another station for further evaluation.

In all settings, I was appalled by the number of women who came to the hospital or clinic and literally gave over their bodies to the system. There was clearly a need to help women become more responsible for their own health and that of their families, despite other pressing priorities in their lives.

By contrast, part of my clinical rotation took place in a new wing of a large medical center. The hospital rooms, which resembled hotel rooms, were in an ultra-modern building that had replaced an older one where only a few years before, my grandfather had been a patient in a large ward in the basement for "colored." Individuals with a full range of health problems were cared for here, but it was clear that the patients were more affluent than any for which I had ever provided care. I resented them, not because of their economic status, but because of the way they treated me. One wealthy widow, for example, ignored all my professional skills and focused on the fact that I was a "single, young thing" whom she wanted to fix up with her butler! Another patient actually treated me like a maid, even though my name tag clearly indicated *SN* for student nurse. Maids don't give injections, nor do they interpret electrocardiograms. Her requests that I tidy her room and run errands for her were offensive, especially since she was only there to have her bunions removed. Others would ask, after a dressing change or suctioning, whether I was a "real" nurse. This question was asked not because I botched the procedure, but rather because they could not believe that a black woman was preparing to become a registered nurse. The ultimate and repeated insult was the experience of assisting individuals to perform basic bodily functions that they ordinarily would do privately and independently, only to have them act in a demeaning or derogatory manner toward me afterwards.

After graduation my first position was staff nurse on a neurosurgical unit. This was a stimulating experience because the opportunities for learning were endless. Every nursing skill that I had learned and ones I hadn't were called upon because of the types of patients we provided for. People from all walks of life, and from different parts of the world, were admitted for head injuries, gunshot wounds, cerebral aneurysms, brain tumors, spinal cord injuries and more. Some patients recovered, sometimes miraculously; some were permanently disabled; and some lives were snuffed out. Although the nurses worked with respirators and cardiac monitors, we lacked other sophisticated technology to assess the neurological status of the patients. It was our constant surveillance at the bedside that enabled us to detect subtle changes that could signal a patient's potential for improvement or sudden deterioration.

During this early phase of my nursing career, I realized the significance of mobilizing family support and prayer to empower the patient and promote self-healing. I recall one nineteen-year-old African-American man who had been in an automobile accident. During his three-month stay in the intensive care unit, he lay motionless in a coma on body support systems and with a tube extending from every orifice. He was given little or no chance of survival and was moved out of the ICU with the expectation that nothing more could be done for him and that he was certain to die. He was provided with supportive care—turning, positioning, suctioning, exercising contracted limbs, and intravenous fluids and antibiotics. At least one family member was present every day of his hospital stay (nearly a year), but every weekend his entire immediate family came to visit—all nine of them, including his estranged wife. They participated in his care, sang, and talked to him while he was comatose. One brother played the guitar and a family prayer was said at the end of each visit. The young man's father came the most often. He would read poetry to his son and carry on a one-way conversation with him for what seemed like hours. Incredibly, the nineteen-year-old regained consciousness and after long, arduous months of relearning to walk and talk, he was finally discharged and returned only as an outpatient for extensive rehabilitation. There is no doubt that the steady stream of love, positive caring and uplifting support had a significant role in this young man's unlikely recovery.

There are many remarkable stories I witnessed about courage, tenacity and love, but there were also too many deaths and too many tragedies. It was disheartening and emotionally taxing to care for youth disabled permanently from motorcycle accidents, or despondent suicidals who had blown out parts of their skull and brain, or energetic individuals who wasted away in a few months from a brain tumor. Equally disconcerting were the inequities in health care delivery that occurred despite the expertise of the health team. It was not uncommon, for example, for an uninsured victim to be moved prematurely from the ICU to make room for an insured patient who often was less critically ill. Coping with dilemmas of this nature and the intensity of care needed by each patient caused me tremendous emotional strain. Moreover, the poor working conditions made it even more difficult to render the best care. Understaffing was usually the major problem. It was often necessary to work up to ten straight days (or nights) without a day off to insure that the unit had adequate coverage. As a new graduate, all these conditions took their toll on me, and I decided to make a change.

I moved to Colorado in search of a different kind of challenge. I accepted a position in the family-centered unit of a major hospital in Denver. The beauty of the Rockies was thrilling, and the change in environment and job was refreshing and invigorating. The opportunity to participate in the birth experience of families was also exhilarating and my enthusiasm for nursing was restored. I was again disillusioned, however, by the subtle and blatant racist attitudes and actions of some of the staff. For example, a large Latino population was served by the hospital where I was employed. On more than one occasion I witnessed physicians approaching Latina women (some of whom understood little English), to have them sign consent forms for sterilization while they were in the most active period of labor or immediately following birth, when they were often exhausted, sometimes still in pain, or heavily medicated. Although the laws regarding informed consent are stringently followed today, thousands of poor and minority women were victimized in the past by doctors who urged them to consent to procedures they did not fully understand and might have refused if they had. It was critical to become an advocate for these women. It was also necessary to intercede on behalf of patients when overzealous medical students and residents repeatedly performed vaginal exams for their own learning and not out of a need to assess a woman's progress in labor.

The African-American population in this community was relatively small, but even then I was aware that these women had a disproportionate number of complications during and after their pregnancies. The nursing staff was generally progressive and provided sensitive care. Nonetheless, I was astounded by their lack of knowledge and misunderstanding of blacks. One time the head nurse called a special case conference to discuss an African-American mother who had called her newborn infant "bad." It was the head nurses's contention that this mother had a problem in bonding with her newborn and might abuse the baby. However, the head nurse had not observed the body language of the mother nor did she understand the full meaning of "bad." The mother was actually bonding wonderfully with her new son. She held him often, talked to him in a soothing voice, handled him gently and breastfed him without difficulty. It was clear to me that she was a loving, attentive, proud mother. She did refer to her son's actions as "bad" but to her, "Oh, he's so-o ba-ad!" meant that he was alert, active and smart. After I provided this explanation to the staff, the mother was spared a visit from the staff psychiatrist and a social service follow-up.

After working in the labor and delivery unit for a little more than a year, I entered the master's program in maternal-child nursing at the University of Colorado and continued to work part-time. Upon completing graduate school, I was recruited to teach in a major university in California. The move to the West Coast was a tremendous leap. There were so many possibilities and so many opportunities. Adjusting to a new city and to academia simultaneously was difficult and extremely trying, however. There were so many lessons to be learned about "the system" and how to survive. Most of my energy was focused on my job teaching maternal-child nursing. Lecturing to students and supervising them in the hospital setting was instructive as well as creative for me. In addition to teaching technical skills and the theoretical foundations of clinical practice, it was possible to help shape their philosophy of caring by providing a model of service: assisting patients to help themselves and advocating for them when they cannot.

After three years of teaching, it became evident that an advanced degree was necessary, and I enrolled in a Ph.D. program in Anthropology. I selected Anthropology because I wanted to explore why cultural groups responded to illness and developmental milestones like birth and death in similar or dissimilar ways. Moreover, I was curious about why certain diseases were prevalent among some groups and not others, and I wanted to broaden my understanding of my own culture. I resigned from my teaching position, moved to a smaller apartment near the campus, and got a part-time job. I enjoyed the rigorous challenge of the Ph.D. program and it was stimulating to be a student again. During my second quarter of classes, however, I became pregnant. Although I was delighted with the prospect of becoming a parent, I was devastated by a shattered relationship and the interruption in my schooling. However, there was never any doubt that I would finish my degree. I completed courses for the first years, and took off only the quarter following the birth of my daughter. Family and friends were invaluable during this time. My immediate family offered support and encouragement long-distance from Illinois, while my so-called "fictive kin" sustained me through some hard times.

I moved again to a more affordable and spacious, yet roach-infested apartment in an area often referred to as "the jungle." The four-unit apartment building presented a tableau of urban ghetto life. Sometimes I could not hear the taps of my typewriter for the commotion of family fighting in the apartment next door. My train of thought was often interrupted by my drug-dealing neighbors across the hall, who transacted business at all hours of the day and night. One night, when my daughter was less than two weeks old, it was necessary to get up repeatedly to quiet her. As I read a chapter from a textbook and breastfed her, I could hear helicopters and sirens outside. Before I knew it, my back door was forced open, and by the time I got to the kitchen, one police officer was in my kitchen and the other was halfway inside. They had seen my light flicker on and off and claimed that they thought I was signaling to the robbery suspect they were pursuing.

Other times were more peaceful. It was delightful to see school-age girls jumping double-dutch on the sidewalk out front. And almost every Saturday morning a neighbor heralded the new day by singing gospel songs, providing the entire neighborhood with an open window invitation to her solo rehearsal. As this sister swung from one octave to the next, many of our troubles were soon forgotten.

After my coursework was finished, my qualifying exam passed and my proposal developed, I was awarded a fellowship which enabled my daughter and me to move to Central America for one year, where I conducted fieldwork for my dissertation. We lived in Belize, a country not much larger than the state of Massachusetts. Because the country had a high percentage of Creoles and Garifuna (both of African descent) and was considered to be the bridge between the Caribbean and Central America, it was an ideal place for me to witness the experience of peoples of African descent who had experienced slavery and the contemporary ramifications of it in a setting other than the United States.

I rented a house in the heart of Belize City and immersed myself in the culture: shopping in the central market, enrolling my four-year-old daughter in a neighborhood school and becoming involved in a number of the social events. Even though the country was beautiful, with coral reefs, white unspoiled beaches and tropical forests, the pervasive poverty was perhaps the most striking feature of our surroundings.

Collecting data was a challenge in this setting. It was necessary to walk to most of my interviews, despite the hundred-degree or higher temperatures and humid weather. Buses were infrequent and crowded. During the rainy season, the streets would sometimes flood, forcing me to wade in knee-deep water to get to a destination. Because of frequent electrical blackouts, the extensive field notes that were a vital part of my research had to be written by kerosene lamp or candlelight. The bombardment of mosquitoes was a constant menace, for an outbreak of dengue fever took place during our stay and malaria was always a threat.

Aside from visiting the families who were part of my study, my contacts with other nurses throughout the country formed one of the most extraordinary experiences I had. The primacy of nursing was evident as I traveled around the country to learn about the health care system. In the cities, nurses had a major role in the actual operation of the hospitals and were the main providers at the bedside, as well. Most of the scattered villages throughout the country had poor access to health care professionals or facilities. Nurses were assigned to geographical areas within districts and were responsible for health care delivery for the several villages in their domain. The commitment of the nurses to the people in their districts was heartening. For example, on one occasion during the rainy season, flooding had caused a bridge to be washed out, preventing the nurse from making a visit to a family in a remote area. The nurse and her assistant camped out for two days on the river's bank until the river subsided and they were able to cross. All the nurses I met wrestled daily with the frustrations of having inadequate refrigeration for vaccines and medications (many of which were outdated), sparse supplies, malfunctioning equipment and poor transportation. Yet they continued to serve with all the expertise and dignity that their circumstances would allow.

When I returned to the United States, I completed my Ph.D. and am now teaching in a school of nursing. My goal is to help produce nurses who are not only technically skilled and knowledgeable about pathophysiology, but who are also sensitive to and have some understanding of the contexts in which illness and life changes occur.

Unlike decades ago, numerous career options are available for today's young people. Partially because of this, fewer men and women are now entering the nursing profession. The numbers are especially low among African-Americans and other ethnic minorities, for they are the ones hardest hit by cutbacks in student loans and the dismantling of affirmative action programs. This trend of minorities forsaking nursing careers is alarming in light of the revolutionary changes occurring in the health care system today—many of which have particular ramifications for African-Americans.

For instance, under the Reagan administration, the health care market was deregulated, prompting competition between public and private health care providers. As the competitive pressures in health care have mounted, the overall health status of African-Americans has declined. Because of dramatic cutbacks in Medicaid and other community health programs, blacks (who are fifty percent more likely than whites *not* to have health insurance) are finding it increasingly difficult to locate private health providers willing and/or able to provide them with care. This situation is exacerbated by the fact that a number of major public hospitals in African-American communities have been closed. Consequently, a growing number of African-Americans are receiving no health care whatsoever. They need all the advocates they can get.

On the positive side, enormous leaps have been made in health technology during the past twenty years. Telematics, which has aligned video, computer and satellite networks, has created almost limitless possibilities for communication and has established data bases for clinical, epidemiological and environmental investigations and discoveries. And most importantly, more Americans are becoming knowledgeable about their health and demanding quality health care. People are living longer, more productive lives in a society that is becoming increasingly ethnically diverse.

Consequently, it is critical that African-Americans become more active in nursing and other health professions. Black nurses can play a pivotal role in helping the African-American community attain greater wellness in an economically constrained but technologically expanding health care system. In short, they can help develop and implement policies that will improve the distribution of health care in this country. Now is the time, with nurses especially in demand, for African-American men and women to step forward and provide this backbone of the health care system.

Nurses, as experts in health, human behavior, and family and community dynamics, can offer the sustenance and continuity sorely needed in our community. We must look to such past leaders as Harriet Tubman and Sojourner Truth, whose contributions as nurses are less well known than their historical actions to free and advance our people. Yet their experiences as nurses were clearly instrumental in their rise to success. In the process of restoring health and revitalizing strength, African-American nurses have the capacity to uplift and give hope. Not only have we experienced discrimination and racism firsthand, we are ourselves also part of the abysmal statistics that weaken our community. We are the experts on our own experience and condition; and with this knowledge, we are a source of immeasurable power.

Although alcoholism prevention efforts have increased in recent years, scant attention has been focused on alcohol and drug abuse treatment in the black community. On the contrary, alcoholic beverage companies have made special efforts to win black consumers by using soul music, black sports stars, black-oriented magazines and inner-city billboards to promote their products. According to the Center for Science in the Public Interest, the alcohol industry spends more than two billion dollars a year on advertising. A significant portion of the seductive, pro-alcohol messages are directed toward the black community.

Prompted by the severity of the problem, many black organizations and individuals are launching educational campaigns about the dangers of alcohol and drug abuse. In the following piece, an expert on substance abuse provides an overview of the problem.

Moving Targets:
Alcohol, Crack and Black Women
Sheila Battle

Drive through any African-American community and what's the first thing you'll see? Chances are it will be numerous billboards advertising liquor and cigarettes. As an African-American social worker employed in health agencies in San Francisco, I have first-hand experience with the negative impact of alcohol and drug addiction in black communities—a problem that must be confronted head-on if we are to alleviate its devastating consequences.

For two years, I worked as an Alcohol Prevention Coordinator for the African-American Community Alcohol Awareness Program in San Francisco. Eighty percent of the clients we served were African-Americans. During the course of my work at this agency it became clear to me that alcohol use has been part of the African-American family system for many generations. Alcohol has been consumed by blacks since the period of slavery to ease the effects and pressures of racism and oppression; to tune out physical and emotional pain. There are also a disproportionate number of liquor stores in most African-American communities. Often store owners are more willing to give credit for alcohol than for food.

Many health problems in the black community are directly related to alcohol use and abuse. Chief among them is cirrhosis of the liver, a chronic disease which causes the liver to degenerate. Another health-related problem in the black community is cancer of the esophagus, which in many cases is aggravated by cigarette smoking, producing a deadly combination. Cardiovascular disease, strokes, diabetes, fetal alcohol syndrome, violent crime and traffic fatalities are all prevalent among blacks and compounded by alcohol.

Recent research on African-American women and alcohol reveals especially troubling data. In a national random sample, thirty-eight percent of black women were found to be heavy drinkers compared to eleven percent of white women. On average, black women enter alcohol treatment programs at age thirty-five compared to age thirty-one for white women.[1] Because of inadequate medical, economic and psychological support, black women are more likely to suffer relapses after completing alcohol treatment. Additionally, studies show a higher prevalence of "escape alcoholism" among black women. In other words, drinking that numbs them from the many griefs, sorrows and disappointments that color black female lives.

In most cases, blacks seek treatment for their alcohol-related health problems before they begin to deal with the underlying issue of alcoholism. Because of the strong sense of denial that is characteristic of alcoholism, people are reluctant to admit that their health is deteriorating because of their drinking. Because they often have full responsibility for their families and feel they must carry on no matter what, black women are even more likely to minimize the negative impact of alcohol in their lives.

Given these circumstances, my agency developed a comprehensive awareness campaign to educate blacks about the harmful effects of alcohol. The program had four major components: 1) organization of a community group composed of residents to address alcohol-related concerns and to work towards solutions such as peer support groups; 2) development of a community training and education program that provided information about alcohol abuse to churches, schools and youth groups; 3) implementation of a community Alcohol Awareness Day; and 4) a community slogan that was a symbol of pride—"We Cannot Stagger to Freedom."[2]

A vital part of this prevention program was to educate various segments of the community through the black churches. Most of the church leaders viewed alcohol as a sin and parishioners as weak if they drank. Through our program we were able to educate the church leaders and help them to see alcoholism not as an evil, but rather as a human response to the very real pain and oppression blacks have suffered beginning with slavery.

At present, I am involved with prevention and treatment programs for pregnant African-American women who use crack cocaine. Most of these women are in their mid-twenties and have been using crack for two to three years.

In this population, prenatal care is sought during the second trimester of pregnancy, if at all. Most women are inconsistent with their prenatal care, miss appointments repeatedly and fail to follow through with prescribed medical care. Because of the seductive and debilitating influence of crack, these women become apathetic about most things.

The highly addictive nature of crack makes it difficult for women who are using it to stop even when they become pregnant and know that the drug poses a great danger to their fetus. For instance, premature births and intrauterine strokes are prevalent among infants whose mothers used crack. There is also a high degree of sexually transmitted diseases (for example, AIDS and herpes) among these women that can directly harm and in some instances kill the baby.

Unfortunately, a high percentage of the African-American women I work with deliver newborns who test positively for cocaine in their blood and urine. Such infants, even if they are full-term, are often much smaller than comparable babies who have not been exposed to cocaine. They are very jittery at birth, are poor feeders and can require prolonged medical treatment, often in intensive care units. The enormous cost of caring for crack babies, which can run into millions of dollars, is straining an already over-burdened health care system.

Crack babies have long-term psychological and physical problems including motor deficiencies, short attention spans and erratic behavior. Because their drug-addicted mothers are unable to care for them, many of these babies are placed in the custody of other family members, often with a grandmother. From what I've seen, this practice makes it more difficult for the mother to seek treatment for her addiction. Because the child is still with a member of her family, the woman does not really feel as if she has "lost" anything by using crack. In most cases, she has regular access to the child and therefore there are no incentives to improve her condition.

While I am not advocating that children be summarily taken away from African-American women who use crack, my experience has shown me that women whose children have been taken from them tend to deal more effectively with their drug problems and are more inclined to seek treatment. Even in the haze of addiction, the bond between mother and child remains strong. Most of the mothers want their children and will consider altering their behavior to increase the probability of having them returned.

Resident programs seem to provide the best overall treatment for black women addicted to crack. Being away from the influence of friends and family members for six to eight months allows the woman to focus more directly on her recovery program. In the new environment the woman is able to concentrate on developing better coping skills and can work on improving her self-esteem. Several women I encountered in residential programs managed to stay off crack for months. But as soon as they returned to their community, the craving for crack returned. The goal of residential treatment is to help women develop skills so that they can build healthy and productive relationships with their communities when they complete the program. I believe that African-American women on crack better their chances for recovery by eliminating feelings of alienation, oppression, despair and low self-esteem from the *inside* out. I've also observed that the most successful of these women experience a spiritual awakening—in themselves, a god of their choosing, or both. These newfound beliefs often motivate the women to take the necessary steps toward recovery.

In my work, I have observed generations of black families on drugs: grandmothers, mothers, daughters; grandfathers, fathers and sons. The only possible hope I see in the face of such comprehensive disenfranchisement is community education, empowerment and alliance building.

To develop successful substance abuse treatment programs for African-Americans, it is critical to consider the culture, lifestyle and attitudes of the black community. Service providers need to know how the community defines its problems, instead of developing treatment plans based on the perceived notions of outsiders. The African-American Community Alcohol Awareness Program I mention earlier was an excellent example of an agency that did not dictate to, but rather served the needs and desires of the black community.

The agency achieved its goal by inviting numerous civic officials to work with us to increase alcohol awareness in the community. Among those who attended regular meetings were representatives from the Department of Public Works; a superintendent from the Department of Public Health; community planners; church and school leaders; store owners and residents; officials from the National Beverage Control Department and executives from major bill-board companies. Working with this powerful coalition was extremely empowering for residents who felt that no one cared about alcohol problems in the black community.

For instance, there were several billboards on the main thoroughfare of this community that advertised tobacco and alcohol. These products were presented as glamorous and necessary components of "the good life." At the coalition meetings, neighborhood residents asked the billboard company officials to replace the signs with advertisements that reflected real community needs—billboards with messages about health education, or for products such as diapers, hair care items or food. The billboard companies agreed to do this.

Residents also met with local liquor store owners to devise strategies to help reduce alcohol abuse in the neighborhood. After presenting a powerful case on the harmful effects of excessive drinking, the neighborhood group persuaded the store owners to: 1) stop selling liquor to customers who were obviously intoxicated already; 2) refuse to sell alcohol to persons who loitered and drank openly on store property; 3) refuse to sell liquor to minors; and 4) open and close their shops at standard business hours. Coming to these agreements was a great victory for the black community.

There also needs to be more culturally sensitive alcohol and drug treatment centers in the African-American community. Highly regarded twelve-step programs such as Alcoholics Anonymous cannot be as effective for blacks until such programs take into account the outlook and experiences of African-Americans. For example, the first step in AA requires alcoholics to admit they are powerless over liquor and that their lives have become unmanageable as a result of alcohol abuse. This is not an earth-shattering or cataclysmic revelation that would immediately propel a black alcoholic into treatment. Powerlessness has been a factor for most people of color all their lives. To my mind, a more culturally sensitive approach would be to address the prejudice and discrimination that have prevented so many African-Americans from fulfilling their dreams. The first step needs to go a step further and delve into the pain, depression, oppression and anger that make so many people of color want to drown their sorrows and escape.

African-Americans and other minorities who are unjustly born into oppression and face it at every turn often expect to be oppressed for the rest of their lives. Alcohol and drug abuse have become the oppressive agents for too many blacks who surely would rise were they not saddled with addiction and all the hopelessness it brings.

The solution to this problem is not easy, but we've got to try. After all, our ancestors are watching.

Footnotes

1.   Fact Sheet, California Women's Commission on Alcohol and Drug Dependencies, 14442 Victory Boulevard, Van Nuys, CA 91411.

2.   We are indebted to Denise Herd and her work, particularly "We Cannot Stagger to Freedom: A History of Blacks and Alcohol in American Politics," in L. Brill and C. Winich, eds., *Yearbook of Substance Use and Abuse*, v. 3 (New York: Human Sciences Press, 1985).

*Proving that one can recover from the most difficult of circumstances,
Lulu F. describes how she conquered her addiction to drugs and alcohol
and has become active in helping others in their recovery process.*

Black, Female and Sober
Lulu F. (as told to Rachel V.)

I was born in the South. There were five of us. I was the baby. My
mother never drank, but my father did. I remember when I was real
young my mother had taken us to church on Sunday morning. My
daddy had been out drinking the night before. We came home and
she put some rolls in the oven. I was out on the front porch playing,
and she was sitting in the big porch swing, talking with some relatives, when I looked up and seen him coming at her with a broom.
He broke that broom right over her because she'd burned the rolls.
He used to beat her quite a bit, but that was the last time. She left.
Next Tuesday we were all in school, all five of us and we got called in
to the principal's office and told to go home immediately. We just
flew out of there.

When we got home, Momma was there to get us. She hired a
man and a truck to help get us and all our things and moved us off to
a big city not too far away, where she'd found work and a place for
us to live. The man who owned the cafe at the bus station where she
was waitressing got real sick and she was able to buy the cafe from
him.

We all had to work. I was the cashier. I must have been all of
eight years old. They would have to stack up those big wooden pop
bottle cases so I could run the cash register. That's when I really
started to learn how to manipulate men for money. I used to dance
real good, and I had long, pretty red hair. It's my natural color, even
though I'm black. The men would give me money to dance, and I'd
just keep the jukebox going, and the more money you put in the
jukebox, the more money was ours. My mother remarried and I did
not get along with my stepfather. I was standing at the kitchen stove
one morning when he walked in with an erection in his pajamas and
said, "If I did something, would you tell your Momma?" I said, "I

wouldn't have to tell her because when I get through pouring this boiling water on you she'd know all about it!" So he never touched me but he made me pay for that. He'd pick fights with me just so he could whip me. We'd fight like two men. Sometimes I'd be beat up so bad I couldn't go to school. My brothers finally beat him up, and I moved out to a cousin's in another town altogether. I started to drink with my brothers when I was ten.

I was real bright, it turned out, so they sent me to a private school, a Catholic school. But I never wanted to be a good student. I just wanted to play hooky and drink. I was the big basketball star, and I loved to play football. I'm a pretty big woman, always was. One of my street names was Big Lu. Well, here I was at this nice Catholic school, and I was always getting in trouble for stuff like teaching some girls how to shoot dice in the bathroom. Finally I got kicked out for drinking.

While I was going to this school, I was living with some other relatives. Moved in with them to go there when I was about twelve years old. My relatives let me drink and smoke. But occasionally I'd have to surrender to one of the men. That was the tradeoff. Incest. It always took alcohol to do that. But finally I got fed up with that situation and that kind of tradeoff, and I left. Fell in love with a baseball player and got pregnant. I drank all through pregnancy. I was so ignorant—about everything. Well, I lost that baby, and then I drank about that. I had started into labor and the baby started coming out on the elevator when the intern who was with me on the elevator pushed the head back in. I finally got up there and delivered. Later on that night they came in and told me that my baby died. He had lived about three hours and I never got to see him. I named him after my favorite saint. That's about the most painful thing I can think of even today all these years later. I left town immediately after that, drinking and running with the ball players. Stayed in North Carolina a while, came back through the South, and ended up with a sister out on the West Coast. That's where I got into drugs.

I'm about eighteen by this time. Got introduced to marijuana. Met a lady at the store. We just started talking, and then I started going over to her house and we'd smoke grass and drink. She was a married lady, and a lesbian. That was my first. It was through going down to visit her sister in the county jail that I met a couple of pimps and that's when the other stuff started. I started picking pockets. I got real good at it. I'd say I was a prostitute to pick up a man, then we'd start toward a room, and by the time we got there I'd have already picked his pocket and had some good excuse why I couldn't go in there. Because I had his money and then I didn't need to go through all that. It was much easier than going in a whorehouse. I started stealing out of stores too, minks and diamonds, all kinds of stuff. Had a new car every year. Went to Vegas a lot, traveled. Of course I was drinking all this time and smoking marijuana too. Sometimes you'd get too hot, and you'd have to leave town. The police knew what you were up to and who you were, so I'd have to cool off somewhere else. I got my first jail time from some checks I got from picking pockets. When I got out of jail, the guys I was running with were selling drugs. I started snorting cocaine with the pimps. They made it look real glamorous. But I wasn't interested in that. I really needed a drink. I couldn't be without alcohol by this time. I always kept a bottle in the glove compartment and a flask in my purse. I remember a girl that nobody wanted to bother with. They called her Boozie. She was a good pickpocket. I liked her because she drank just like I did. We would just drink and fight. She was my kind of girl.

I got involved with a dealer who was on a run bringing back some cocaine and heroin from Mexico. We got busted. I got off and he had to do time. They brought me back to the town where I'd been living because there were three bench warrants out on me for picking pockets. I had to stay in jail a while more. When I got into court, the judge said that I was a menace to society and the only way he'd let me out of jail was if I left the state entirely. So I did. That's when I moved on and really began to get into heroin.

No more pimps. I was too slick for them. I had a Chinese man now. I was his mistress. That didn't last long. A girlfriend introduced me to her man, and we went off and got married. He was a heroin dealer. Every husband I've had, and that's four, has been an alcoholic-addict. I knew from what I saw with my daddy that that was bad, but that's always who I ended up with. Funny thing was, they never wanted me to drink or use drugs. Here's this guy cutting up heroin, snorting it all the time, and he doesn't want me to use. I'm still drinking, and I start sneaking the heroin. Finally he let me start snorting it. Three days later he locked me up in that apartment, and when he came back I had torn the place apart looking for more. This stuff was real pure, came from the Orient. He was a merchant seaman so he could get it. I was really hooked. Alcohol wasn't enough any more. Then I started selling it with him. We got busted, so we left town.

At this point I hadn't started shooting yet, I was just snorting. That's how we could tell ourselves we weren't bad, that we weren't dope fiends. I still couldn't go anywhere without a drink. By this time we've been all over the country, and we're in Colorado. I told my husband that I was going to the store to get some groceries and that's really what I meant to do. But I had to walk past a bar on the way, so I thought I'd have just one drink, then I'd get the groceries. I hadn't picked pockets in years, but there's a guy in there who buys me a drink, and when he opens his wallet and I see all the money he has I end up picking his pocket, getting caught by the police and taken to jail. That pattern just continued and got worse. Got out of jail, went to Frontier Day in Cheyenne, Wyoming. Everybody was just getting drunk and having a time. Now I was picking pockets in blackouts. I went into a bar, and the next time I looked I had five wallets and I didn't even remember picking them. I went into the bathroom and looked, and four of them were sheriffs. They were going to this bar after duty and getting drunk with the girls. The next morning my husband and I are sitting down to eat breakfast when the sheriff drove up. They were real nice about it, and they just sat in the car and waited till we finished breakfast, and then I went to jail. After that we went up north. I started shooting heroin. Still smoking marijuana and drinking and using cocaine. More blackouts, busted again. This time I got sent out of state because there was no federal prison for women there. I got in trouble there. I shot drugs, sold drugs while I was in prison. We made hooch and drank. I smoked grass. The police brought us drugs. I played softball and helped coach the team. That was the first time I ever went to an Alcoholics Anonymous meeting or started hearing about AA in prison. But I'd go there to laugh at their drunk stories and eat donuts. I'd hang around and drink coffee, but I didn't get it.

Then something happened. When I had been arrested for smuggling years before and was in jail waiting for trial, there was a lady that they put in the tank with us who got busted for drunk driving. She was real drunk, and everybody laughed at her and didn't want to bother with her. She woke up with the shakes and I could see myself in her, but I couldn't admit that to myself or anyone else at the time. She was an older woman, a professional woman, and I took care of her. Here it is now years later and I'm in prison again, and I'm walking into one of the AA meetings and I saw that lady come in. That got my attention. I was scared to death. She was in AA and she was bringing the program into the prison. I sat down and really listened, and a seed got planted. We hugged. I was so glad to see her. I was so glad for her that she was sober, because God knows she needed it. I was still denying how much I needed it, too.

When I got out of prison, it was going to be different this time. The insanity of this disease! I swore I'd never do any drugs again. It was that man's fault, wasn't it? If I just stayed away from him and drugs I'd be okay. It was the drugs that made me so crazy, not the alcohol. I tried to go back south, but even my home state wouldn't accept my parole, so I went back north. Despite all intentions, in less than a week's time I'd sold everything I could for drugs. I did not want to go back out on the streets. I knew something bad was happening. I talked to my parole officer but he couldn't really help me get a job. I couldn't tell him about the drugs but I asked him to please help me get work. There was no halfway house. I was real frustrated. They always told us in prison that if we would just get a job, get you a family, and get married then everything will be all right. But they didn't tell you about how you're going to feel or why I had to have alcohol to get up in the morning. It was everybody's fault but mine what was happening. I just couldn't see it, and no job was going to help what was wrong with me.

No job, addicted to everything, and so my husband and I are dealing again. Another dealer calls us up, wanting drugs to sell that we won't front him. He gets mad and threatens us, tells us to be ready, he's out for us. Everything's getting real crazy. We're walking down the street one night, and he walks up to us with one hand behind his back. We thought he had a gun. I pulled a pistol out of my boot and handed it to Merril—and he killed him, shot him. Threw the gun in the ocean. We didn't know he didn't have anything until he fell. In the street they call it "selling wolf tickets," bluffing like that. We got arrested and beat the case.

I met a guy in the military, dumped my husband, and left town with him to get married in his home state in the Midwest. I got out of jail, went straight to the airport as the judge had ordered, and was drunk by the time I arrived. When I got there I discovered that his mother was an alcoholic too and that was all I needed. I really want to make this marriage work. I am sick of my life. He wants me to stay home and be a wife, and I'm trying, and I'm going nuts. My parole officer was a former captain in the service and we drank together. He gave me some leads and I got a job in a chicken factory; but between my asthma and my drinking I couldn't keep a job. I'd keep a bottle in the car and was out there every break. My drinking was a lot worse now because I was trying to be good and wasn't doing any drugs. It was drugs that were the problem. If I just stayed off the drugs, I'd tell myself, I could just drink a little and it would be okay. I'd drink, and I'd go for a loaf of bread at the store and might not come home for two or three days. My husband was a nice guy, but he was alcoholic too.

Finally I met a dope lady at the bootleg house one day and started snorting again. This kept me away from home a lot. He swore I had another man, and one day when we were in the car he was drunk and mad and decided he was going to kill us both. He wrecked the car, but it didn't kill us. Broke my jaw, cut my throat, broke my leg. I just laid there. I had a spoon of dope in my bra. I managed to put it in my purse, wouldn't throw away any dope. The woman I got the dope from came to the hospital when I first got there. I told her the heroin was in my purse, and she got it out and fed it to me. Even with all the medication they gave me when the doctor got there I never passed out, that's how bad my tolerance was.

I end up going home to Mother to get well. I'm just getting worse but I don't know how to let loose of all this. So it's one year later, and I'm sitting at a red light, me and some girls that had been out stealing and drinking and drugging all day, when a truck comes up from behind and totals the car. I had just started to walk from the year before when this happened. Next day I'm hurting and I call my mother and ask for help for the first time. She said, "I'll take you to my neighbor. This man used to go outside naked and fall down all the time and he went somewhere for two to three months and he came back okay, and he's been all right ever since." I said, "You don't understand, that's not what I'm talking about. I have this physical problem from this accident. I don't know why you're talking about this neighbor." I know that neighbor had gone to treatment and is now in AA. I got referred to a doctor who examined me, and I finally said, "I think I have another problem. Alcohol and drugs." He knew all about it and arranged for me to go into a women's halfway house after I got out of the hospital, where I'd ended up again. We called AA, and somebody came down to the hospital to see me. That's when I really got the message.

AA people are the only people in the world that had come to me for anything, and they gave me something and I didn't have to do anything. Just be me. I really used to act up. My mouth was real bad, foul. I only knew the way of the streets, and that's the only way I knew how to express myself. They tolerated me at any and all levels. They brought AA to the hospital, and they took me to meetings when I got out. That's the first time I remember saying a prayer since I was a child except when I was drunk. People made me feel like I belonged, no matter what I had done.

There was a speaker at the first meeting I went to out at the hospital that I could identify with. I started hearing about feelings. I didn't know anything about feelings, I had drowned them with alcohol and drugs so long ago I didn't know I had any anymore. I didn't know anything about resentment. I didn't "resent" people, I just didn't like them. I didn't take the time to just "resent" you, you know. I did not know that anger motivated me to function all my life. And I didn't know that anger is a form of fear. I learned all this in this program. I didn't know what those knots were when I woke up in the morning—the ones that feel like donuts in your stomach they're so big. I didn't know that was fear. I didn't know that I was always scared of what was going to happen that day and by the time I got through with that day, something *had* happened. I sure didn't know that I was my problem. I thought it was everyone else. I didn't know that every single problem I had, I had in some way or another created. It's my attitude toward a particular situation that makes it a problem for me. I'm a crisis junkie, most alcoholics and addicts are. If I didn't have a crisis in my life, I'd go out and create one, then I'd be fine. I had you to blame for the way that I was feeling, then I could get drunk, get loaded, and it was somebody else's fault. I didn't know that I didn't have to worry about everything. Today the God of my understanding shows me that I don't have to worry, that all I have to do is get my ego out of the way, and that I'll be taken care of. Any problem I have, I don't care how upset I was with it, if I just let go of it long enough and ask God to take care of it for me and help me, it always turns out better than anything I could have made of it.

When I came to AA—eight years ago now—there were only two other black women coming to meetings. Now this is a big city. One of them was dropping pills, so I couldn't turn to her. The other one was too damn nice for me. She had over twelve years in the program, but I couldn't relate to her, our experiences were so different. She was middle-class. I came off the street. So here I am a black woman in this big old town, and the only people I got to identify with are the people they told me were fucking me over all my life, and that's white people. Keeping me without nothing. Even when I go to meetings now, there often aren't black people unless I bring them with me. But it just doesn't bother me. I talk and share just the same because AA works no matter what the color of your skin. I was never taught to be prejudiced. But when you're looking for an excuse not to change, the first excuse the black person has is "I can't identify with or relate to those white people." I heard Betty Ford talk one time, and we felt exactly the same way; she just had more money to spend than

I did. Thank God I didn't have it or I would have been dead. That's just an excuse, saying, "I can't identify, I can't relate, this is a white folk's program." I took a young woman into a meeting with me and she said, "Oh, but look at all those white people!" And I said to her, "Where did you see a sign that says, 'No Niggers are supposed to be here'? Did anybody ever tell you that in AA?" After the meeting she couldn't get over how nice everybody was and how many white friends I had that had come up and hugged me, wanted to know how I am. I can't tell you how good I have been made to feel in the program of Alcoholics Anonymous.

I went to an AA convention not too long after I came into the program. I was sitting in the hotel lobby talking to a lady from that town, telling her that AA was different in her town, that back at my home people were really friendly. She asked me how many people I had gone up to and introduced myself to, and she was right on. I wasn't reaching out to anybody. I thought because I was one of the six blacks out of six hundred people that they were supposed to make me special and come up to me.

I've learned how to have friendships with men in this program, that means without sex being involved, just as people. You know, it made me feel real good to understand that I have a disease and that it took being a drunk and a dope fiend to take advantage of people and do the things I did because I can't do that sober. I have changed so much through working this program that it's almost like talking to another person to tell all this.

My way of staying sober is continuing to work with drunks and addicts. I started a residential treatment program. That business about sharing and giving away was imbedded in me. People and God have given me so much that I have to keep giving it away. So I just went out and got a building and some drunks and started working with them. I've always wanted to give to people; we all do, I just never knew how before, too busy doing myself in. All I've got is me and my experience, strength, and hope, and that's enough today. God loves me just like he loves you, and he has forgiven me for what I did. It's today that counts.

Today we don't turn anybody away here. We're getting involved with kids. We've taken the parolees, all sorts of folks that nobody else knew how to handle, but I do. The elderly alcoholic woman. Nobody wants her. But we take them. If we don't have room, we make room. I didn't have anywhere to go when I got out as a parolee and I haven't forgotten where I come from. The elderly woman has nowhere to go either. Nobody wants to mess with you when you get old. Regardless of why they end up here, the bottom line is almost all of them had some kind of alcohol problem or they're hooked on pills. We see so many now of the elderly hooked on pills. Pain medication. It's more loneliness, sometimes, than anything.

I hope I never go back out again and drink or use, because I don't think I'd make it back. I'd wind up dead. God has been so good to me. Everything that I need as a human being to be happy again has been given to me through this program, just like people told me, if I would just be patient. I'm happily married, I have a child. One day at a time. I just got a big award for outstanding community service, can you believe that!

Smoking-related illnesses kill nearly a thousand people a day in America. Smoking has been scientifically linked to cancer, heart disease, emphysema, bronchitis, spontaneous abortions, birth defects, infant mortality and high blood pressure. According to medical experts, cigarettes have a far worse addictive potential than either alcohol or heroin.

Nearly thirty-eight percent of African-Americans smoke. A large proportion of the nearly seven million dollars in advertising the tobacco industry spends each day is targeted at the black community.

Stopping smoking is perhaps the single most important step a black woman can take toward achieving a healthier and longer life. In the following piece, the author offers hope to all who are trying to give up cigarettes.

Look for Guidance: How I Stopped Smoking
Mary Lou Lee

I started smoking when I was twenty-one years old. I had seen other young ladies smoking and I thought they really looked good. I made up my mind to look good, too. I was grown, why not? No one had warned me of the dangers of tobacco. This was in 1933.

I suffered three weeks trying to inhale and look all grown-up. Because of self-consciousness, I decided never to smoke while walking in the streets.

Smoking is a progressive type of habit. At first, one package of cigs would last at least three days. Toward the end of my smoking career, I was using two packs a day. I found myself having special reasons for smoking, such as getting up in the morning, after each meal or after finishing any type of task. Yes, in the middle of the night on my way to the bathroom, I would reward myself with a cigarette. The sight of someone else smoking or sitting in my car as it warmed up, brought me a reason or an opportunity to light up.

Back in the old days, very few friends would ask you not to smoke. Consequently, after social activities their homes would smell like public bars. My body, hair and breath reeked with the smell of old tobacco mixed with fine perfumes. I did not realize how awful smokers smell until I stopped smoking.

My clothes were burn-spotted. My furniture, both wood and cloth, also had burn marks. I smoked around my friends even though I knew some of them had respiratory ailments. This smoking addiction went on for the next fifty-four years. I raised a child, worked with girl scouts and my church, all the time puffing away.

Then came the warnings—chest pains, hacking cough, trouble breathing. I was afraid! I tried many times to stop smoking, sometimes I even made it for a whole day. The longest I ever quit was for two months. I did that by using nicotine gum. I'd say to myself, "Oh boy, I deserve a treat. I haven't smoked for two months." I'd light up and one cigarette would have me addicted all over again.

I had asked God to remove this nasty habit from me. My family begged me to stop smoking. I did not heed their words until I had a heart attack in 1987. I'll never forget it.

The doctor sat across from me in the intensive care room and asked slowly and softly, "Mrs. Lee, do you smoke?" "Yes," I replied, feebly. "It is imperative that you stop!" He did not have to explain why. I have not had a desire to smoke since.

I damaged my lungs only to the extent that they are now subject to frequent respiratory afflictions. But I have managed to avoid the big-C (cancer)—thank God!

I truly regret having abused my body in such a manner. It must have been a strong healthy body in the beginning for I am now seventy-seven years old and except for the heart attack, I have yet to suffer a serious disease of any kind.

Now I can detect a smoker a mile away. My house no longer reeks of smoke, there are no burns on my furniture and my dresses do not have little tobacco-inflicted holes in them.

The sweetest words I have heard since my great victory over tobacco are, "Smoking or non-smoking?" "Non-smoking, please," I reply, while thinking, "and I thank you Jesus."

I realize now that no one can really help smokers unless the desire to quit comes from within. They must be willing to stop puffing either because of fears of medical problems or simply because smoking is increasingly frowned upon by society.

I remember praying many times for God to remove the cross of smoking from me. I actually waited for the miracle to happen. I thought I would just wake up one day without the desire to smoke.

As the years rolled by, I began to notice the disgust in the faces of family and friends as I continued to smoke one cigarette after another. By now the dangers of smoking were known to everyone. "Bad vibrations" were being directed at smokers. I wasn't "cute" any more.

My advice to anyone who wants to stop smoking is to search and hunt for your way out. Sometimes getting another person to support you in your efforts can help.

To guide me, I used Abraham, one of my favorite heroes from the Bible. Abraham was about to make a burnt offering of his son Isaac to please God. Seeing Abraham's willingness to sacrifice his beloved son, God told him to look in the brush where he would find a ram to sacrifice instead. I know now that our higher power will always have a ram in the bushes for us. In other words, an option. My ram turned out to be an opportunity to live free of being a hostage to tobacco.

In February 1987, I was healed of the smoking addiction that had plagued my life for fifty-four years. The habit left me because I know I love life. I came very close to losing this precious gift because of a stupid habit.

I sympathize with all those who have not yet been healed of the smoking addiction and my advice to you is the same that God gave to Abraham. Look for guidance.

In the past two decades American women have gotten increasingly heavier. This trend has been even greater for black women. According to researchers, nearly thirty-five percent of all black women between the ages of twenty and forty-four are overweight, or twenty percent above the ideal body weight for their height, frame and age. An alarming fifty percent of black women forty-five to fifty-five years of age weigh far more than they should. Excess weight puts people at higher risk for heart disease, diabetes, high blood pressure and other conditions that are prevalent in the black community. Researchers believe that social factors including self-image, career and marital expectations, education, images in the media and role models can influence weight gain.

In the piece that follows, the author tells her personal story of dealing with obesity.

Coming Home: One Black Woman's Journey to Health and Fitness
Georgiana Arnold

I was not a fat child. My earliest photos depict a big-eyed, brown-skinned girl with a shy smile and slim arms and legs. And I just loved walking to school; for me, it was like being invited to a progressive party. I would set out eagerly from my Seattle home and then quickly accumulate friends along the way. Our conversations revolved around sports, games, Davy Crockett and hushed references to classmates who had caught polio. I remember Glenda so well—she was blond, beautiful, serious and very articulate. "Now Georgiana," she would admonish after I had volunteered some unsolicited advice, "this is not your affair." Properly chastised, I would follow her to school in silent adoration, anyway. Then there was Kathy, the undisputed queen of our second-grade class. Her honey-olive skin, dark curly hair and rich, silky laugh clinched her celestial status. Even then she had the easy assurance of those who are born to beauty, power and popularity.

From my self-selected and/or designated hiding place, I soon realized that I was different—not white, rich or beautiful. I was humored, I was tolerated, I was patronized, but not loved, like Kathy or Glenda.

When I was in fifth grade, my mother, who had separated from my father when I was five, moved us in with the Thorn family. Shared accommodations made it easier for my mother, the sole breadwinner to provide for her five children. Florence "Polly" Thorn was a large, beautiful woman who liked to cook and loved to eat. Fried chicken, smothered steak, and rice served with gravies and sauces were on her menu every day. I ate heartily and soon began to lose the trim, athletic physique that helped me excel at track, tether-ball, kickball and other sports. It never occurred to me that my ravenous hunger might be connected to my father's absence and subsequent death. To silence my grief, anger and rage, I sought solace in eating. Food became my best friend.

By my eleventh birthday, I had gained a substantial amount of weight. I still played baseball and basketball, but I was beginning to lose some of my speed and agility. Truth is, I was more perplexed than disturbed by my increasing girth. But that changed forever after one of my classmates referred to me as a "tub." We had just finished eating glazed donuts (I would eat one or two to everyone else's four or five and yet they were skinny and I was not). I still remember the blood rushing to my face and the thunder of my heart beat. I laughed with everyone, but the humiliation I experienced was indescribable. All of my life I had strived to fit in or fade in and now here I stood, exposed to the derision of my friends. If I needed further confirmation of my "tub"-like status, it was soon forthcoming.

After exhausting the largest sizes in the girls' section of the local department store, my mother, over my strenuous objections, began purchasing my clothes in the "chubette" salon. I painfully remember the outfits as shapeless sacks, but what other options were there for a twelve-year-old girl who wore a size 18? The "chubette" salon was the final public confirmation of my difference and prompted my retreat to the sidelines of life in earnest. From then on, I hid out in big coats and oversized blouses. I buried myself in school, films and music, especially rock and roll because the liveliness of the music made me feel alive and connected.

My mother voiced her feelings about my rapid weight gain in the fleeting and inconsistent admonitions that characterized our communication and through the diet school lunches she prepared for me during my elementary and high school years. My struggles with food and body image were mirrored by my sisters and brother who also gained weight during puberty. In our home, food was a source

of nourishment, a sign of love, a reward and the heart of family cele-
brations. It was also a source of ambivalence, guilt, shame and conflict. Our "family fat" issues descended into the same cavern of silence that housed my father's alcoholism, gambling, and willful dis-
appearance from our lives. There was no talking about it and there
were no tears.

As an "A" student at the predominantly white Holy Names Academy, I attained the recognition and acceptance reserved for excep-
tional black youngsters. But the newfound attention confused and
frightened me. Isolated from my culture, I felt like a fraud. But instead of reaching out for help (after all, I was only fifteen), I continued my flight into food, books, films and music. A box of Good 'N
Plenty was my treat for my walk home from school, Milk Duds and
Rollos my movie candy, a quart of Coke my incentive to walk home
from church, and gigantic bologna sandwiches slathered in mayonnaise my late-night snack.

Recurring episodes of depression which had blanketed my
childhood like the rain over Seattle were now more noticeable. One
night as I lay in bed, I said a desperate prayer—"God, surely black
people must dream. I have dreams and I'm black." But at Holy
Names, the history books taught me about the degradation of slavery instead of the majestic empires of Ghana or Mali. As I sat in the
midst of my white classmates, this information made me feel
ashamed of black people. I didn't want to be associated with happy
slaves singing in the fields!

It was at this point during my teen years that I was introduced to
Dr. Clinton, crash diets and diet pills. Reports of his success had
spread to every social strata of Seattle, including the city's small
black community. At my enthusiastic insistence, my mother enrolled me in Dr. Clinton's regime of amphetamine pills and injections. After several weeks of the program, I'd lost twenty-seven
pounds and was gloating over my swan-like neck and trim arms. My
drug-induced euphoria lifted me above my constant food cravings.
But knowing nothing about nutrition, moderation or maintenance,
the effects of Dr. Clinton's program soon wore off. In a short time, I
was fat again and had retreated back into my inner universe. At the
movies, I became mesmerized by the pristine beauty of Grace Kelly
and the aristocratic elegance of Audrey Hepburn. They were everything that I longed to be: beautiful, slender, white and loved!

As one of three hundred blacks out of 23,000 students at the University of Washington, I felt isolated and totally overwhelmed. The
academic competition was fierce and there were no people of color in

sight. In four whole years, I never encountered a professor, instructor or employee of color (except janitors and gardeners). My grades were good, but with no role models I felt like an imposter and lived in abject fear of failing. In the university but not of it, I sought out food as my comfort and friend. I began to eat before, during and after studying. I would eat and ache and eat again.

When I was twenty, I had my first physical exam (believe it or not, I never had one when I was in the clutches of the diet doctor). During the course of the examination, the doctor informed me that I had dangerously high blood pressure. Suddenly the copious and inexplicable nose bleeds made sense. "They may have saved your life," he said. Toward the end of the exam, he announced that he wanted to record my height and weight. I hesitated, but finally got on the scale and watched in utter mortification as the nurse adjusted the weights from 175 to 190, then 200 and finally to 220 pounds. I was stunned, horrified and immobilized with self-loathing. Soon afterward, I was asked to serve punch at a friend's wedding. The only suitable dress I had was a lovely gown I'd worn to a formal dance during my senior year in high school. The dress was still beautiful, but I was 50 pounds heavier. I cringed at my reflection in the mirror. It was this distressing apparition far more than my impaired health that propelled me into action. I got down to 210.

To celebrate my graduation from college, I decided to go to Europe with three of my girlfriends. Imagine—four black women from Seattle travelling to Europe in 1967. It was unheard of, but we got jobs, saved our money and did it.

In the late 1960s, a post-graduate trip to Europe was considered a rite of passage for millions of American students. Back then, international travel was exhilarating, chic and inexpensive. We arrived in London's Heathrow Airport on a cool, rainy June day. After a whirlwind tour of London, we picked up our rental car in Belgium and began a journey that would take us through Luxembourg, Germany, Switzerland, Austria, Italy, Spain, France, Monaco, Portugal and the Netherlands.

It was an extraordinary trip and it transformed my life in ways that were not immediately apparent, even to me. In retrospect, I realize that this was my first encounter with politicized people of color. We met Africans, Indians, Pakistanis and Jamaicans during the trip. Their ideas and their lives challenged my erroneous and circumscribed perceptions of people of color. I was profoundly disturbed to realize that I had looked at Africa and myself through the distorted prism of racism. For the first time in my life, I had a seed of hope. I could sense but not yet see the possibilities of my life. I still lacked the encouragement and self-esteem to transform my hope into desire, then into vision and finally reality.

When I returned to Seattle in September, I was energized, tanned and thirty pounds lighter. The weight loss was pleasant but short-lived because I was still totally ignorant of nutrition, food preparation, portion control and exercise.

My first permanent job as an employment counselor with the Washington State Employment Security Department did not help matters. My freedom-loving spirit was completely throttled by the numbing sameness of the place. Everyone reported to work at 8:00 a.m. EXACTLY; coffee breaks were at 10:00 a.m. and 2:00 p.m. EXACTLY; the work day concluded at 5:00 p.m. EXACTLY. In light of this deadening situation, the comforting allure of my old "friends" became irresistible. I ate to get myself to work, I ate to get myself through the work day, and I ate to reward myself for surviving until five o'clock. Taking refuge in Vienna sausages, donuts, jelly beans, Good 'N Plenty, Snickers, Oreos with ice cream, and of course giant bologna and mayonnaise sandwiches, I was soon back to my pre-European weight of 210 pounds.

I don't remember how I heard about the Stillman Program, but I do know that I was young, eager and hell-bent on being thin. I purchased the book and went on the diet. One week later I was weak, exhausted and thirteen pounds lighter. I was delighted with the weight loss and determined to achieve a thin, attractive body. Eventually headaches, heart palpitations and other symptoms forced me to modify the all-protein diet by including fruits, vegetables and other low-calorie carbohydrates. But I continued to lose weight and by the time I left for a teaching job in the Bahamas in the early 1970s, I weighed 156 pounds.

Isolated and with few friends, my first year on the island was fraught with disappointments. I solved them as I always had—with food. But my pride and tenacity eventually paid off, ultimately making my time in the Bahamas very rewarding. "Hi slim!" someone called out as I returned from an errand one evening, after getting down to a svelte 135 pounds. I was astounded. "Someone called me slim," I repeated to myself. But slim didn't stay for long. Unhappiness and calories soon crept back into my life again.

My post-Bahamas malaise was alleviated by exposure to the arts and my decision to get a masters degree in public health education. Unlike my undergraduate years, I flourished in this demanding yet challenging, exciting and relevant course of study.

In September 1977, I decided to lose weight... again. By that time I'd been a disciple of Weight Watchers, the Stillman Diet, the Cambridge Plan, the grapefruit and egg diet, the Scarsdale diet and many others. This time, I'd develop my own regimen consisting of a 1,200-calorie meal plan and exercise, especially jogging. It worked. I went from 168 pounds to 135 in seven months.

A viral disorder dropped me down to 133 pounds just in time for graduation. At my commencement I looked thin and hopeful in my purple and gold robe. I had completed my graduate studies with a near-perfect grade-point average, written a challenging thesis and regained the trim physique of my early childhood. It was one of the happiest moments of my life.

I was thrilled with my slender appearance. Unfortunately, it was just that, the appearance of thinness. Success still terrified me, and within weeks, my scale began to reflect this unresolved conflict. I soon got a job in the Health Education Department of Group Health Cooperative of Puget Sound. I should have been ecstatic, but instead I was riddled with self-doubt. The aching emptiness and insecurity returned and soon I was on the run again from the challenge and the scrutiny. Despite my desperate efforts, the frightened child in me edged back to the comfort of her devoted "friends." My weight crept back up to 138, then 140 (I started an exercise class), 145 (I exercised three times a week), 148! I was the only one who knew about the broken promise, but every retreat pierced my spirit. My easily damaged self-esteem began to quiver, quake, then collapsed.

In 1980, I got a job with the Seattle-King County Department of Public Health. It was a challenging position that offered me visibility and an unprecedented opportunity to apply the skills I had accumulated during the previous twelve years. But when I reported for work, I was consumed by fear and insecurity. My sensors were on red alert and the smell of failure was in the air. I gradually settled into my new routine and, as usual, gained weight.

Unable to reach out to my predominantly white colleagues for help, I floundered in silence. My retreat from professional associates increased my sense of isolation and infuriated some of my co-workers. In a misguided attempt to bring stability into my unhappy and chaotic life, I purchased a condominium. It quickly devoured my tiny paychecks and thrust me into the burgeoning ranks of America's house poor. When previous depressions had threatened to overwhelm me, I would take "fix it" trips to California or my favorite department store. Now shopping and travel were out of the question. I was imprisoned by an insistent mortgage and a deepening emotional malaise.

Memories of that period are still too painful to fully share, but I knew that something was terribly wrong. My perpetually polite public face began to crumble and my rage erupted at embarrassing and inopportune moments. For example, a fellow bus rider's rude remarks and behavior one day triggered an outraged response from me that silenced the boisterous passengers. I will never forget the heat of my fury nor the abject fear that I read on the woman's face. All I recall is her neck and her terrified eyes, which stilled my screaming curses and readied fists. The void that I had sensed all my life had finally overtaken me. I crashed into a black hole that snuffed out all of my hope. Ironically, no one clearly recognized the depths of my despair. All my life I had been described as an "intelligent, together sister." No one expected to see me on my knees, so when I fell, everyone was looking up . . . at the image.

In 1982, I met a woman named Marilyn Thadden at her Adventures in Healthy Living Weekend in West Seattle. She introduced me and my fellow escapees to visualization, nutrition, exercise, relaxation techniques, reflexology and long, leisurely walks. Marilyn cooked wonderful low-fat, low-sodium meals and allowed us to draw, write and discuss our dreams. My drawing depicted a figure (me) imprisoned in chains and surrounded by storm clouds. "I want to break out of my chains," I volunteered, "and reach up to the light and love that await me." The retreat was the first ray of hope that I had experienced in a long time. The two-day respite from depression was my first tentative step away from painful family memories and back home . . . to me.

The following year, I attended the First National Conference on Black Women's Health Issues at Spelman College in Atlanta, Georgia. The black women who participated were there to share and speak the truth. We discussed the tough issues: internalized racism, low self-esteem, alcohol/drug abuse, sexual abuse, family violence and empowerment. Those four glorious days were the most loving response to my prayer of long ago. They showed me that, yes, black people do dream and achieve.

After a failed attempt to stave off gall stones with a change in diet, I found myself desperately ill in 1987. Though my weight plunged from 163 to 150 pounds, I was not pleased. One Saturday afternoon, as I lay half asleep on my mother's couch, a soft Southern accent coming from the television brought me back to consciousness. "If that's another evangelist... ," I hissed to no one in particular. As I opened my eyes and listened, I discovered he was not an evangelist, but a therapist, teacher and healer named John Bradshaw. He began to talk about children and dysfunctional families and the healing power of speaking and sharing the truth.

For me, both his message and his presentation were magnetic. I made a commitment to take his ten-week course and to keep a journal. I had just finished reading M. Scott Peck's *The Road Less Traveled* and knew that this was the next step of my long-delayed journey into my inner universe. It was an excruciating trip. I sobbed my way through the course, confronting my most deeply repressed traumas of family loss and disappointment. I eventually had to have surgery for my gall stones. I continued Bradshaw's program through my hospitalization and recuperation. I had prayed for health and healing and now I was receiving both.

Through my healing, I discovered that empowerment is a risky business. You have to come out of hiding, acknowledge your pain and then examine it. You have to shed your carefully cultivated public face, a process which can be especially terrifying for black women. You have to dig around in the muck that made you sick in the first place and you can't wear rubber gloves.

I recovered from my surgery and at last was on the road to recovering myself. With the return of my physical and spiritual health, I began to make plans to travel to Africa. I followed Professor Ali Mazrui's telecourse "The Africans: The Triple Heritage" and devoured every travel book, article and brochure on Africa that I could find. After months of study, I finally decided to visit Senegal, The Gambia and Togo. As the dream of returning to Africa became a reality, I set out toward another more elusive goal: permanent weight loss.

On May 5, 1987, I began a weight reduction program that included a balanced, very-low-calorie diet, daily weigh-ins, counseling, nutrition education and vigorous exercise. It was a grueling regimen. The diet-binge cycles of my twenties and the cyclical weight loss-weight gain patterns of my thirties had severely damaged my body and my self-confidence. But my family's history of adult onset diabetes, high blood pressure and cancer of the colon gave my quest for health an added urgency. I also discovered that I had fluctuating blood sugar, a subtle dysfunction that produces fatigue, intense hunger and a feeling of being out of control. My lifelong addiction to sugar was, in part, an inappropriate response to this condition.

In my single-minded pursuit of thinness, I put my body through a punishing routine, but by mid-July, I had reached my weight goal of 135 pounds. I had lost thirty-two pounds in eleven weeks and Africa was just two weeks away.

My girlfriend Sandy and I arrived in Dakar in early August. As our plane touched down, many of the black Americans on board began to weep. Our African companions were perplexed and a bit surprised, but we knew that this homecoming was the fulfillment of the broken dreams of our great, great, great, great-grandparents. Yes, indeed, black people do achieve their dreams.

Epilogue

I completed my weight loss program in July 1987. Since then, I have maintained a weight of 135 pounds (to within five pounds) by continuing the inner healing and empowerment process I initiated in 1983 and by adhering to a program that includes frequent aerobic exercise (four to six times a week) and a balanced, low-fat, high complex-carbohydrate diet. My weight loss was the result rather than the cause of my inner healing. Hence I am reluctant to share diet or exercise "tips." However, I realize that everyone is different and, for some women, weight loss may be the catalyst for other behavioral changes including empowerment.

Weight reduction is an exhilarating, but temporary state. Maintenance is forever. It requires vision, perseverance, creativity, assertiveness and a sense of humor. You will have to experiment to determine which techniques work best for you. I have found the following blueprint to be especially helpful for me.

Aerobic exercise, which burns calories and reduces stress, is the cornerstone of my maintenance program. In addition to my aerobic classes, I often walk to work (twenty-five minutes), in rain or shine, and continue to walk as often as I can during the day. To improve the tone and definition of my upper body, I also do weight training at least two times a week. In addition to these broad outlines, I would like to share the following recommendations with black women who are trying to lose weight. All exercise and diet programs should be supervised by a licensed physician.

1. Learn to monitor and control your reaction to stress. You may not be able to control the number and/or intensity of the stressors in your life, but you can control your reaction to them. Incorporate relaxation techniques into your daily schedule. They don't have to be elaborate. A few moments of prayer, meditation and/or deep

breathing will usually suffice. Stress management takes very little time but a lot of practice. Be patient and keep practicing your new skills.

2. Visualize how you look, feel and think in your healthier, slimmer body. Visualize in the present tense: for example, I am a trim, toned woman.

3. Incorporate aerobic exercise into your life. Aerobic exercise reduces body fat and strengthens your heart and lungs. You need a minimum of three twenty-minute sessions (within your target range) each week. Begin slowly. Aerobic exercises include brisk walking, high- and low-impact aerobic dancing or exercise classes, cycling, swimming, rowing, jogging and cross-country skiing. There are machines available which make it possible to do many of these activities in your home.

4. Eat more complex carbohydrates including whole grain breads, cereals, crackers, beans and lentils, brown rice, fruits and vegetables. Complex carbohydrates should be the most substantial part of your diet.

5. Reduce your consumption of fat to twenty percent or less of your daily calories. Read labels carefully and remember that one gram of fat has twice the calories contained in one gram of protein or carbohydrate. Eat more fish (baked or broiled) and poultry (without the skin) and less red meat and whole-fat dairy products. Bake, steam, or broil your fish, poultry and meat.

6. Cut down on salt, especially if high blood pressure runs in your family. Use lemon, garlic, ginger and other spices to season your food.

7. Give yourself periodic rewards as reminders that you are worth the effort. Self-care gifts may include a fitness magazine or book (check your local library), a master exercise class, music from one of your favorite artists, an article of clothing in a style and size appropriate to the new you, a haircut or treatment at your favorite salon, a facial, a massage, or a weekend at a health spa. Use your imagination!

8. Eat on time. This is critical if you have low or fluctuating blood sugar. Always carry an emergency "stash" of fresh fruit, fresh vegetables, low-fat yogurt, whole grain bread/crackers, or low-fat cottage cheese. A ready supply of these items will help you resist the unhealthy foods and beverages that no longer fit your new life.

9. Plan ahead and be prepared. Remember you, and no one else, are in control of your body. Organization is the foundation of discipline and discipline is the touchstone of successful weight maintenance.

Finally, be realistic. What size is your body frame? How old are you? Did you gain weight as an adult or have you been obese for many years? All of these factors will influence your weight loss and maintenance programs. If you have the muscular build of a Jackie Joyner-Kersee, you will never have the willowy appearance of a Naomi Sims. No amount of diet/exercise will transform a statuesque body into a model-thin one. Strive to achieve *your* best body, not someone else's. Good luck and keep reaching for your dreams!

Self-love and a positive self-image are likely to enhance one's health. Unfortunately, society's mirror presents all too many negative images of black women.

For black women with visible or hidden disabilities, it can be especially difficult to learn how to love oneself and celebrate being different. In the following piece, Pulitzer Prize-winning author Alice Walker writes of losing her right eye in a childhood accident and discovering that true beauty emanates from the spirit, not from outward appearances.

Beauty: When the Other Dancer is the Self
Alice Walker

It is a bright summer day in 1947. My father, a fat, funny man with beautiful eyes and a subversive wit, is trying to decide which of his eight children he will take with him to the county fair. My mother, of course, will not go. She is knocked out from getting most of us ready: I hold my neck stiff against the pressure of her knuckles as she hastily completes the braiding and then beribboning of my hair.

My father is the driver for the rich old white lady up the road. Her name is Miss Mey. She owns all the land for miles around, as well as the house in which we live. All I remember about her is that she once offered to pay my mother thirty-five cents for cleaning her house, raking up piles of her magnolia leaves, and washing her family's clothes, and that my mother—she of no money, eight children, and a chronic earache—refused it. But I do not think of this in 1947. I am two and a half years old. I want to go everywhere my daddy goes. I am excited at the prospect of riding in a car. Someone has told me fairs are fun. That there is room in the car for only three of us doesn't faze me at all. Whirling happily in my starchy frock, showing off my biscuit-polished patent-leather shoes and lavender socks, tossing my head in a way that makes my ribbons bounce, I stand, hands on hips, before my father. "Take me, Daddy," I say with assurance; "I'm the prettiest!"

Later, it does not surprise me to find myself in Miss Mey's shiny black car, sharing the back seat with the other lucky ones. Does not surprise me that I thoroughly enjoy the fair. At home that night I tell the unlucky ones all I can remember about the merry-go-round, the man who eats live chickens, and the teddy bears, until they say: that's enough, baby Alice. Shut up now, and go to sleep.

It is Easter Sunday, 1950. I am dressed in a green, flocked, scalloped-hem dress (handmade by my adoring sister, Ruth) that has its own smooth satin petticoat and tiny hot-pink roses tucked into each scallop. My shoes, new T-strap patent leather, again highly biscuit-polished. I am six years old and have learned one of the longest Easter speeches to be heard that day, totally unlike the speech I said when I was two: "Easter lilies/ pure and white/ blossom in/ the morning light." When I rise to give my speech I do so on a great wave of love and pride and expectation. People in church stop rustling their new crinolines. They seem to hold their breath. I can tell they admire my dress, but it is my spirit, bordering on sassiness (womanishness), they secretly applaud.

"That girl's a little *mess*," they whisper to each other, pleased.

Naturally I say my speech without stammer or pause, unlike those who stutter, stammer or worst of all, forget. This is before the word "beautiful" exists in people's vocabulary, but "Oh, isn't she the *cutest* thing!" frequently floats my way. "And got so much sense!" they gratefully add... for which thoughtful addition I thank them to this day.

It was great fun being cute. But then one day, it ended.

I am eight years old and a tomboy. I have a cowboy hat, cowboy boots, checkered shirt and pants, all red. My playmates are my brothers, two and four years older than I. Their colors are black and green, the only difference in the way we are dressed. On Saturday nights we all go to the picture show, even my mother; Westerns are her favorite kind of movie. Back home, "on the ranch," we pretend we are Tom Mix, Hopalong Cassidy, Lash LaRue (we've even named one of our four dogs Lash LaRue); we chase each other for hours rustling cattle, being outlaws, delivering damsels from distress. Then my parents decide to buy my brothers guns. These are not "real" guns. They shoot "BBs," copper pellets my brothers say will kill birds. Because I am a girl, I do not get a gun. Instantly I am relegated to the position of Indian. Now there appears a great distance between us. They shoot and shoot at everything with their new guns. I try to keep up with my bow and arrows.

One day while I am standing on top of our makeshift "garage"— pieces of tin nailed across some poles—holding my bow and arrow and looking out toward the fields, I feel an incredible blow in my right eye. I look down just in time to see my brother lower his gun.

Both brothers rush to my side. My eye stings, and I cover it with my hand. "If you tell," they say, "we will get a whipping. You don't want that to happen, do you?" I do not. "Here is a piece of wire," says the older brother, picking it up from the roof; "say you stepped on one end of it and the other flew up and hit you." The pain is beginning to start. "Yes," I say. "Yes, I will say that is what happened." If I do not say this is what happened, I know my brothers will find ways to make me wish I had. But now I will say anything that gets me to my mother.

Confronted by our parents we stick to the lie agreed upon. They place me on a bench on the porch and I close my left eye while they examine the right. There is a tree growing from underneath the porch that climbs past the railing to the roof. It is the last thing my right eye sees. I watch as its trunk, its branches, and then its leaves are blotted out by the rising blood.

I am in shock. First there is intense fever, which my father tries to break using lily leaves bound around my head. Then there are chills: my mother tries to get me to eat soup. Eventually, I do not know how, my parents learn what has happened. A week after the "accident" they take me to see a doctor. "Why did you wait so long to come?" he asks, looking into my eye and shaking his head. "Eyes are sympathetic," he says. "If one is blind, the other will likely become blind too."

This comment of the doctor's terrifies me. But it is really how I look that bothers me most. Where the BB pellet struck there is a glob of whitish scar tissue, a hideous cataract, on my eye. Now when I stare at people—a favorite pastime, up to now—they will stare back. Not at the "cute" little girl, but at her scar. For six years I do not stare at anyone, because I do not raise my head.

Years later, in the throes of a mid-life crisis, I ask my mother and sister whether I changed after the "accident." "No," they say, puzzled. "What do you mean?"

What do I mean?

I am eight, and, for the first time, doing poorly in school, where I have been something of a whiz since I was four. We have just moved to the place where the "accident" occurred. We do not know any of the people around us because this is a different county. The only time I see the friends I knew is when we go back to our old church.

The new school is the former state penitentiary. It is a large stone building, cold and drafty, crammed to overflowing with boisterous, ill-disciplined children. On the third floor there is a huge circular imprint of some partition that has been torn out.

"What used to be here?" I ask a sullen girl next to me on our way past it to lunch.

"The electric chair," says she.

At night I have nightmares about the electric chair, and about all the people reputedly "fried" in it. I am afraid of the school, where all the students seem to be budding criminals.

"What's the matter with your eye?" they ask, critically.

When I don't answer (I cannot decide whether it was an "accident" or not), they shove me, insist on a fight.

My brother, the one who created the story about the wire, comes to my rescue. But then brags so much about "protecting" me, I become sick.

After months of torture at the school, my parents decide to send me back to our old community, to my old school. I live with my grandparents and the teacher they board. But there is no room for Phoebe, my cat. By the time my grandparents decide there *is* room and I ask for my cat, she cannot be found. Miss Yarborough, the boarding teacher, takes me under her wing, and begins to teach me to play the piano. But soon she marries an African—a "prince," she says—and is whisked away to his continent.

At my old school there is at least one teacher who loves me. She is the teacher who "knew me before I was born" and bought my first baby clothes. It is she who makes life bearable. It is her presence that finally helps me turn on the one child at the school who continually calls me "one-eyed bitch." One day I simply grab him by his coat and beat him until I am satisfied. It is my teacher who tells me my mother is ill.

My mother is lying in bed in the middle of the day, something I have never seen. She is in too much pain to speak. She has an abscess in her ear. I stand looking down on her, knowing that if she dies, I cannot live. She is being treated with warm oils and hot bricks held against her cheek. Finally a doctor comes. But I must go back to my grandparents' house. The weeks pass but I am hardly aware of it. All I know is that my mother might die, my father is not so jolly, my brothers still have their guns, and I am the one sent away from home.

"You did not change," they say.

Did I imagine the anguish of never looking up?

I am twelve. When relatives come to visit I hide in my room. My cousin Brenda, just my age, whose father works in the post office and whose mother is a nurse, comes to find me. "Hello," she says. And then she asks, looking at my recent school picture, which I did not want taken, and on which the "glob," as I think of it, is clearly visible, "You still can't see out of that eye?"

"No," I say, and flop back on the bed over my book.

That night, as I do almost every night, I abuse my eye. I rant and rave at it, in front of the mirror. I plead with it to clear up before morning. I tell it I hate and despise it. I do not pray for sight. I pray for beauty.

"You did not change," they say.

I am fourteen and baby-sitting for my brother Bill, who lives in Boston. He is my favorite brother and there is a strong bond between us. Understanding my feelings of shame and ugliness he and his wife take me to a local hospital, where the "glob" is removed by a doctor named O. Henry. There is still a small bluish crater where the scar tissue was, but the ugly white stuff is gone. Almost immediately I become a different person from the girl who does not raise her head. Or so I think. Now that I've raised my head I win the boy-friend of my dreams. Now that I've raised my head I have plenty of friends. Now that I've raised my head classwork comes from my lips as faultlessly as Easter speeches did, and I leave high school as valedictorian, most popular student, and *queen*, hardly believing my luck. Ironically, the girl who was voted most beautiful in our class (and was) was later shot twice through the chest by a male companion, using a "real" gun, while she was pregnant. But that's another story in itself. Or is it?

"You did not change," they say.

It is now thirty years since the "accident." A beautiful journalist comes to visit and to interview me. She is going to write a cover story for her magazine that focuses on my latest book. "Decide how you want to look on the cover," she says. "Glamorous, or whatever."

Never mind "glamorous," it is the "whatever" that I hear. Suddenly all I can think of is whether I will get enough sleep the night before the photography session: if I don't, my eye will be tired and wander, as blind eyes will.

At night in bed with my lover I think up reasons why I should not appear on the cover of a magazine. "My meanest critics will say I've sold out," I say. "My family will now realize I write scandalous books."

"But what's the real reason you don't want to do this?" he asks.

"Because in all probability," I say in a rush, "my eye won't be straight."

"It will be straight enough," he says. Then, "Besides, I thought you'd made your peace with that."

And I suddenly remember that I have.

I remember:

I am talking to my brother Jimmy, asking if he remembers anything unusual about the day I was shot. He does not know I consider that day the last time my father, with his sweet home remedy of cool lily leaves, chose me, and that I suffered and raged inside because of this. "Well," he says, "all I remember is standing by the side of the highway with Daddy, trying to flag down a car. A white man stopped, but when Daddy said he needed somebody to take his little girl to the doctor, he drove off."

I remember:

I am in the desert for the first time. I fall totally in love with it. I am so overwhelmed by its beauty, I confront for the first time, consciously, the meaning of the doctor's words years ago. "Eyes are sympathetic. If one is blind, the other will likely become blind too." I realize I have dashed about the world madly, looking at this, looking at that, storing up images against the fading of the light. *But I might have missed seeing the desert!* The shock of that possibility—and gratitude for over twenty-five years of sight—sends me literally to my knees. Poem after poem comes—which is perhaps how poets pray.

> *On Sight*
>
> I am so thankful I have seen
> The Desert
> And the creatures in the desert
> And the desert Itself.
>
> The desert has its own moon
> Which I have seen
> With my own eye.

There is no flag on it.

Trees of the desert have arms
All of which are always up
That is because the moon is up
The sun is up
Also the sky
The stars
Clouds
None with flags.

If there *were* flags, I doubt
the trees would point.
Would you?

But mostly, I remember this:

I am twenty-seven, and my baby daughter is almost three. Since her birth I have worried about her discovery that her mother's eyes are different from other people's. Will she be embarrassed? I think. What will she say? Every day she watches a television program called "Big Blue Marble." It begins with a picture of the earth as it appears from the moon. It is bluish, a little battered-looking, but full of light, with whitish clouds swirling around it. Every time I see it I weep with love, as if it is a picture of Grandma's house. One day when I am putting Rebecca down for her nap, she suddenly focuses on my eye. Something inside me cringes, gets ready to try to protect myself. All children are cruel about physical differences, I know from experience, and that they don't always mean to be is another matter. I assume Rebecca will be the same.

But no-o-o-o. She studies my face intently as we stand, her inside and me outside her crib. She even holds my face maternally between her dimpled little hands. Then, looking every bit as serious and lawyerlike as her father, she says, as if it may just possibly have slipped my attention: "Mommy, there's a *world* in your eye." (As in, "Don't be alarmed, or do anything crazy.") And then, gently, but with great interest: "Mommy, where did you *get* that world in your eye?"

For the most part, the pain left then. (So what, if my brothers grew up to buy even more powerful pellet guns for their sons and to carry real guns themselves. So what, if a young "Morehouse man" once nearly fell off the steps of Trevor Arnett Library because he thought my eyes were blue.) Crying and laughing I ran to the bathroom, while Rebecca mumbled and sang herself off to sleep. Yes indeed, I realized, looking into the mirror. There *was* a world in my eye. And I saw that it was possible to love it: that in fact, for all it had taught me of shame and anger and inner vision, I *did* love it. Even to see it drifting out of orbit in boredom, or rolling up out of fatigue, not to mention floating back at attention in excitement (bearing witness, a friend has called it), deeply suitable to my personality and even characteristic of me.

That night I dream I am dancing to Stevie Wonder's song "Always" (the name of the song is really "As," but I hear it as "Always"). As I dance, whirling and joyous, happier than I've ever been in my life, another bright-faced dancer joins me. We dance and kiss each other and hold each other through the night. The other dancer has obviously come through all right, as I have done. She is beautiful, whole and free. And she is also me.

New Bones
Lucille Clifton

we will wear
new bones again.
we will leave
these rainy days,
break out through
another mouth
into sun and honey time.
worlds buzz over us like bees,
we be splendid in new bones.
other people think they know
how long life is
how strong life is
we know.

FIVE: SOON AND VERY SOON

In contrast to our glorious diversity of skin color, size and other physical traits, there is one characteristic that far too many black women share—our suffering from uterine fibroid tumors. Because many of us have them, it is important that we have a wealth of information about this widespread health problem.

The Fibroid Epidemic
Evelyn C. White

Fibroids are benign, nonmalignant tumors that grow in the uterus of forty percent of women in their mid-thirties to early forties. Bundles of smooth muscle and connective tissue with their own blood supply, fibroids are usually found in one of three locations: within the muscle layer of the uterus (intramural); outside the uterine wall (subserous); and inside the uterus (submucous). Often changing their size and shape, the single or multiple growths can range from the size of a pea to as large as a grapefruit.

While no one knows what causes fibroids, researchers believe the tumors thrive on the hormone estrogen because they seem to enlarge during childbearing years and usually shrink after menopause when the production of estrogen decreases. Medical experts also know that black women have a seventy-five percent chance of developing the tumors, compared with a thirty-three percent chance for white women. In fact, it is not uncommon for several generations of black women in the same family to suffer from the disease.

While there may appear to be an hereditary factor in the prevalence of fibroids among African-American women, there is no medical evidence to support the theory that black women are genetically predisposed to the growths, says Ezra C. Davidson, Jr., M.D., president of the American College of Obstetricians and Gynecologists. Rather, he and others believe that black women suffer a higher rate of fibroids and more complications from the tumors because we do not get routine checkups early or often enough. "Far too many black women delay getting basic gynecological exams," says Dr. Davidson. "By the time they get into a physician's office, their presentation of fibroids is often dramatic."

How to Recognize Fibroids

Often detected during a routine gynecological exam or by a pelvic ul-trasonic scan (which produces a sound-wave picture), most fibroids are small, harmless growths that cause no symptoms and require no treatment at all. However, if left unchecked, the tumors can create a domino-like effect of reproductive health problems ranging from ex-cessive bleeding to infertility to hysterectomy—the surgical removal of the entire uterus.

Heavy or prolonged menstrual bleeding is one of the early warn-ing signs of fibroids. Some women complain of bleeding so heavily that they go through pads and tampons by the boxful. For others, the bleeding is so severe that they become anemic and have to be trans-fused to get their low blood counts back to normal. "We're not just talking heavy periods; some women hemorrhage so badly that they go into shock," according to Dr. Billie Jean Pace, a sister who practices gy-necology in Orlando, Florida. "It's dangerous because anemia leaves a woman susceptible to all kinds of infectious diseases. And in this AIDS era, no doctor wants to give a patient a transfusion if it can be avoided."

In addition to heavy bleeding, large fibroids can cause abdominal swelling (many women mistake large fibroids for unexplained weight gain), lower-back pain, painful intercourse, fatigue due to iron defi-ciency and a sensation of pressure on the back, legs or lower abdomen. A large tumor can also exert pressure on the bladder and/or bowel, causing frequent urination or constipation.

For women trying to conceive, fibroids can interfere with the im-plantation of the egg in the womb. For pregnant women, the growths can distort the uterine cavity, leading to recurrent miscarriage or com-plicated delivery.

Preventing and Shrinking Fibroids

The best protection against fibroids is to pay close attention to your body and get regular gynecological exams. Many experts also say that improvements in diet can help women avoid or shrink fibroids. Eating healthily means cutting down on caffeinated drinks (coffee, tea, choco-late, cola drinks) as well as red meat, fried and sugary foods, whole-milk dairy products and processed food items. Many women have found success by eliminating all meat and chicken from their diets.

Some holistic practitioners speculate that the hormones injected into animals cause or worsen fibroid tumors. Try substituting soy products for dairy and fish for meat. You should also eat plenty of fresh vegetables, fruit, potatoes, pasta and whole-grain rice to help keep fibroids at bay.

Daya, a holistic-health consultant and director of Daya Associates in Harlem, treats fibroids by detoxifying the body through nutrition counseling and colonic irrigation, which clears the bowel tract of impurities. She bluntly states the importance of a healthy diet: "About seventy percent of my female clients have fibroids, which I believe are an accumulation from high-fat, high-cholesterol diets. Black women need to spend their money on juicers and organic vegetables. You either pay now to prevent fibroids or pay later for surgery that might prevent you from having a child."

Building a healthy relationship between your mind and body can be critical in the prevention and management of fibroids. Like fatty, cholesterol-packed foods, stress and negative mental attitudes, studies suggest, contribute to illness. For black women, learning how to deal positively with racism and sexism can help reduce the stress many of us live with. Meditation, yoga and regular exercise such as walking, aerobic dancing and running are some of the holistic techniques African-American women can use to "chill."

In addition to vitamins A, B and E, which help balance estrogen levels, many women include herbal-medicine treatments in their battle plan against fibroids. Wild yam, chaste berry, raspberry leaf and damiana are all herbs that have proven effective in the reduction of fibroids, according to experts. (While a variety of vitamins and herbs are widely available, don't self-medicate without the supervision of a health-care professional.)

How to Treat Fibroids

Your fibroids may shrink on their own and require no treatment at all, especially if you are following a healthy diet and exercise regimen. But even if you have small fibroids that are not growing or not growing rapidly, you must visit a gynecologist who will monitor them. Though you may notice some positive signs (such as lighter menstrual periods), only a health-care professional can tell you for sure the exact state of your fibroid tumors.

If your fibroids are large and causing major health problems, chances are you will have to consider undergoing some form of surgery to remove the growths. But before you go under the knife, be sure to ask your doctor about the numerous alternatives to hysterectomy, which is a drastic measure of last resort. Hysterectomy will forever rid your body of fibroids, but also ends the possibility of giving birth.

Every year physicians perform some 650,000 hysterectomies, making this operation the second most frequent major surgery performed in the country; only Caesarean sections are performed more often. Doctors in the United States perform hysterectomies more than physicians in European countries, and they remove ovaries in greater numbers than they did twenty years ago. Hysterectomies are most often performed for fibroid tumors.

Yet a number of experts believe that many, if not the majority, of hysterectomies may be unnecessary. Black women undergo a disproportionate number of hysterectomies, and the mortality rate for the operation is twice as high for black women than for white women.

If a doctor tells you that you must have a hysterectomy to rid your body of fibroids, consult another physician. Some doctors will automatically recommend hysterectomy out of "tradition," or because they are unaware of or not proficient in some of the newer techniques to treat fibroids.

For smaller fibroids (less than the size of a twelve-week pregnancy), microsurgery can be performed with a laser. In this procedure, which is known as **laparoscopy**, a doctor uses tiny instruments to vaporize or remove fibroids through a small incision just above the navel.

With **hysteroscopy,** an instrument is inserted through the vagina and cervix to remove fibroids inside the womb. The physician uses a wire loop to shave the fibroid from the uterine wall. Both laparoscopy and hysteroscopy can be performed on an outpatient basis. Not only are they far less invasive and costly than a hysterectomy (these operations end up costing much less than the $3,000 to $6,000 average cost of a hysterectomy), but they also require a much shorter recovery time. In addition, because the procedures eliminate the need for a major abdominal incision, the likelihood of postoperative complications is decreased.

If the fibroids have caused the uterus to swell to the size it would be in a twelve-week pregnancy or larger, **myomectomy** might be recommended. In this procedure, the physician surgically removes the fibroids while leaving the uterus intact—which means that a myomectomy shouldn't affect your ability to conceive. Myomectomy is a more complicated procedure than hysterectomy with a greater risk of blood loss, which prompts many physicians to disregard it as a treatment option. (Remember that not all doctors are created equal: Skill level and experience makes a big difference when it comes to myomectomy, so don't be afraid to ask your physician how many of the procedures she or he has performed.) Five to thirty percent of women who undergo myomectomies also report subsequent problems because of regrowth of the tumors. The best way to find out if myomectomy is for you is to openly discuss all the advantages and disadvantages with your physician.

Studies show that a drug called **GnRh analog** (gonadotrophin-releasing hormones), can reduce fibroids by temporarily shutting down the body's production of estrogen, the hormone that feeds fibroid growth. Taken by injection or nasal spray for three to six months, the medication shrinks the fibroids, so that physicians are better able to monitor them or to remove them using less invasive procedures.

GnRh analog is not without drawbacks. At several hundred dollars a treatment, the drug can be much too expensive for most women. Also, because it inhibits the release of estrogen it can induce a temporary menopausal state with such side effects as hot flashes, vaginal dryness and mood swings.

You Can be Healed

One of the most important things for black women to remember about uterine fibroid tumors is that we can avoid or manage them, and we don't have to do it alone. Though there hasn't been enough research conducted on the cause, growth, treatment and prevention of fibroids (given how widespread the problem is, especially among sisters), you can find information about natural healing, surgery and other treatment options that are available to you. If you have been diagnosed with fibroids, talk to other black women friends and family members about the problem. And most important, choose health-care providers who treat you as a partner and allow you to determine your medical destiny. If you have fibroids, here are some questions to ask your doctor:[1]

1. Do you think my fibroids should be removed? Why?

2. What diagnostic tests have you done to rule out other causes for my symptoms?

3. If the fibroids aren't causing any problems, what are the risks if I don't have surgery?

4. Is there a way to treat this without surgery?

5. Can I shrink the fibroid with medication? Would the resulting smaller fibroid lessen the complications of surgery?

6. If surgery is required, are you comfortable doing the procedure?

How many times have you done it before? Can you recommend someone else?

7. What are the risks if I decide to postpone or rule out surgery? How often should I monitor the fibroid with checkups?

8. If I decide to have surgery, what is the estimated cost and recovery period?

One Woman's Story[2]

In the following piece, an African-American woman describes her experience with fibroids. If you have any of the symptoms that she mentions—heavy menstrual bleeding, painful cramping or fatigue—see your doctor.

Several years ago, while having my tubes tied, my doctor discovered that I had fibroids. Because I always scratch out the line on the pre-surgery sheet that gives medical staff the right to do whatever they feel is "appropriate" in these circumstances, I was told about them during recovery after surgery.

When I questioned my doctor about the implications of his findings, he said not to worry about the fibroids—they weren't serious yet. But during my first post-surgery menstrual period, I had the misfortune of leaving a large bloodstain in a front row chair during a business-related meeting. I was both surprised and embarrassed because I had put in a tampon *and* a maxi-size sanitary napkin not thirty minutes before.

Following my usual pattern of educating myself on topics of which I'm relatively ignorant, I immediately began to ask questions of everyone who knew anything about fibroids. Without exception, the response that I received was, "You're going to have a hysterectomy, just like my sister, cousin, mother, aunt, daughter, etc."

Though I wasn't interested in having more children at that time, I had no intentions of having a hysterectomy either. So I did the only thing I knew to do at the time: gather more information while being extra careful during my periods.

From reading about fibroids, I learned that the hormones in chicken and dairy products may induce them to grow, so I *kind of* cut down. Then I began to read about various barks and herbs that were said to decrease the menstrual flow or dissolve tumors. I went to a health food store and stocked up on some of those.

These different herbs, however, remained in my cupboard untouched. My hectic lifestyle and the daily stress in my life, along with my unfamiliarity with the herbs themselves, seemed to prevent me from ever using them.

Meanwhile, my menstrual periods were getting longer. They began lasting fourteen to eighteen days with unexpected spotting in between. Plus, they were becoming unbearably heavy. During each cycle, I always experienced at least one night of changing maxi-pads every forty to sixty minutes. This was both physically and emotionally draining, not to mention expensive. It was also beginning to affect my social life because I was afraid of having an "accident." Despite these problems, my approach to my condition continued to be somewhat lackadaisical—partly because I always felt so tired. I didn't press my doctor for more information, and though I had cut down, I still ate chicken and dairy products, and I stayed away from healthier foods because they seemed hard to prepare, and the ingredients were expensive.

This probably would have gone on indefinitely had I not had a simple phone call from my aunt. During our conversation I happened to mention the fibroids and tell her about the heavy bleeding and fatigue.

"You're going to have to have surgery," she said, "like my friend."

"I'm not having surgery," I fired back.

"Yes, you are," she insisted.

"No, I'm not," I repeated in the firmest, most adult voice I could respectfully give to an elder.

"We'll see," she replied in a tone that seemed both self-righteous and condescending.

That conversation, as annoying as it was, jarred something in me. I wasn't angry at my aunt, I was angry at myself for doing almost nothing during these increasingly debilitating menstrual cycles.

I went on a three-day cleansing diet, which consisted mainly of fruit, vegetables and water. Then I began taking herbs while eating only healthy foods. No meat, sugar, white flour, or processed foods touched my lips. The herbs—white oak, witch hazel, slippery elm bark and yellow dock—tasted strong and bitter to me, so I put them into capsules rather than drinking them as teas.

Soon I began to feel better. During my next period, I bled for only eight days, and conspicuously absent were the huge clots, heavy flow and unpredictable spotting that had plagued me in months past.

Today, I feel like a new woman. Still, I consider this only phase one of my healing. I plan to stick to my healthy eating habits and pay close attention to my body and its changes.

After what I went through, I'd like pass on a few words of advice to sisters who would like to consider a holistic approach to shrinking fibroids. Remember that every woman's body is different. These tips should not be a substitute for a doctor's advice.

1. Don't begin a new regimen at the beginning of a menstrual cycle. Wait until your flow has stopped to allow maximum healing time.

2. Take it easy. Realize that rest is an important component of the healing process.

3. Monitor your physical and emotional symptoms so you know as much as possible about your body and its responses.

4. Allow yourself time to heal. Consider this a wellness vacation that you have earned. Otherwise, your regimen could turn into just another stressful problem.

5. Compare the cost of good, healthy, vital food to that of extra sanitary pads, painkillers, possible surgery and your own pain and suffering. Healthy food is sometimes more expensive and more time-consuming to prepare than fast food and highly processed food items, but taking other "costs" into consideration, it's worth the time and expense. And don't forget: You're worth it.

6. Keep a journal. Healing is an empowering experience which you will want to remember and possibly share with other sisters.

Footnotes

1.   Sources: Dr. Alan Johns, medical director of the GYN Laparoscopy Center at Harris Methodist Fort Worth Hospital; Dr. Sidney Wolfe, director of Public Citizen Health Research Group, Washington, D.C.

2.   A slightly different version of this story appeared in *Vital Signs,* news from The National Black Women's Health Project, October 1991.

There is a long legacy of natural healing in the African-American community. In the following piece, the author discusses her personal journey as a practitioner of non-Western medicine and offers advice for black women in search of natural healers.

Notes From a Non-Western Healer
Francesca A. Jackson

In an ancient land in a faraway time, our ancestors associated health maintenance with the phases of the moon, the seasons of the year and even with the positions of the planets, which were known to affect the human body and its functioning. Our ancestors understood that spring was the best time to clean the system and that winter was a time of slowing down and turning inward.

A variety of roots, herbs, oils, powders and rituals played an important role in people's daily lives. Communities often relied on the "village healer," whose sphere of influence extended over the physical, spiritual and emotional well-being of people.

The notion that the mind, body, soul and heart might be separate entities, disconnected and unrelated to each other, was unknown to our ancestors. Natural health and healing practices survived the diaspora and many of us have memories of hearing about the "root doctor" during our childhood.

As society has become more "advanced," many of the simple ways have been forgotten. We need to heed the call of our ancestors and include their knowledge and power in our lives.

The Journey

From a very young age I considered the traditional medical model to be the alternative. It was a rainy afternoon in Tokyo. I was five years old and attending a small school for military children. Miss Wise, a middle-aged woman with intense blue eyes, had asked her first grade class to sit in a circle. As she walked around the circle she asked, "What are you going to be when you grow up?" When it was my turn the words flew out of my mouth, "I'm going to be a doctor."

I had formed this thought the previous year while in kindergarten. I had broken my arm and was put in a large hospital room by myself while the doctor and nurse watched through a small window. They were taking an x-ray and stood behind a lead door to protect themselves from radiation, but I was too young to understand this at the time. I do remember thinking that if what they were doing was not going to hurt me, then why weren't they in the room, too?

Another time, I remember going to the hospital when my grand-mother was very ill. I wasn't allowed to see her, nor was my sister, be-cause we were too young. I remember the energy coming from the building and saying to my sister, "People die here." I was very sensi-tive as a child.

I also remember my younger brother's asthma attacks; the many times he would be rushed to the hospital in the middle of the night. I have memories of being terrified that he would never come back home.

We were a family of seven juggling life on a meager Air Force sal-ary. I remember my mother talking about the expense of getting sick and having to go to the doctor. She said repeatedly, "If you have your health, you have everything."

In my response to Miss Wise's question, I was voicing my desire to become the kind of doctor who helped people "have everything." Not with x-rays, but with sensitivity, spirits and touch.

My journey toward becoming a doctor continued through dance and theater, both of which I studied in college. Dancers were offered an anatomy class with a required lab. I remember the first time I went to the lab. There on the table was the cadaver of a child, less than a year old, with its brain, spinal cord and nerve systems intact and exposed. I went to the lab often and looked in awe at this child as I began to un-derstand how tiny nerve systems, no bigger than threads, carry all of our power and human ability.

As I danced, I became fascinated with the idea of the "thinking body" and how our body functions are interwoven and linked with our minds. I learned to watch people and to "see" places in their bod-ies where emotions were stored. Later I studied massage and discov-ered that touch releases not only physical pains, but also old thought patterns and emotional injuries. I began to study meditation. I studied chakras (subtle energy centers). In the early 1980s I went to India, and with the guidance of my spiritual teacher, learned about metaphysics. I returned to California and through a myriad of circumstances, de-cided to attend chiropractic school. After four years of full-time study, I passed my board exams and was awarded a license as a Doctor of Chiropractic.

Chiropractic Care and Homeopathy

There are five billion people on Earth and therefore, five billion ways to get to Heaven. Chiropractic and homeopathy are the roads I chose. Chiropractic is a science and art that recognizes and approaches the body as a self-regulating, self-healing and integrated organism. The major premise of chiropractic healing is that a Universal Intelligence is in all matter and manifests itself in the body. The body has the innate intelligence to adapt and direct all forces toward optimum conditioning and functioning. Physiology teaches us that all of our abilities—mental, physical, emotional—are governed either directly or indirectly through our nervous system, which is housed in the spine.

Energy flows effortlessly through a clear spine. In the absence of clear passages, our "back hurts." The underlying goal of chiropractic care is to maintain open channels in the spine. By doing so, all levels of our being can be impacted positively.

Classical homeopathy is the science of respecting the individual. Here it is understood that it is not the "disease" that is being treated, but rather the individual person who carries it. Homeopathy evaluates the individual as a total organism—a reservoir of not only mental, physical and emotional stimuli—but also as one that has reactions to weather, sleep patterns, certain foods, and so on.

The homeopath does not hand out standard medicines for lupus or fibroids, for example. Instead she works with the individual to elicit a healing response and move toward a cure. The remedies, which are prepared from plant, animal or mineral substances, have all been tested on human beings and are diluted to get to the essence of their curative powers and to eliminate toxicity. Homeopaths believe that the "energy" of the curative substance carries healing knowledge directly to the person taking it. It is a practice which requires a team approach. The homeopath's job is to find the remedy that resonates with the totality of symptoms presented by the patient. The patient's job is to practice careful self-observation in order to help the homeopath respond accurately and effectively to the symptoms.

Other Healing Practices

Chiropractic and homeopathy are the methods that have worked most powerfully in my life and helped me to heal others. There are other forms of non-Western medicine you might wish to try.

Acupuncture is a system of care that comes to us from the Chinese and is thousands of years old. With acupuncture, very fine, sterile needles are inserted at specific points in the body. For most, the procedure is painless. Acupuncture balances the body's energy—chi- and clears blockages that can cause pain and organ dysfunction. As the body's energy flow is unblocked, organ systems function more effectively, leading to improved well-being. Acupuncturists often use Chinese herbs in treatment plans. Dietary changes might also be suggested.

Ayurveda is a holistic system of medicine that is indigenous to and widely practiced in India. For the past decade, it has been practiced, with increasing frequency, in the United States. "Ayu" means life, "veda" means knowing. Thus ayurveda becomes "the science of life." Ayurveda practitioners assess people according to body types or constitutions and make recommendations for improving health. Pulse and tongue diagnosis are used to help develop the course of treatment. Advice about diet, herbs and exercise are individualized to one's body type.

Breath is the elixir of life! I often recommend breathing exercises to my patients. We can go for days without food, a little less without water, some people live for years without touch but *no one* lives longer than six minutes without air. Correct breathing not only aids in improving posture, but it sends a flood of oxygen (food) to all tissues. Deep diaphragmatic breathing helps to eliminate stress, lowers the heart rate and gives the whole body a sense of renewal.

Naturopathic medicine is a distinct system of primary health care that uses natural forces such as botanical medicines, light, heat, air, water and massage to promote healing.

Massage therapy improves muscle functioning by relaxing the musculo-skeletal system. As the muscles relax, so does the sense of "armoring" that so many of us carry—leaving us feeling much lighter and open-hearted. The invisible walls of protection begin to crumble and a space is created for greater goodness to enter our lives.

In my years of practice I have discovered that there are many black women who have never had a full body massage. Many of us equate massage with sex because we are so unaccustomed to having our bodies touched for any other purpose. Professional massage therapy does not and should not involve sexual interaction. During massage therapy, do not hesitate to leave and report anyone who touches you improperly.

Beginning the Holistic Partnership

So great, you say, how do I go about finding a non-Western healer? The most direct and practical way is to get a recommendation from a friend you trust. She may say "so and so really helped me . . . why don't you call her? Here's the number." Don't let that piece of paper stay in your pocket and go through the wash cycle—use it! If you do not have a direct referral, you might pick up a "new age" newspaper in your area. Many holistic health practitioners advertise in such papers. You can also let your fingers do the walking through the yellow pages. Check listings under *chiropractic, health* and *licensed massage therapy.*

Always keep in mind that you are looking to begin a partnership with a person you are employing to assist you in your journey toward greater health. It is perfectly legitimate for you to question practitioners about their background, education, experience and methods of working with people. Shopping around is fine—call a few people and assess how you feel about what they've told you. Get an idea of what you can expect and decide if it sounds right for you. *Trust your intuition.* There have been times when I passed over the person with the largest office and the most famous name for another practitioner with whom I resonated more deeply.

Remember that no one is going to "heal" you. Showing up passive in a practitioner's office won't do the trick. You must be prepared to get fully involved and examine all aspects of your life in ways you may not have thought of before. Your journey will not be complete in five minutes! I cannot stress this enough. If your goal is long-term healing, the instant gratification offered by over-the-counter cures will not apply here. Know that if you choose the holistic path, the journey will take time. Be patient, with yourself, your practitioner and the process.

Take the Step

African-American women are called upon daily to deal with situations that create stress. These situations make it difficult for us to come into balance. They leave us drained and without the energy to even think about being healthy. For those of us with limited resources, a therapeutic massage can be viewed as an expensive "luxury." Even those of us with well-paying jobs can place our health concerns fairly far down the line. If you are wondering whether you can afford to take care of your health, please remember my mother's words, which ring true to me to this day, nearly forty years after she first uttered them: *It is more expensive to get sick than to take care of yourself.*

I've had countless conversations with sisters who, once they discover what I do, tell me how much they know they need to see a chiropractor, but it's so expensive, they don't have time to make an appointment or their insurance won't cover it. I have been black and female

my entire life. I know the pressures on us. I understand and I sympathize. But we all make choices. In making choices about your health,
remember that an ounce of prevention is worth a pound of cure. Facing
a health problem in its earliest stages, rather than just ignoring it and
hoping that it will go away, will save you time, money and emotional
turmoil further down the line. The longer you wait, the higher the cost
to your mental, physical and spiritual well-being. As a black woman
dedicated to the health of my sisters and my community, I ask you to
love yourself. You are worth the investment. Take the step. Now.

Often the centerpiece of our festivities, the culinary tradition of African Americans is rich indeed. In the following essay, the author traces the evolution of our diet as we made the passage from our African homeland to the United States. Major components of good health, fresh produce and natural ingredients long have been a part of our cooking heritage, even as we suffered the oppressive conditions of slavery. As primary caretakers, black women historically have been responsible for nourishing our families and communities. This piece can help us reclaim our healthy eating traditions as we savor the foods that remind us of "home."

Celebrating Our Cuisine
Jessica B. Harris

Nutritionists have been saying, "you are what you eat" for years. No culture bears this out more than ours. The history of Africans in this hemisphere is in our food. The tendency to eat soupy stews over a starch, the taste for succulent meats, the love of okra and leafy greens, the desire to "dunk" and the appetite for such New World ingredients as corn, chiles and potatoes, all have roots in our old African world.

Our entire culinary heritage has been tempered with a history of slavery and hardship that influences our traditional choices of poorer cuts of meat and of slow-cooked foods that could be put on the stove while we did other people's work. It is simmered in the heavy cast iron cauldron of deprivation and second-class citizenship and at the same time savored with the joy of communion with others. Our foods are very much us. They are so much us that it sometimes surprises us to realize the extent of our influence on American taste in general.

African influence is the great unknown in the American cooking pot. Everyone knows it's there, but no one is quite sure when it begins, when it ends, or how to trace its octopus-like grasp on much of the country's cooking. It's a subtle process—in which ingredients are transformed into something other, something different and savory, with the turn of a wooden spoon or with the addition of another chile or a mixture of fresh thyme, onions and garlic. It's as familiar as the heady aroma of a mess of greens stewing in a heavy iron pot, or the smoky perfume of a slab of barbecue grilling over hickory charcoal. It is as exotic as dried smoked shrimp or cassava meal.

In much of the American South, it has become such an integral part of the culinary ethos that even the most adept researchers are hard pressed to distinguish where Africanisms end and Southern cooking begins.

African Roots

It's clear that the Africanization of American taste began during slavery. In the antebellum period in the American South and throughout the hemisphere, most of the cooking in the Big House kitchens, the plantation Great Houses, etc., was done by African Americans, some recently arrived from Africa. Scholars argue about the importance of the influence of the mistress on the food. However, as any cook knows, when recipes are transmitted from one cook to another, whether by oral or written instruction or by demonstration, the results are different from the original, transformed by the culinary inventiveness of the receiving cook. This then was the beginning of the Africanization of Southern cooking, an influence so prevalent that historian Eugene Genovese in his book *Roll Jordan Roll: The World The Slaves Made*, speaks of, "the culinary despotism of the slave cabin over the big house."

This is the period that saw the European tradition of overcooking vegetables and discarding the cooking liquid transformed by the Africanism of conserving and consuming the "pot likker" as the savory essence of the vegetables came to be called. The period also saw the West African habit of eating thick soups and stews over a starchy mash develop into the habit of "sopping" savory gravies and sauces with biscuits, hoecakes, ashcakes, cornbreads and even plain old white bread.

At this time numerous ingredients indigenous to Africa arrived on these shores and became a part of the taste of first the South and eventually the entire country. Southerners crave their black-eyed peas and rice. Yet we do not always recognize Africa's hallmark. How many of us realize that the black-eyed peas that are the main ingredient of the Hoppin' John are African in origin and arrived with the slaves? Arab chronicles from the Middle Ages tell us that these peas and other peas and beans were eaten in Western Africa prior to the arrival of the Europeans. Very few of us know that the links are ongoing and that a dish similar to Hoppin' John—Thiebou Niebe—is served in Senegal, West Africa today.

Okra, the West African pod, is a major totem of African-American cooking; where its green tip can be seen, Africa has passed. The classic example of this is Louisiana's gumbo—the very name of the dish tells the tale. Gumbo is a derivation of Tchingombo, one of the Bantu words for okra. It's used throughout Africa from Egypt to Angola in soups and stews as a thickener. Frequently it is teamed up with leafy greens and with hot chiles, a New World addition. The main ingredient and thickener in many southern Louisiana gumbos, okra also pops up in Charleston, South Carolina's Okra Soup, also called Carolina Gumbo by some. It is also used in numerous okra, corn and tomato dishes that appear annually at our barbecues, fish fries, and picnics throughout the South—dishes that are craved and savored nostalgically in the North.

Leafy greens are another hallmark of our cooking and they turn up throughout the African-Atlantic world in a variety of soupy stews that are virtually one-pot meals. The use of nuts and seeds to thicken and enhance dishes is another indicator of our African culinary heritage.

Pigs' Feet and Potato Salad

The conditions of slavery combined with African culinary techniques such as fritter making, roasting in ashes, grilling, frying and stewing with New World ingredients resulted in the creation of numerous dishes which African Americans can truly claim as our own: ash-baked sweet potatoes, banana fritters, spoon breads, candied sweet potatoes, smothered cabbage and more.

The New World also introduced the pig to many of us for good and for ill. And whatever our position today on the ubiquitous porker, it was, for many, love at first sight. For centuries and even today, many of us ate and still eat everything on the pig but the "oink." (However, the tenets of Islam forbid all practitioners to eat pork).

Pigs' feet, one of the numerous parts that we consume, are considered a delicacy. Not braised or grilled as in Europe, but simply boiled, they're considered a treat by many. At family dinners, each little knuckle or joint is sucked clean of meat and fat and the sticky gelatin is wiped on reams of paper napkins. The feet are usually savored with hot or cold potato salad prepared according to the house's traditional recipe. In fact, potato salad itself has become so much a part of summer menus that many a barbecue has ended in a heated debate as to whether or not chopped sweet pickles or hard boiled eggs are admissible ingredients. Our love of pig does not end with pigs' feet.

There are also innards—hog maws and chitterlings. Cleanliness is a prime requirement for preparation of these and the eating of another's chitterlings becomes a sign of confidence and friendship. Head cheese is consumed by the slabs and each summer in our neighborhoods North and South, barbecue fires are fanned into a veritable orgy of grilling. The expression "high on the hog" comes from this period and testifies to our desire for a better life. (Think about moving up from the feet to the ham, from chitterlings to chops!)

This desire for a better life sent thousands of us northward and westward via rivers and along railroad track lines in search of our share of the American dream. We settled ourselves in the inner cities and outer suburbs of the nation's largest cities. These northern migrations which began in the years following the Civil War and continued up to the period of World War II mark the second phase of the Africanization of American taste: one in which our foods moved northward and westward and became national.

An undeniable reality of any migration is nostalgia, and a longing for the cooking of our Southern homes marked and still marks many families. Our neighborhoods could and still can be recognized by the wealth of leafy vegetables displayed at produce markets: collard, turnip, kale and mustard greens, with dandelion greens and poke salad if you're really lucky. There are also numbers of root vegetables which we have adopted from northern Europe such as turnips and rutabagas. The array of pork products available in the butcher shops is mindboggling and enough to give a nutritionist a coronary. In some neighborhoods, such as my own in Brooklyn, small but savvy entrepreneurs cash in on the nostalgia for our Southern homes by driving trucks up from the South and selling products that speak of Southern fish fries and country picnics. In my neighborhood, the change of seasons can be marked by these vendors' transition from the watermelons of summer to greens and sweet potatoes of fall and winter.

While this food has always existed in our households, the cultural revolution of the 1960s and 1970s brought it to national attention and baptized it "Soul Food." The home-cooked tastes of pork chops smothered in brown gravy, the slightly sweet tang of green cabbage fried with smoky bacon, the divine combinations of barbecued ribs and potato salad, of chicken and dumplings, or of spicy fried chicken served with hot buttered biscuits touched something basic in us and brought back fond memories of family reunions, Sunday school picnics and summer fish fries.

For those who had not grown up in our kitchens, this was the first hint of the wealth of our food experience. The world learned how foods, even basic ones, could taste if prepared thoughtfully with love, for that too is a main ingredient in much of our cooking. We are a sociable people and whatever the dish, part of the experience of the food is the communion in the savoring of it: the gathering, the conversation, the guests.

Passages

As the twentieth century comes to a close, our culinary history enters its third phase. New tastes of Africa are being added to the American cooking pot, tastes that have migrated with new Americans from the Caribbean, from Brazil and from the African continent itself.

While savory and rife with memories of home and comfort, the new and the old Africanized foods cannot and should not be made a steady part our diet. We no longer have the active lives of our forebears. Moreover, we have new threats to survival to combat—hypertension, diabetes, high cholesterol and other diseases. If we look back to the West African diet and to our cousins in this hemisphere we will discover that we can improve our diets. For just as there is much in our African-influenced diet that is not nutritionally sound, there is much good also.

Traditionally our diets placed the emphasis on vegetables with small, less tender cuts of meat used for seasoning. Seasonally selected fresh fruits and vegetables have also been a centerpiece of our diet. When fruits and vegetables were canned, the process was usually done at the peak of freshness to guarantee flavor. We could identify the taste of an ear of corn picked straight from the garden and the flavor of greens after the first frost. Our taste buds were among the most sophisticated in the country. Although it takes planning and perhaps a little extra effort, it is not impossible for us to get back to our more natural ways. We can serve fresh fruit instead of sugar-rich desserts at the end of a meal. A dash or two of hot sauce or a seasoning squeeze of lemon can replace salt in a dish.

These bountiful foods, in their traditional servings or in their new forms, speak to our journey, as African Americans, to these shores. They speak of our dreams, our hardships, our feasts and hopes for the future. Our food is why we are here. It enabled our ancestors to survive so we can be here today to do better. Our survival is in each flavor, in the humble ingredients that recall the past need to make the best of a bad situation and the flair that shows our desire to live "higher on the hog." Our food is filled with the love that got us through.

Filled with nutrients that strengthen their immune systems from the moment infants leave the womb, mother's milk is vital to the growth and development of healthy babies. Research shows that breastfed babies have fewer problems with infections, diarrhea, constipation, rashes, allergies, upset stomachs and future dental problems than bottle-fed babies. The physical closeness between mother and infant during breastfeedings is beneficial to the baby's emotional health. While it is a totally natural process, successful nursing requires practice, patience, commitment and support. In the following piece, the author provides encouragement and information that will help mothers give their newborns a healthy start.

The Magic of Mother's Milk: Breastfeeding Your Baby
Joyce Gardner

I knew from the moment I found out I was pregnant that I was going to breastfeed my baby. The thought of formula feeding never crossed my mind. When I became pregnant, more than a decade ago, I was a graduate student majoring in Foods and Nutrition at Oregon State University. Because of my major, I knew that breast milk was the ideal food for newborns. As a pregnant woman, I wanted to provide the best for my baby.

Soon after I became pregnant I visited relatives in Los Angeles. One of my cousins was breastfeeding her young baby. Although I planned to breastfeed, I had never seen anyone actually nurse a baby. I talked with my cousin about pregnancy, birth and breastfeeding. We also discussed the challenges I would face as a single parent who was enrolled in graduate school full time and working part time. I honestly did not know how I was going to support myself and stay in school with a new baby. So it was helpful to talk with my cousin who assured me that breastfeeding my baby would make it easier to manage my very hectic life.

My cousin encouraged me to take Bradley Method Natural Childbirth Education classes (for information call 1-800-42-BIRTH). The Bradley Method helps expectant parents approach childbirth with a positive attitude. Among the topics covered in the course are: natural breathing, nutrition, exercise, the stages of labor, postnatal care and breastfeeding.

The course taught me how to become an advocate for myself in a health-care system that is not designed to support nursing mothers. I learned that hospital policies and practices with regard to nurseries, pacifiers, glucose water and feeding schedules actually hinder breast-feeding. The Bradley Method helped me develop the support systems I needed to successfully nurse my new baby. While the quality of in-structors varies, you might want to consider taking Bradley Method classes or another childbirth education course.

Immunity, Artistry and the Importance of Support

I knew about the nutritional, psychological and immunological bene-fits of breastfeeding when I began childbirth education classes. By the time I completed the course, I understood the "art of breastfeeding."

As I gained a greater understanding of the obstacles nursing moth-ers face in the traditional health-care system, I knew I would have to find other sources of support. Living proof that it is never too late to stand up for yourself and your baby, I left a team of obstetrician/ gynecologists during my seventh month of pregnancy because they were not as supportive of my childbirth plans as I would have liked for them to be. I began seeing Mabel Dzata, an African midwife from Ghana who provided excellent prenatal care and who was a strong ad-vocate of breastfeeding. I knew how important it was to start nursing as soon as possible after delivery.

Upon her birth, the first tactile experience my daughter enjoyed was the feel of the midwife's hands; then my hands; and next my breast. After she was cleaned up and had overcome the shock of leav-ing the cozy "home" she had lived in for nine months, she slept, nursed frequently and had regular bowel movements—all positive signs that we were off to a healthy start. I loved it!

During the first few days of nursing, breasts secrete the thin amber or yellow fluid *colostrum*, not milk. Often called "liquid gold" colos-trum contains nutrients and antibodies that protect newborns from a variety of infections and illnesses.

I knew instinctively when my milk came in because my breasts be-came tender and engorged with milk. I was uncomfortable, but I knew that the discomfort would only last a couple of days. I also knew that it was important for me to connect with experienced breastfeeders who would give me guidance and encouragement.

I often think about how different my experiences as a new mother would have been without the support of my family and friends. I especially appreciated the support of my mother. While she is not a lactation expert, my mother knows about infant care and wanted a healthy grandchild. Without hesitation, she supported my efforts to become a successful breastfeeder.

Sisters *Should* Be Doing it For Themselves

As I became more knowledgeable about breastfeeding and its positive impact on mother, infant and society, I began to notice that the majority of newborns are bottlefed, not nursed. As I examined maternal and child health more closely, I was saddened to discover that very few African-American women breastfeed their babies.

When I talked to my mother about this problem she told me that she had breastfed me for about a month. She said that she had planned to continue nursing me but she stopped when our family doctor told her that formula was just as good as breast milk. The eldest of four children, I vaguely remember my mother breastfeeding my youngest sister Donna. She was breastfed for about two weeks before my mother switched to formula. I clearly remember my mother boiling bottles and preparing formula with canned milk and Karo syrup. During my pregnancy, I knew only three other black women in my age group who nursed their babies: my sister, my cousin and a very close friend.

The Benefits of Breastfeeding

The American Academy of Pediatrics endorses breastfeeding as the ideal method of feeding healthy, full-term babies. Academy experts recommend that such babies be breastfed for at least the first year of life. I believe that more black women would nurse their babies (which have an infant mortality rate 2.3 times higher than that of white babies) if they had a greater understanding of the benefits of breastfeeding which:

- promotes optimal growth and development of the baby
- protects against illness and disease and contributes to better development of dental arch and jaw structure
- is inexpensive and convenient
- promotes strong bonding between mother and infant
- helps women get back into shape because nursing mothers burn about 1,000 calories a day and more readily expel excess fluids and tissue gained during pregnancy

- decreases stress because many women report feeling more re-laxed while breastfeeding

- improves self-esteem of both mother and infant

- decreases costs for postnatal health care

Breastfeeding clearly has many advantages. Given the high infant mortality rates in our community, why aren't more African-American women nursing their newborns?

Breastfeeding in America

Women have breastfed their babies since the beginning of time. How-ever, there has always been a need for other infant feeding methods. Among the reasons for alternatives to breastfeeding are: the death of the mother, the absence of the mother, the lack of desire or inability of the mother to nurse.

Before the 1850s wet nursing was the primary option for mothers who could not or would not breastfeed. During this era, multitudes of black women nursed white infants and then their own. The Industrial Revolution brought societal and lifestyle changes that ushered in the artificial feeding of newborns. Women began to work outside the home and thus were separated for longer periods from their babies. Infants began to be fed unsanitized and unprocessed milk.

Numerous factors led to the decline of breastfeeding between the 1880s and the 1920s. Among them were:

- advances in technology which increased the availability of pas-teurized milk, glass bottles, rubber nipples, refrigeration and sanitary water

- the women's movement for social and political freedom

- sociocultural focus on women's breasts as "sexual objects"

- "scientific" and business interest in the development of alterna-tives to breast milk

Formulas and Sociocultural Pressures

By the 1930s formula companies had used advances in microbiology to "duplicate" breast milk and began marketing their products directly to the public. Because the formula companies were successful in per-suading the public that their products contained enough proteins, fats, carbohydrates, vitamins and minerals to meet the nutritional needs of babies, it became a popular trend among mothers and their physicians to choose bottlefeeding over breastfeeding.

However, breastfeeding remained the primary method of infant feeding until the mid-1950s. Seventy-seven percent of all infants born between 1936-1940 were breastfed; black infants were more likely to be nursed than whites.

During the 1950s, when there was great pressure on women to stay at home and fulfill "traditional" female roles, breastfeeding declined rapidly. Influenced by a culture that encouraged them to emulate the lifestyle and behavior patterns of white America, many black women stopped nursing their babies. By 1960, for the first time in American history, white women were more likely to breastfeed than black women. Between 1966-1970 fourteen percent of black babies were breast-fed compared to twenty-nine percent of white babies.

Raised to consciousness by the feminist movement, many educated, middle-class white women rediscovered breastfeeding in the 1970s. Aware of the immunological, mother/infant bonding and other benefits of breastfeeding, many of these women began to choose natural childbirth and quickly embraced nursing as part of the shift toward natural health and healing.

However, the majority of black women (perhaps influenced by their alienation and isolation from the 1970s feminist movement) did not return to breastfeeding. Today, women most likely to breastfeed are white, college-educated, married and live in the Western United States. Women least likely to breastfeed are black, single and live in the South. Black women most likely to breastfeed match their white counterparts in that they tend to be older, college-educated and married.

Challenges for Black Women

There are many barriers within the social, cultural and health care systems that make it difficult for black women to breastfeed their infants. Among them are:

- embarrassment, modesty, shame—feelings which are heightened by the societal view of breasts as sex objects

- loss of freedom/incompatibility with lifestyle

- lack of support in job/school setting

- concern that milk supply is inadequate

- high-tech marketing by formula companies

- lack of support from partner

- concern with figure

- lack of adequate and accurate information about breastfeeding

- lack of support from health care providers, family and friends

- limited or no postpartum assistance

- few or no role models

African-American women can begin to overcome these barriers by seeking—as I did—adequate support, encouragement and advice about breastfeeding. Husbands and partners of black women who wish to breastfeed need to be educated about the importance of breast-feeding. People who are offended by women who nurse in public be-cause they view the breast primarily as a sexual object need to under-stand that it is also a biological organ that provides the best possible nourishment for infants.

La Leche (Spanish for "the milk") is an organization that provides advice, literature and support for breastfeeding mothers. You can obtain information about the group by contacting La Leche League International, 9616 Minneapolis Avenue, Franklin Park, Illinois 60131, 1-800-LA-LECHE.

Successful Breastfeeding

First and foremost, breastfeeding is a mother's personal choice. Women should not be pressured, made to feel guilty or treated as fail-ures for not breastfeeding. Many women who know that breastfeeding is best stop nursing their babies, not because they are "bad mothers," but rather because of lactation problems and lack of support. What ap-pears to be common knowledge about breastfeeding is not common at all. Women who are successful at nursing their newborns have accu-rate information, support and encouragement *before* delivery. The fol-lowing hints can help you increase your chances of having a rewarding breastfeeding experience:

- Eat healthy and nutritious foods during your pregnancy. A good diet will help you establish and maintain a good milk supply. Work with your practitioner to create a healthy food plan.

- Avoid sudden and drastic weight loss. The extra pounds women gain during pregnancy help improve milk production. Through breastfeeding you will shed the added pounds naturally.

- Drink plenty of fluids—water, juice or milk—every time you nurse. Many African Americans have a lactose intolerance (inability to digest milk or milk products efficiently). Consult your health care provider if you have this condition.

- Get plenty of rest. It is easier for your body to keep the milk supply flowing when you are calm, rested and relaxed.

Reasons Not to Breastfeed

More than ninety-five percent of women can successfully breastfeed. A small percentage of women cannot because of physiological reasons. The breast is a biological organ that can malfunction and fail to produce adequate milk for an infant's healthy growth and development.

Despite its benefits, not every woman can or should breastfeed. Among those who should not breastfeed are women for whom nursing would pose a medical risk to herself or to her baby. Medical risks may exist with the following conditions:

- mothers who test positive for HIV, the virus that causes AIDS

- tuberculosis

- use of drugs that may be harmful to the infant. Whatever a mother consumes will be passed onto the baby via the milk supply

- serious contamination of food, air or water with substances that will pass to the infant through the mother's milk

Promoting Mother's Milk

The promotion of breastfeeding in the African-American community is critical for the health and well-being of our infants and young children. As students, professionals, wives, mothers, friends, partners, sisters, health care providers and activists, we must help ensure that the oldest, safest and best method of infant feeding once again becomes the norm in our community. We must embrace the philosophy of Chilean poet Gabriela Mistral who writes:

> We are guilty of many errors and many faults, but our worse crime is abandoning the children, neglecting the foundation of life. Many of the things we need can wait. Children cannot. Right now is the time their bones are being formed, their blood is being made, and their senses are being developed. To them we cannot answer "Tomorrow." Their name is Today.

One Woman's Story

Following is an account of a woman's experiences with breastfeeding. It reveals some of the obstacles facing black women who wish to nurse and provides information that can help make the health-care system more responsive to breastfeeding.

Diane Roberts (not her real name) is originally from Mississippi. She is the youngest of nine children, all of whom were breastfed. Diane's mother nursed her for more than a year.

In 1976, Diane was twenty-three and on active duty in the military in Washington State. She gave birth to her daughter that year in a military hospital.

Diane's obstetrician never discussed infant practices with her during the course of her pregnancy. He did not offer encouragement or support for breastfeeding. After a routine delivery, Diane and her daughter spent three days in the hospital. While there the baby was kept in a nursery, given a pacifier, glucose water and was fed formula every three to four hours. When Diane left the hospital she was given a free package of infant formula.

During the three days Diane and her baby were in the hospital, her daughter ate very little and cried most of her waking hours. For the next three months, the baby cried constantly, suffered from diarrhea and had severe vomiting episodes. Alarmed, Diane took her baby to the doctor several times. He always told her that there was nothing wrong with the infant. Saying that the problem was all in her head, he dismissed her concerns calling her an "overprotective" mother.

At the end of her rope, trying to care for a crying baby who was obviously in pain, Diane went home to Mississippi for a visit and to get much needed help with the baby. While there she made an appointment with the family doctor who had delivered Diane and all her siblings. The doctor knew immediately that the baby was allergic to the milk-based formula she was being fed. He put her on a soy-based formula that also caused problems. He then switched her to an expensive formula specifically for babies with severe allergies, which solved the problem immediately.

Diane had a family history of severe allergies. She and all her siblings experienced allergic reactions to milk and milk products. But because they had been breastfed, they did not develop the allergies until later in life. Had Diane been encouraged to nurse her daughter, chances are high that the baby would have been likewise protected from illness. Research shows that bottlefed babies have a greater incidence of allergic disorders than infants who are breastfed.

Diane did not nurse her daughter because she was unaware of the benefits of breastfeeding. As a young mother she came face to face with the barriers that exist in the health-care system—namely a doctor who did not promote breastfeeding, hospital procedures that interfered with successful breastfeeding and the marketing efforts of formula companies deadset on getting new mothers hooked on their products before they are barely out of the hospital bed.

Today Diane is a nutrition educator working to increase the rates and duration of breastfeeding among low income and African-American women. She has received advance training in breastfeeding education and is part of an interdisciplinary health team dedicated to helping black women nurse successfully. Because she was denied the opportunity to breastfeed her daughter, she wants to make sure that other sisters have the chance to give their babies a healthy start.

The World Health Organization projects that by the end of the decade, forty million people will be infected with the human immunodeficiency virus (HIV) that causes AIDS. A disproportionate number of AIDS sufferers are black and female. This article takes a look at the impact of the disease on black women and outlines prevention and treatment strategies.

HIV Infection, AIDS and Black Women
*Janet L. Mitchell, Patricia O. Loftman
and Betty W. Carrington*

Acquired immune deficiency syndrome, or AIDS, was first identified as a health problem in 1981, when it appeared among a cluster of white gay men in Los Angeles and New York. Since then it has spread around the globe, becoming the most serious infectious disease identified in the late twentieth century.

HIV—which is spread *only* through infected blood, semen, vaginal secretions, mother-to-fetus contact and possibly through breast milk—attacks and weakens the body's immune system. Once HIV destroys the immune system, the body becomes susceptible to all sorts of infections that healthy people can routinely fend off. These "opportunistic infections" may eventually trigger AIDS-related illnesses that can lead to death.

Complications from AIDS is one of the leading causes of death in African-American women between the ages of twenty-five and forty-four. For black women of that age group in New York and New Jersey, it is the primary cause of death. To stem the tide of this devastating epidemic, it is critical that black women assume positions of leadership and advocacy in formulating AIDS education and prevention strategies. We cannot abdicate our responsibility to our sisters, brothers, children and ourselves. We must fight this battle with the dedication, determination and care that we have fought all the battles that have come before.

A Legacy of Neglect
The AIDS epidemic has focused much needed attention on the long-standing neglect of women's health concerns in this country. Typically,

the medical establishment has not considered gender an important factor in disease. Results from research studies done primarily on white men have been applied with minimal modification to women. This same "blind" approach had long ago been abandoned as it pertained to illness and children, who are no longer considered just "little adults." In more recent times, racial differences have been examined with regard to their influence in the manifestation and prevalence of certain diseases, most notably hypertension in the African-American community. Unfortunately, not enough attention has been given to the particular way HIV impacts women.

Obstacles to Care

The lack of information about women and HIV is steeped in sexism, classism, racism and invisibility. The women most likely to be infected with HIV are generally poor, minority, drug users or partners of drug users. Original interest in HIV-infected women centered on their relation to pediatric AIDS and mother-to-fetus transmission—the tragedy of the so-called "AIDS babies." HIV-infected women were viewed as "vectors or vessels" of transmission to their babies and to others; very little attention was given to them as HIV-infected themselves or to the care and treatment they needed.

At the end of 1992, African-American women accounted for over half (fifty-three percent) of all women infected. Of that number, fifty-four percent reported that they are intravenous drug users. Thirty-six percent reported having practiced unsafe sex. Three percent were infected through contaminated blood products and the source of infection either had not been established or could not be established for seven percent of African-American women.

Access to health care and services historically has been marginal for women who are poor, minority or drug users. Thus HIV-infected women, many of whom fall into one if not all of these categories, have been unable to get adequate care. Moreover, because of the pressures, strains and stresses in their lives, many HIV-infected women are crisis-oriented in their "health-seeking behaviors." The overwhelming need to survive takes precedence over other concerns. Health—even if one is HIV-infected—finds itself far down the list of priorities after food, shelter and personal safety.

Education and Prevention

The following illnesses are prevalent among HIV-infected women, according to The Centers for Disease Control in Atlanta: pelvic inflammatory disease, frequent and recurrent yeast infections, abnormal Pap smears, cervical cancer.

Women concerned about their HIV status should consider having a test at an anonymous test site. Contact an AIDS agency in your area for information or the National AIDS hotline at 1-800-342-2437.

Despite the increased level of awareness about HIV disease, especially modes of transmission and prevention, infection rates in African-American women continue to rise. According to a New York State report that examined infection rates in childbearing women from 1988 to 1992, AIDS infection rates decreased in white and Latina women ages twenty-four to twenty-nine, but increased in black women of the same age groups. We are compelled to ask "why?"

As previously noted, the initial focus on HIV-infected women was driven by the increasing numbers of infected infants. Agencies in federal, state and local governments have had to grapple with fact that the "M" in MCH—maternal and child health—programs had been lacking long before the AIDS epidemic. The reluctance to deal with HIV infection in women independent of their childbearing potential may stem from an inability and uneasiness within the medical establishment to address issues of diversity, sexuality and drug use. Caring for and having to counsel intravenous drug users about their sexual practices is something most health-care providers have not been trained to do.

Getting Involved

Programs must deal with these issues and develop culturally appropriate prevention and education strategies. In addition to providing information about condoms, safe-sex practices and the dangers of intravenous drug use, health-care providers must examine and learn to understand the total needs of HIV-infected women. Compassionate attention must be given to the importance of childbearing and the need for all women to make their own decisions about their reproductive life. A recommendation that HIV-infected women should delay childbearing and consider abortion may not be well received in African-American communities where a high premium is placed on children—REGARDLESS. Health-care providers cannot make decisions in a vacuum that does not include the sociocultural practices of the community.

For a black woman who uses intravenous drugs, a pregnancy may boost her self-esteem and give her hope for the future. Numerous studies have indicated that pregnancy prompts such women to try to get off drugs and begin recovery. As with most pregnant women, they hope that their children will thrive. This sense of hope is such a strong motivator that many HIV-infected women choose to continue their pregnancies despite the nearly twenty-five percent odds that their infant will be born HIV-infected. Hope prompts them to carry the baby to term nonetheless.

For those who wish to terminate the pregnancy, the option is not available in many states. Those of us who claim we want women to have choices about their bodies, must thus work for reproductive freedom. We must also be aware of our attitudes. Poor and minority women have long been legitimately leery of the individuals and institutions that have been insensitive and unresponsive to them.

African-American health-care providers must be especially mindful of the messages we relay to HIV-infected women in our care. It is important to take note that we are perceived as authority figures; women can fear that if they do something to "displease" us, they will be penalized. We must understand and respond to their vulnerability, always. As is our heritage and tradition, we must extend our best selves, as we try to stem the tide of this frightening health crisis that is ravaging our communities.

Eunice Rivers was a pivotal figure in the infamous Tuskegee Syphilis Study. In this landmark essay, the author examines the pressures Nurse Rivers faced as she tried to perform her duties in a milieu both racist and sexist.

Your Silence Will Not Protect You: Nurse Eunice Rivers and the Tuskegee Syphilis Study[1]
Evelynn M. Hammonds

I've been afraid to know more about this story. I sat in the library over an hour killing time—flipping through magazines, talking with a friend, making several trips to the water fountain. I stared at her picture on the poster from the Schlesinger Library's Black Women's Oral History Project.

Her face has always looked so familiar to me. The reddish-brown skin and the gray hair brushed back from her forehead in the style worn by many of the women from the central part of Georgia where she and my family were reared. Her hands were large and looked as if they were used to hard work. She had a shy smile on her face. When I could not postpone it any longer, I sat down to read the words of Eunice Rivers, the black woman who had been a major character in an ugly episode in American history, the Tuskegee Syphilis Study.

In July 1972, the world first learned that for forty years the United States Public Health Service had been conducting a study of untreated syphilis on almost four hundred black men in Macon County, Alabama. From 1932 to 1972, 399 men who had syphilis and another 201 who were free of the disease serving as controls, were a part of what became known as the Tuskegee Study. While whites reacted with shock at the exposure of such scientific abuse in their own country (which was for many of them comparable to the crimes of the Nazis against Jews during World War II), African Americans almost universally saw the study as just one of the more blatant acts of genocide long perpetrated against our communities by whites.

As the indifference of the medical and public health establishment has allowed the slow, steady increase of AIDS in African-American communities to continue unabated, many black people have likened the tragic AIDS epidemic to the Tuskegee Study. In the case of AIDS, many African Americans feel that we have little reason to trust public health experts, still largely white, who were part of an agency that used a group of poor black men as their guinea pigs for forty years. But there is another lesson we need to learn from the Tuskegee Study as we enter the second decade of the AIDS epidemic, and that is about our own responsibilities as black women to speak about the ravages of this disease in our communities. The story of the Tuskegee Study and particularly Nurse Eunice Rivers' role in it, should remind us of the ways in which we can be made complicit in the suffering of our own people.

What's Done in the Dark is Revealed in the Light

While historians have known the detailed story of the Tuskegee Study since 1981, when white male historian James H. Jones published his book, *Bad Blood: The Tuskegee Syphilis Experiment*[2], most people have only recently learned of the event from articles in *Essence* magazine. There have also been television programs about the study (a NOVA special and a segment on the news show PrimeTime Live) and a play, *Miss Evers' Boys*, which was written by David Feldsuh, a white man. In the play, the character of Miss Evers is based on the black public health nurse who worked on the Tuskegee Study, Nurse Eunice Rivers. It was Nurse Rivers' job to serve as a liaison between the white doctors who designed and ran the Tuskegee Study and the black men who were its subjects. She kept track of the men in the study, visited with them and came to know their families. She tried to protect them from the racist behavior of the doctors and consoled their families when the men died of the disease. By all accounts, it was the men's trust in Nurse Rivers that kept them in the study. Yet, despite her performance of her duties and the care and concern she displayed toward the men in the study, Nurse Rivers has been depicted in Jones' book and Feldsuh's play as a problematic figure—carrying the weight of the questions: Did she knowingly participate in deceiving the men? Or was she herself a victim of the study?

Furthermore, while she was the only female officially involved in the study, Nurse Rivers was not the only woman who had to deal with its consequences. In addition to the above questions, we need to ponder: What of the wives of the men? How many of them were put at risk because of the failure to treat the men? And most importantly, what are we, as African-American women, to make of various attempts to cast Nurse Rivers as a collaborator in one of the most unethical medical studies of this century?

Eunice Verdell Rivers

Eunice Verdell Rivers was born in 1899 in Early County, Georgia.[3] With her father's encouragement and support, she decided to study nursing. She graduated from the nursing school at Tuskegee Institute in 1922. Her first job was with the Movable School, which was a specially built bus that traveled across Alabama providing hands-on demonstrations of canning, mattress-making, carpentry, animal husbandry and midwifery to black folks with no access to formal education. Following a short stint as a night nursing supervisor at the John A. Andrew Hospital on the Tuskegee Institute campus, Nurse Rivers was recruited in 1932 to join the public health project on the study of venereal disease in Macon County. She remained on the project for the next thirty-three years. In addition to her work on the syphilis study, she also collected information and recorded data on births and deaths in the black population. She often had to travel alone to do this work, going from plantation to plantation in the southern part of the state. Nurse Rivers also taught midwifery for a number of years and worked on other issues related to infant and maternal health among the poorest blacks in Macon County.

In April 1958, Eunice Rivers became only the third recipient of the Oveta Culp Hobby Award, the highest commendation given to an employee of the Department of Health, Education and Welfare. The citation read, "for notable service covering 25 years during which through selfless devotion and skillful human relations she has sustained the interest and cooperation of the subjects of a venereal disease control program in Macon County, Alabama."[4] The irony of her receiving this award for her work on the Tuskegee Study would only become apparent more than a decade later when the details of the study were revealed to a wider public.

Always Mindful

Since the troubling details of the Tuskegee episode have come to light many people have asked the following question: How could a black woman, educated and trained as nurse, willfully participate in a study that ultimately harmed so many of her people? I believe that part of the answer lies in the way Jones depicted Nurse Rivers in *Bad Blood*, which is perhaps the most widely cited text on the study.

From the opening pages of the book, Jones displays a great deal of moral outrage about the study. Noting the pivotal role that Nurse Rivers played in the experiment, he writes, in the book's acknowledgements: "I owe an enormous debt to Eunice Rivers (Laurie) for spending several days with me and helping me to see the experiment through her eyes. More than any other principal of the Tuskegee Study, she increased my tolerance for ambiguity."[5] On the contrary, it is clear from the manner in which Jones renders the story that his vision was skewed. He did not understand nor convey the complexity of the study through Nurse Rivers' eyes.

Eunice Rivers knew firsthand the world of poor black people living in Alabama during the Depression. She could not fail to see how segregation sat like a heavy boot on the backs of all blacks in the South. Though she was an educated woman and one of the few black nurses in Alabama, Nurse Rivers too felt the weight of segregation and oppression on her back. She knew she had to be careful as she traveled around the state collecting birth and death records. She had to be mindful always that her job put her close to white people who were threatened by her professional status. At the same time, she had to consider and attend to the feelings of blacks who might have been disdainful toward her because of her close working relationships with whites. In short, she straddled two worlds.

Early in her career, white supervisors praised Nurse Rivers for her ability to win the trust of the black community, wherever she was dispatched. On one occasion, a white nurse suggested that she might follow Nurse Rivers to learn the secret of her success. But she would have none of that. "You tell me what you want me to do in the office and I'll go and do it," Nurse Rivers replied. "But you're not going to follow me there. The first thing the Negroes would say was that I had been framing them."[6] Nurse Rivers walked this line throughout her career.

Because of our national amnesia about the conditions black people lived under before the civil rights movement, it is difficult for us to remember the world of the segregated South. Black women nurses, social workers, teachers and the few clerks who worked in white-owned stores, played a much more central role in the lives of black people than they do today.

For example, I can remember as a small child, going on Saturday shopping trips with my mother and sister to a major department store in downtown Atlanta. My mother always took us to this particular store because she had a black woman friend who worked as a clerk, not a saleslady (in those days the title "saleslady" was reserved for white women) in the girls' and women's department. My sister and I liked going to this store because my mother was always less tense and anxious when we shopped there. Her friend would help pick out clothes for us and then stand guard at the one dressing room we were allowed to use. She wouldn't let the white salesladies talk down to my mother and even at a young age, my sister and I understood the importance of her protection. And certainly, when our friend was home on the weekends, as a valued member of her church and community, the role she played was validated by all. These women were seen as muting the force of a system of apartheid that at any moment could turn a simple shopping trip—during which a black child might innocently touch a pretty dress on a rack—into an ugly and dangerous racial incident.

It is within this context that Nurse Rivers carried out the duties of her job. She had no ambitions to be a doctor, she wanted to be a nurse because she was, in her own words, "interested in the person, and it just never occurred to me that I wanted to be a doctor . . . the nurse plays an important part there. She's closer to the patient. Patients would get to the point where if they're not sure, they're going to ask you. They get you in the middle."[7]

"These Are Grown Men"

When Nurse Rivers became involved in the Tuskegee Study, she fiercely protected the men, making sure that the young white doctors who gave them their yearly checkups understood that the men were human beings. "They're human," she told the doctors, who often treated the men insensitively. "You don't talk to them like that. . . . If anything happens that you can't get along; that you can't get it through their head, just call me. We'll straighten it out. But don't holler at them. These are grown men."[8]

To the white physicians conducting the study, the men were nothing more than experimental "subjects." To Nurse Rivers, men like Charles Pollard and Lester Scott (two in the study who are mentioned by name in Jones' book) were deserving of courtesy and respect. Her duties included keeping track of the men in the study, driving them to the hospital for their annual blood tests and checkups and providing them with medicine and tonic throughout the year. The most difficult part of her work was obtaining permission from the men's families to allow the government to perform autopsies after their deaths. She sat with the families and talked them through their fears about the autopsies and at the urging of the widow of the first man in the study to die, she requested that the Public Health Service provide burial stipends of fifty dollars for each family. The autopsies were difficult for her. She attended every funeral. "I was expected to be there," she said. "They were part of my family."[9]

At the Crossroads of Race and Gender

While Nurse Rivers was protective of the men in the study and provided care to them and their families, she also knew that they were being denied treatment for syphilis.[10] In her response to questions about this matter, she reiterated what the doctors had told her about the study: that its purpose was to make a comparison with a similar study that was being conducted on white men in order to determine if syphilis manifested itself differently in black people. The devastating nature of the late stages of syphilis was visible to all. It is a condition characterized by tumors and ulcers on the skin, bone deterioration and often severe damage to the cardiovascular and central nervous systems. Syphilis could cause blindness, progressive paralysis, and in those whose spinal cord nerves were affected, it impaired movement of legs, producing a stumbling gait.

As Jones noted, all these complications were known to medical science before the Tuskegee Study began. Eunice Rivers was not alone in accepting the Public Health Service physicians' view that a study of the late stages of syphilis in black people was needed. Dr. Eugene Dibble, the black medical director of the Tuskegee Institute and head of its hospital, had given his approval to the study from its inception and had also performed some of the spinal punctures and autopsies on the men. Dr. William Perry, a black physician from the Harvard School of Public Health, sanctioned the study and participated in it. Dr. Jerome J. Peters, a staff physician at the Veterans Hospital in Tuskegee, likewise performed spinal punctures and autopsies on the men. In 1969, nearly thirty-seven years after the study began, most in the predominately black medical establishment in Macon County had sanctioned the study.

Nurse Rivers perceived the study and its impact this way: While the men did not get treated for syphilis, they did get "good medical" care—care they would not have received otherwise because of their socioeconomic status. Neither Tuskegee Institute nor other local hospitals had provided adequate care for the poor black people in Macon County. As Nurse Rivers saw it, the fact that the men were given cardiograms and other expensive tests over the course of the study, meant they had access to quality care that few of their station ever received. Nurse Rivers consistently mentioned care when questioned about the ethics of the study. Nonetheless, she did not refrain from addressing the overriding problem of the research, "The doctors didn't tell the patients they had syphilis."[11]

Who Shall Be Called to Account?

While some might construe Nurse Rivers' response as a casting aside of her own responsibility and complicity in the study, I think her answer reflects the complexities in the experiment, the majority of which have been largely ignored. Jones devotes a major portion of *Bad Blood* to describing Nurse Rivers' work and the trusting relationships she established with the men in the study. He spends far too little time documenting her relationship with the black and white male physicians who supervised her. Castigating her for "ethical passivity," Jones seems almost personally aggrieved that Nurse Rivers was unable to stop the experiment. He does not call to account the male physicians who had much more power and authority than she.

Thus, in his rendering of the story, the black woman nurse becomes the center of the ethical dilemmas raised by the Tuskegee Study. The person who in fact had the least amount of power to resist or question the study is blamed. Eunice Rivers was in no position based on her education or her work to evaluate the scientific merits of the study. And to be sure, the white physicians who supervised her were extremely adept at masking the ethical issues raised by the study. Despite their approval of the study, neither the black male medical establishment nor the administrators (again black and male) of Tuskegee are depicted as central figures in Jones' book. All these men, both black and white, are spared the censure Eunice Rivers receives.

"We're Sick Too"

The Tuskegee Study is a story of the betrayal of poor black men and women. The men in the study and their mates were betrayed by both black and white male physicians who cared little about their lives because the people were black and poor. In the beginning of the study, the black physicians who lent their support to it, saw in the project a way to enhance their standing with the white medical establishment. These men knew full well the implications of the study and the system of racialized medical research from which it had emerged.

They put their professional interests above the medical needs of their people. They put their well-being above that of the fifty unnamed women and children who contracted syphilis because of the government's failure to treat the men.[12] We know nothing of the plight of these women or their children.

Eunice Rivers was also betrayed. Praised for her work with the men in the study by white physicians who noted her skill at warning the physicians of "eccentricities" of the patients, Nurse Rivers stood in the middle. She watched black male physicians cooperate with and validate a study controlled by white men.

She was called upon to console, but was powerless to advocate for the wives of the men who asked her why only men could be in the study. "We're sick too, Nurse Rivers," they said. As a middle-class, educated woman who interacted with both black physicians and the poor black men who were subjects in the study, Nurse Rivers lived in two communities. She saw herself as at least trying to do something for people others had forsaken.

Silent No More

Eunice Rivers died at age eighty-seven in Tuskegee, Alabama. Her obituary noted that she had been a member of the Greater St. Mark Missionary Baptist Church for forty years. She organized the church's nurses' guild, taught women's Bible classes, was a member of the sisterhood, Trustee Board, Women's Missionary Board and Religious Education Board.[13] She lived a life of service to her community, but no one was served by her silence.

I wish that Nurse Rivers had been able to see that the Tuskegee Study was wrong. I wish that she had been able to speak. But I will not ask her to carry the weight for what was a failure on the part of the entire black community. I will not ask a lone black woman to carry the moral obligations of our community by herself.

This is a burden we must all bear. Black people face the same dilemma today as AIDS continues to spread unchecked in our families and neighborhoods. The toll AIDS is taking on African-American women and children is as ignored as the plight of the women in the Tuskegee Study.

Too few black physicians, nurses and public health workers are talking about the multitudes of black men, women and children with AIDS who are languishing in hospital beds. Too few historians, social scientists, community activists, religious and political leaders are speaking out. Because of homophobia and shame, too few black families are revealing the cause of death of the many young men and women they are laying to rest.

But listen up. Our silence will not stop the AIDS epidemic. Nor will our acceptance of the medical establishment's inertia and racism exonerate us from our responsibility to our sisters and brothers. We must speak about the failures to stop AIDS. The African-American community must deal with the sensitive issues that are at the heart of this matter—all unsafe sexual practices, but especially unprotected homosexual and bisexual relations and intravenous drug use. If we do not speak out, then another generation will be perfectly justified in asking us, as we today ask those involved in the Tuskegee Study, why blacks stood silent while our people died.

Footnotes

1.   The title is taken from a line in Audre Lorde's essay, "The Transformation of Silence into Language and Action," in *Sister Outsider: Essays and Speeches*. (Freedom, CA: The Crossing Press, 1984)

2.   James H. Jones, *Bad Blood: The Tuskegee Syphilis Experiment* (New York: The Free Press, 1981).

3.   The biographical information on Nurse Rivers is taken from the interview conducted by Lillian A. Thompson for the Black Women's Oral History Project. It is published in *The Black Women's Oral History Project* (Westport: Meckler Publishing, 1991), volume 7, pp. 213-242. In 1952, Eunice Rivers married Julius Laurie and took his surname. However, in published works, she is most often cited as Nurse Eunice Rivers.

4.   Jones, p. 169.

5.   Jones, op. cit., p. xi.

6.   *The Black Women's Oral History Project*, op. cit., p. 230.

7.   Ibid., pp. 240-241.

8.   Ibid., p. 233.

9.   Jones, op. cit., p. 154.

10.   Eunice Rivers, Stanley Schuman, Lloyd Simpson and Sidney Olamsky, "Twenty Years of Followup Experience in a Long-Range Medical Study," *Public Health Reports*. vol. 68. No. 4, April 1953, pp. 391-395. This paper, which lists Eunice Rivers as co-author, unabashedly opens with the statement, "One of the longest continued medical surveys ever conducted is the study of untreated syphilis in the male Negro."

11.   Jones, op.cit., p. 219.

12.   Jones, op.cit., p. 255.

13.   Program from the funeral service of Eunice Verdell Rivers Laurie, September 1, 1986. Tuskegee University Archives. My thanks to Wellesley College Professor Susan Reverby for her assistance.

Without question, our physical, spiritual and emotional health is enhanced by the transformative power of love. However, many black women have yet to achieve the loving relationships we would like. In the following piece, excerpted from her book, Sisters of the Yam, *the author examines the sociocultural influences that have blocked black women's road to intimacy. Moreover, she shows us how to keep moving toward the healthy relationships we deserve and desire.*

Living to Love
bell hooks

Love heals. We recover ourselves in the act and art of loving. A favorite passage from the biblical Gospel of John that touches my spirit declares: "Anyone who does not love is still in death."

Many black women feel that we live lives in which there is little or no love. This is one of our private truths that is rarely a subject for public discussion. To name this reality evokes such intense pain that black women can rarely talk about it fully with one another.

It has not been simple for black people living in this culture to know love. Defining love in *The Road Less Traveled* as "the will to extend one's self for the purpose of nurturing one's own or another's personal growth," M. Scott Peck shares the prophetic insight that love is both an "intention and an action." We show love via the union of feeling and action. Using this definition of love, and applying it to black experience, it is easy to see how many black folks historically could only experience themselves as frustrated lovers, since the conditions of slavery and racial apartheid made it extremely difficult to nurture one's own or another's spiritual growth. Notice, that I say, difficult, not impossible. Yet, it does need to be acknowledged that oppression and exploitation pervert, distort and impede our ability to love.

Given the politics of black life in this white-supremacist society, it makes sense that internalized racism and self-hate stand in the way of love. Systems of domination exploit folks best when they deprive us of our capacity to experience our own agency and alter our ability to care and to love ourselves and others. Black folks have been deeply and profoundly "hurt," as we used to say down home, "hurt to our hearts," and the deep psychological pain we have endured and still endure affects our capacity to feel and therefore our capacity to love. We are a wounded people. Wounded in that part of ourselves that would know love, that would be loving. The choice to love has always been a gesture of resistance for African Americans. And many of us have made that choice only to find ourselves unable to give or to receive love.

Slavery's Impact on Love

Our collective difficulties with the art and act of loving began in the context of slavery. It should not shock us that a people who were forced to witness their young being sold away; their loved ones, companions, and comrades beaten beyond all recognition; a people who knew unrelenting poverty, deprivation, loss, unending grief, and the forced separation of family and kin; would emerge from the context of slavery wary of this thing called love. They knew firsthand that the conditions of slavery distorted and perverted the possibility that they would know love or be able to sustain such knowing.

Though black folks may have emerged from slavery eager to experience intimacy, commitment, and passion outside the realm of bondage, they must also have been in many ways psychologically unprepared to practice fully the art of loving. No wonder then that many black folks established domestic households that mirrored the brutal arrangements they had known in slavery. Using a hierarchical model of family life, they created domestic spaces where there were tensions around power, tensions that often led black men to severely whip black women, to punish them for perceived wrongdoing, that led adults to beat children to assert domination and control. In both cases, black people were using the same harsh and brutal methods against one another that had been used by white slave owners against them when they were enslaved. We know that life was not easy for the newly manumitted black slaves. We know that slavery's end did not mean that black people who were suddenly free to love now knew the way to love one another well.

Slave narratives often emphasize time and time again that black people's survival was often determined by their capacity to repress feelings. In his 1845 narrative, Frederick Douglass recalled that he had been unable to experience grief when hearing of his mother's death since they had been denied sustained contact. Slavery socialized black people to contain and repress a range of emotions. Witnessing one another being daily subjected to all manner of physical abuse, the pain of over-work, the pain of brutal punishment, the pain of near-starvation, enslaved black people could rarely show sympathy or solidarity with one another just as that moment when sympathy and solace was most needed. They rightly feared reprisal. It was only in carefully cultivated spaces of social resistance, that slaves could give vent to repressed feelings. Hence, they learned to check the impulse to give care when it was most needed and learned to wait for a "safe " moment when feelings could be expressed. What form could love take in such a context, in a world where black folks never knew how long they might be together? Practicing love in the slave context could make one vulnerable to unbearable emotional pain. It was often easier for slaves to care for one another while being very mindful of the transitory nature of their intimacies. The social world of slavery encouraged black people to develop notions of intimacy connected to expedient practical reality. A slave who could not repress and contain emotion might not survive.

Repressed Emotions: A Key to Survival

The practice of repressing feelings as a survival strategy continued to be an aspect of black life long after slavery ended. Since white supremacy and racism did not end with the Emancipation Proclamation, black folks felt it was still necessary to keep certain emotional barriers intact. And, in the worldview of many black people, it became a positive attribute to be able to contain feelings. Over time, the ability to mask, hide and contain feelings came to be viewed by many black people as a sign of strong character. To show one's emotions was seen as foolish. Traditionally in Southern black homes, children were often taught at an early age that it was important to repress feelings. Often, when children were severely whipped, we were told not to cry. Showing one's emotions could lead to further punishment. Parents would say in the midst of painful punishments: "Don't even let me see a tear." Or if one dared to cry, they threatened further punishment by saying: "If you don't stop that crying, I'll give you something to cry about."

How was this behavior any different from that of the slave owner whipping the slave by denying access to comfort and consolation, denying even a space to express pain? And if many black folks were taught at an early age not only to repress emotions but to see giving expressions to feeling as a sign of weakness, then how would they learn to be fully open to love? Many black folks have passed down from generation to generation the assumption that to let one's self go, to fully surrender emotionally, endangers survival. They feel that to love weakens one's capacity to develop a stoic and strong character.

"Did You Ever Love Us?"

When I was growing up, it was apparent to me that outside the context of religion and romance, love was viewed by grown-ups as a luxury. Struggling to survive, to make ends meet, was more important than loving. In that context, the folks who seemed most devoted to the art and act of loving were the old ones, our grandmothers and great grandmothers, our granddaddys and great granddaddys, the Papas and Big Mamas. They gave us acceptance, unconditional care, attention and, most importantly, they affirmed our need to experience pleasure and joy. They were affectionate. They were physically demonstrative. Our parents and their struggling-to-get-ahead generation often behaved as though love was a waste of time, a feeling or an action that got in the way of them dealing with the more meaningful issues of life.

When teaching Toni Morrison's novel *Sula*, I am never surprised to see black female students nodding their heads in recognition when reading a passage where Hannah, a grown black woman, asks her mother, Eva: "Did you ever love us?" Eva responds with hostility and says: "You settin' here with your healthy-ass self and ax me did I love you? Them big old eyes in your head would a been two holes of maggots if I hadn't." Hannah is not satisfied with this answer for she knows that Eva has responded fully to her children's material needs. She wants to know if there was another level of affection, of feeling and action. She says to Eva: "Did you ever, you know, play with us?" Again Eva responds by acting as though the question is completely ridiculous:

> Play? Wasn't nobody playin' in 1895. Just 'cause you got it good now you think it was always this good? 1895 was a killer girl. Things was bad. Niggers was dying like flies. . . . What would I look like leapin' round that little old room playin' with youngins with three beets to my name?

Eva's responses suggest that finding the means for material survival was not only the most important gesture of care, but that it precluded all other gestures. This is a way of thinking that many black people share. It makes care for material well-being synonymous with the practice of loving. The reality is, of course, that even in a context of material privilege, love may be absent. Concurrently, within the context of poverty, where one must struggle to make ends meet, one might keep a spirit of love alive by making a space for playful engagement, the expression of creativity, for individuals to receive care and attention in relation to their emotional well-being, a kind of care that attends to hearts and minds as well as stomachs. As contemporary black people commit ourselves to collective recovery, we must recognize that attending to our emotional well-being is just as important as taking care of our material needs.

It seems appropriate that this dialogue on love in *Sula* takes place between two black women, between mother and daughter, for their interchange symbolizes a legacy that will be passed on through the generations. In fact, Eva does not nurture Hannah's spiritual growth, and Hannah does not nurture the spiritual growth of her daughter, Sula. Yet, Eva does embody a certain model of "strong" black womanhood that is practically deified in black life. It is precisely her capacity to repress emotions and do whatever is needed for the continuation of material life that is depicted as the source of her strength. It is a kind of "instrumental" way of thinking about human needs, one that is echoed in the contemporary song Tina Turner sings—"What's love got to do with it?"

If We Would Know Love

Love needs to be present in every black female's life, in all of our houses. It is the absence of love that has made it so difficult for us to stay alive, or if alive, to live fully. When we love ourselves we want to live fully. Whenever people talk about black women's lives, the emphasis is rarely on transforming society so that we can live fully, it is almost always about applauding how well we have "survived" despite harsh circumstances or how we can survive in the future. When we love ourselves, we know that we must do more than survive. We must have the means to live fully. To live fully, black women can no longer deny our need to know love.

If we would know love, we must first learn how to respond to inner emotional needs. This may mean undoing years of socialization where we have been taught that such needs are unimportant. Let me give an example. In her recently published book, *The Habit of Surviving: Black Women's Strategies for Life*, Kesho Scott opens the book sharing an incident from her life that she feels taught her important survival skills:

> *Thirteen years tall, I stood in the living room doorway. My clothes were wet. My hair was mangled. I was in tears, in shock, and in need of my mother's warm arms. Slowly, she looked me up and down, stood up from the couch and walked towards me, her body clenched in criticism. Putting her hands on her hips and planting herself, her shadow falling*

*over my face, she asked in a voice of barely suppressed rage, "What hap-
pened?" I flinched as if struck by the unexpected anger and answered,
"They put my head in the toilet. They say I can't swim with them."
"They" were eight white girls at my high school. I reached out to hold
her, but she roughly brushed my hands aside and said, "Like hell! Get
your coat. Let's go."*

Straight-away it should be evident that Kesho was not learning
that her emotional needs should be addressed at this moment. In her
next sentence she asserts: "My mother taught me a powerful and enduring lesson that day. She taught me that I would have to fight back
against racial and sexual injustice." Obviously, this is an important
survival strategy for black women. But Kesho was also learning an unhealthy message at the same time. She was made to feel that she did
not deserve comfort after a traumatic painful experience, that indeed
she was "out-of-line" to even be seeking emotional solace, and that her
individual needs were not as important as the collective struggle to resist racism and sexism. Imagine how different this story would read if
we were told that as soon as Kesho walked into the room, obviously
suffering distress, her mother had comforted her, helped repair the
damage to her appearance, and then shared with her the necessity of
confronting (maybe not just then, it would depend on her psychological state whether she could emotionally handle a confrontation) the
racist white students who had assaulted her. Then Kesho would have
known, at age thirteen, that her emotional well-being was just as important as the collective struggle to end racism and sexism—that indeed these two experiences were linked.

Many black females have learned to deny our inner needs while
we develop our capacity to cope and confront in public life. This is
why we can often appear to be functioning well on jobs but be utterly
dysfunctional in private. You know what I am talking about. Undoubtedly you know a black woman who looks together, in control on the
job, and when you drop by her house unexpectedly for a visit, aside
from the living room, every other space looks like a tornado hit it,
everything dirty and in disarray. I see this chaos and disorder as a reflection of the inner psyche, of the absence of well-being. Yet until
black females believe, and hopefully learn when we are little girls, that
our emotional well-being matters, we cannot attend to our needs. Often we replace recognition of inner emotional needs with the longing
to control. When we deny our real needs, we tend to feel fragile, vulnerable, emotionally unstable and untogether. Black females often
work hard to cover up these conditions.

Let us return to the mother in Kesho's story. What if the sight of her wounded and hurt daughter called to mind the mother's deep unaddressed inner wounds? What if she was critical, harsh, or just downright mean, because she did not want to break down, cry, and stop being the "strong black woman?" And yet, if she cried, her daughter might have felt her pain was shared, that it was fine to name that you are in pain, that we do not have to keep the hurt bottled up inside us. What the mother did was what many of us have witnessed our mothers doing in similar circumstances—she took control. She was domineering, even her physical posture dominated. Clearly, this mother wanted her black female presence to have more "power" than that of the white girls.

A fictional model of black mothering that shows us a mother able to respond fully to her daughters when they are in pain is depicted in Ntozake Shange's novel *Sassafrass, Cypress and Indigo*. Throughout this novel, Shange's black female characters are strengthened in their capacity to self-actualize by a loving mother. Even though she does not always agree with their choices she respects them and offers them solace. Here is part of a letter she writes to Sassafrass who is "in trouble" and wants to come home. The letter begins with the exclamation: "Of course you can come home! What do you think you could do to yourself that I wouldn't love my girl?" First giving love and acceptance, Hilda later chastises, then expresses love again:

> You and Cypress like to drive me crazy with all this experimental living. You girls need to stop chasing the coon by his tail. And I know you know what I'm talking about . . . Mark my words. You just come on home and we'll straighten out whatever it is that's crooked in your thinking. There's lots to do to keep busy. And nobody around to talk foolish talk or experiment with. Something can't happen every day. You get up. You eat, go to work, come back, eat again, enjoy some leisure, and go back to bed. Now, that's plenty for most folks. I keep asking myself where did I go wrong? Yet I know in my heart I'm not wrong. I'm right. The world's going crazy and trying to take my children with it. Okay. Now I'm through with all that. I love you very much. But you're getting to be a grown woman and I know that too. You come back to Charleston and find the rest of yourself. Love, Mama.

Loving What We See

The art and practice of loving begins with our capacity to recognize and affirm ourselves. That is why so many self-help books encourage us to look at ourselves in the mirror and talk to the image we see there.

Recently, I noticed that what I do with the image I see in the mirror is very unloving. I inspect it. From the moment I get out of bed and look at myself in the mirror, I am evaluating. The point of the evaluation is not to provide self-affirmation but to critique. Now this was a common practice in our household. When the six of us girls made our way downstairs to the world inhabited by father, mother and brother, we entered the world of "critique." We were looked over and told all that was wrong. Rarely did one hear a positive evaluation.

Replacing negative critique with positive recognition has made me feel more empowered as I go about my day. Affirming ourselves is the first step in the direction of cultivating the practice of being inwardly loving. I choose to use the phrase "inwardly loving" over self-love, because the very notion of "self" is so inextricably bound up with how we are seen by and in relation to others. Within a racist/sexist society, the larger culture will not socialize black women to know and acknowledge that our inner lives are important. Decolonized black women must name that reality in accord with others among us who understand as well that it is vital to nurture the inner life. As we examine our inner life, we get in touch with the world of emotions and feelings. Allowing ourselves to feel, we affirm our right to be inwardly loving. Once I know what I feel, I can also get in touch with those needs I can satisfy or name those needs that can only be satisfied in communion or contact with others.

Where is the love when a black woman looks at herself and says: "I see inside me somebody who is ugly, too dark, too fat, too afraid—somebody nobody would love, 'cause I don't even like what I see;" or maybe: "I see inside me somebody who is so hurt, who is just like a ball of pain and I don't want to look at her 'cause I can't do nothing about that pain." The love is absent. To make it present, the individual has to first choose to see herself, to just look at that inner self without blame or censure. And once she names what she sees, she might think about whether that inner self deserves or needs love.

I have never heard a black woman suggest during confessional moments in a support group that she does not need love. She may be in denial about that need but it doesn't take much self-interrogation to break through this denial. If you ask most black women straight-up if they need love—the answer is likely to be yes. To give love to our inner selves we must first give attention, recognition and acceptance. Having let ourselves know that we will not be punished for acknowledging who we are or what we feel can name the problems we see. I find it helpful to interview myself, and I encourage my sisters to do the same. Sometimes it's hard for me to get immediately in touch with what I feel, but if I ask myself a question, an answer usually emerges.

Sometimes when we look at ourselves, and see our inner turmoil and pain, we do not know how to address it. That's when we need to seek help. I call loved ones sometimes and say, "I have these feelings that I don't understand or know how to address, can you help me?" There are many black females who cannot imagine asking for help, who see this as a sign of weakness. This is another negative debilitating world view we should unlearn. It is a sign of personal power to be able to ask for help when you need it. And we find that asking for what we need when we need it is an experience that enhances rather than diminishes personal power. Try it and see. Often we wait until a crisis situation has happened when we are compelled by circumstances to seek the help of others. Yet, crisis can often be avoided if we seek help when we recognize that we are no longer able to function well in a given situation. For black women who are addicted to being controlling, asking for help can be a loving practice of surrender, reminding us that we do not always have to be in charge. Practicing being inwardly loving, we learn not only what our souls need but we begin to understand better the needs of everyone around us as well.

Black women who are *choosing* for the first time (note the emphasis on choosing) to practice the art and act of loving should devote time and energy showing love to other black people, both people we know and strangers. Within white-supremacist capitalist patriarchy, black people do not get enough love. And it's always exciting for those of us who are undergoing a process of decolonization to see other black people in our midst respond to loving care. Just the other day T. told me that she makes a point of going into a local store and saying warm greetings to an older black man who works there. Recently, he wanted to know her name and then thanked her for the care that she gives to him. A few years ago when she was mired in self-hate, she would not have had the "will" to give him care. Now, she extends to him the level of care that she longs to receive from other black people when she is out in the world.

When I was growing up, I received "unconditional love" from black women who showed me by their actions that love did not have to be earned. They let me know that I deserved love; their care nurtured my spiritual growth.

Many black people, and black women in particular, have become so accustomed to not being loved that we protect ourselves from having to acknowledge the pain such deprivation brings by acting like only white folks or other silly people sit around wanting to be loved. When I told a group of black women that I wanted there to be a world where I can feel love, feel myself giving and receiving love, every time I walk outside my house, they laughed. For such a world to exist, racism and all other forms of domination need to change. To the extent that I commit my life to working to end domination, I help transform the world so that it is that loving place I want it to be.

Love Heals

Nikki Giovanni's "Woman Poem" has always meant a lot to me because it was one of the first pieces of writing that called out black women's self-hatred. Published in the anthology, *The Black Woman*, edited by Toni Cade Bambara, this poem ends with the lines: "face me whose whole life is tied up to unhappiness cause it's the only for real thing i know." Giovanni not only names in this poem that black women are socialized to be caretakers, to deny our inner needs, she also names the extent to which self-hate can make us turn against those who are caring toward us. The black female narrator says: "how dare you care about me—you ain't got no good sense—cause i ain't shit you must be lower than that to care." This poem was written in 1968. Here we are, decades later, and black women are still struggling to break through denial to name the hurt in our lives and find ways to heal. Learning how to love is a way to heal.

I am empowered by the idea of love as the will to extend oneself to nurture one's own or another's spiritual growth because it affirms that love is an action, that it is akin to work. For black people it's an important definition because the focus is not on material well-being. And while we know that material needs must be met, collectively we need to focus our attention on emotional needs as well. There is that lovely biblical passage in "Proverbs" that reminds us: "Better a dinner of herbs, where love is, than a stalled ox and hatred therewith."

When we as black women experience fully the transformative power of love in our lives, we will bear witness publicly in a way that will fundamentally challenge existing social structures. We will be more fully empowered to address the genocide that daily takes the lives of black people—men, women and children. When we know what love is, when we love, we are able to search our memories and see the past with new eyes; we are able to transform the present and dream the future. Such is love's power. Love heals.

The inadequate treatment of black women in the health care system reflects the suffering disenfranchised people experience in the general society. In the following piece, the author writes of the circumstances surrounding her grandmother's death and offers important insights about the responsibility of medical institutions to the communities they serve.

In Emergency
Elizabeth Lorde-Rollins

The day was especially sticky, one of those August days in New York when anyone with a little money and freedom is out of town. I was in town because medical school was to begin in a week. My Aunt Helen, a social worker for the city, was in town as well. We were both worried about my grandmother Linda, who had been in bed with a cold for about a week. When I'd visited a couple days before, she hadn't felt up to listening as I read the Sunday comics aloud, one of her favorite weekend activities.

At the age of ninety-one, she was living a simple life. A couple of home attendants lived with her: Enid stayed five days a week and Mrs. Morgan came for the weekends. My Aunt Helen visited every afternoon, sometimes coming by in the morning as well with prescription refills or food. Linda enjoyed talking with Enid and Mrs. Morgan (all three hailed from the Caribbean, and although they rarely talked about "home" they shared a certain view of this crazy place called New York); seeing her children and grandchildren; listening to the radio; saying her prayers in the morning; holding her ancient leather bible as if she could still read the tiny print; having a scotch and ginger ale before Sunday supper. She also had pain—arthritis in her back and hands and difficulty walking. She was old and her life wasn't easy, but it was a life worth living. She had things she wanted to see yet. One of these was to see me graduate from medical school.

When my aunt called that August afternoon, I was enjoying one of my last chances to watch "All My Children" without feeling that there were more important things I should be doing. Helen said that Grandma had a fever—could I come down to the apartment? When I got there, we took her temperature again; it was 104 degrees. We decided to take her to the hospital. Carol, a friend who had just finished her first year of medical school, said she'd meet me at the hospital after her classes. After waiting for almost an hour, an ambulance arrived and whisked us to Columbia Presbyterian Medical Center, the closest hospital. When we got to the emergency room, I found myself wishing that Carol had come with me. My grandmother was wheeled to Area A, through two large brown doors. I kept trying to get inside to see her. When the doors opened, I could see her on a gurney in the hall. However, the guards wouldn't allow me to go inside and they repeatedly told me to get back to my seat. Other ambulances arrived almost every ten minutes; people on the edge of death were wheeled to the back immediately; women about to deliver were told to walk two blocks to Babies' Hospital; all others sat in plastic bucket seats in a dirty, crowded room and waited. Young men with blood pouring down their faces and crusting over their eyes waited. Babies with rashes and small children whose arms hung from their bodies at weird angles waited. A young woman with two bloody towels around her cut wrists waited.

We had arrived at the emergency room at about 2:30 p.m. My aunt and I spent some time calling St. Croix and speaking with my mother and then we settled in to wait. At 8:30 p.m. Carol came. I don't think I've ever seen anything as beautiful as the sight of my friend in her white coat with her stethoscope around her neck and her ID cards dangling. She was an "innie" not an "outie" like my aunt and me. She could help us. She could get me in to see my grandmother. Sure enough, with Carol towing me along, we had no trouble walking past the abusive guards who stood at the entrance to Area A as if we were all in prison. Grandma was on a stretcher, exposed, in a hallway littered with bandage wrappings and plastic syringe covers.

"Grandma?" I said, covering her with a sheet and taking her hand from the stretcher bar.

"Is that you, bamsy?"

"Yes, it's me. How are you feeling now? Is it still hard to breathe?"

"Not too bad," she said, although it sounded as if her lungs were coming loose.

"Has a doctor seen you?"

"Yes. They took some blood from me."

Carol leaned towards me. "They took some blood cultures in addition to the regular labs, probably, and she's waiting now for an x-ray." In the flurry of activity around us, no one noticed me, and I was able to stay with my grandmother for almost two hours. Back in the waiting room, my aunt and I talked. My mother had been contacted, but we really didn't know what to tell her. My aunt was scheduled to leave for vacation in the morning.

A continuous flood of people arrived at the ER as we sat and waited. Both accident victims and people whose medical problems had just gone too far without the benefit of a doctor's care came and filled the seats. Kids with firecracker injuries, an overdosed twelve year old, a few homeless folks with a range of medical problems, and a wire-thin young woman with AIDS and her father, who she was leaning on for support, walked in on their own. The guards got louder and kicked one man's leg off of an adjacent seat (the man had an open sore on the leg and was trying to elevate it). The television, hanging from the wall at a threatening angle, continued to blare sitcoms about little white kids. The TV was definitely transmitting messages from another planet, a planet where hospitals are clean places, where no one gets kicked when they can't sit up straight, where people have their own doctors to go to when they're sick instead of a faceless stream of interns and residents. The people behind the door, attending physicians, residents, and medical students were almost exclusively white. In fact, Carol was the only black med student in the ER that night. The nurses were mixed—white, black, Latina. Most of the clerks behind the glass (it reminded me of the liquor stores in my neighborhood) were black and Latina women, but there were a couple of white women and one white man. The security guards were almost all black men, and the patients and families in the ER were almost all black and Dominican.

Around eleven, a guard finally let me back in to see my grandmother. A nurse told me that Dr. Borman had seen my grandmother, and she asked me a few questions. My grandmother had Parkinson's disease, had it since the mid-1960s; she had a cold, and had been wheezing for about a week; she was blind, and had been since 1976; she lived in her own walk-up apartment, had a live-in home attendant, and used a walker to get around. Many things that I wanted to tell her about my grandmother wouldn't fit a history; how she'd gone to the Center for Independent Living in 1977 after losing her eyesight and learned how to maneuver around her apartment, identify bills of different denominations, and boil water for tea; how she, a light-skinned black woman, newly arrived from Grenada, had passed for white and worked as a maid at the Waldorf to help support her family during the Depression; how she fought to get to church every Sunday, even with her mobility impairments, and then, when that became impossible, she had the priest come to her to give her sacrament; how she'd had two mild heart attacks in the 1970s and had come back from both of them; how she was a proper, no-nonsense West Indian lady, and call her Mrs. Lorde or call her nothing at all.

At around midnight, Dr. Borman came and presented Aunt Helen and me with a form authorizing a lumbar puncture for Linda Lorde. ("What's that?" my aunt whispered. "A spinal tap," I said.) He volunteered no information about her condition, but when it became clear that we were not going to sign the form without being told what was going on, he said, "She had an x-ray that showed nothing. The culture will not be done for a couple of days. In the meantime, with her fever, we have got to rule out meningitis. The only way to do that is to perform the spinal tap. It's really quite safe. This is pretty routine."

"But what about the cough? She's had a cough for ten days," I asked.

"The same bacteria that make you cough can cause meningitis," he responded.

I looked at my aunt. She looked nervous. I felt nervous. I was tired and enraged at these people. My aunt said, "Whatever you think, Bethie-Poo. You're the medical person. I don't really know much about this." I didn't know *anything* about it, but I did know that I didn't think my grandmother had meningitis. It seemed more like something mundane, like a cold that had gotten really bad, or pneumonia, or something like that. I mean, she'd been coughing for ten days. We thought she'd get better. If it were meningitis, wouldn't she be dead by now? And a spinal tap. With her arthritic back? How was she ever going to be able to bend enough for them to put a needle in between her spread vertebrae? Most of them were fused anyway.

"I don't think she should have it," I told my aunt.

The intern spent a little more time explaining that he really thought I was being foolish. "It doesn't hurt as much as people think it does. We pass a small needle into the sac that holds the spinal cord and we see if there are any bacteria there." I refused to give consent. "Fine," said the intern. "Wait outside."

I convinced my aunt to go home and pack for her trip the next morning, assuring her I'd call if there were any further developments. Carol and Deborah came over from our house to keep me company. I got back in to see my grandmother at around midnight after being very nice to one of the guards. She was in a cubicle now, and I was delighted. Deborah and I pulled a curtain around the bed and hid out in Area A so we could stay with her. At around 12:30 a.m., Dr. Borman came back. He asked me if I had "thought long and hard" about giving consent for the lumbar puncture. I told him I had, and that I still didn't think it was necessary, and that it would probably cause my grandmother a great deal of pain. He left and returned five minutes later with two other doctors. They asked me to step outside. I was only introduced to Dr. Bass, the chief of service. I asked Dr. Bass about my grandmother's wheezing. Her lungs sounded full of fluid. Did Dr. Bass think she had pneumonia? The x-rays were negative, Dr. Bass repeated.

"If you don't have this procedure done, your grandmother could die. A lumbar puncture is the only way we can find if there's infection. If you don't give consent, and she dies tomorrow, are you willing to live with that?"

I thought about my mother in St. Croix, and my Aunt Helen, and my Aunt Phyllis. What if she *did* have meningitis? These doctors had to be smart to get to where they were. On the other hand. . . .

"I just think it's a lot of pain for someone who's ninety-one to go through," I said. "She hasn't shown any signs of meningitis these past two weeks, and she has an arthritic back."

"There may be some discomfort, but pain is minimal, especially if the back doesn't move much, as seems to be your grandmother's case." The three doctors were staring at me, waiting for me to give consent for the "necessary," "life-saving" procedure. I signed the form. Deborah and I went back in to wait.

At 2:30 a.m. Dr. Borman came in with a lumbar puncture kit under his arm. He walked right up to my grandmother. "Sweetheart? Are you awake? Wake up, Sweetheart!" My grandmother opened her eyes.

"Do you know where you are? Do you know why you're here? Sweetheart?"

"Dr. Borman?" I couldn't take this anymore. "She's blind, but she hears very well. Could you please call her Mrs. Lorde?"

"Mrs. Lorde?" he said in a slightly lower voice. "Do you know where you are?"

"Columbia Presbyterian Hospital," she said.

"Do you know why you're here?"

"Well, I've been feeling poorly lately."

"OK, now if you can help me roll you over, Swee—Mrs. Lorde—." Dr. Borman went to work. He asked me to step outside.

At 6:00 a.m. they told us the tap was negative. My grandmother could go home. I asked Dr. Bass, then Dr. Borman and even another doctor to admit her to the hospital. That didn't work, so I called Dr. Evertze (my grandmother's regular doctor at CPMC) and left a message with her service. I asked Dr. Bass again about my grandmother's breathing, because it didn't sound any better to me. "We'll prescribe ampicillin for that." I even had to ask for a prescription for the pain my grandmother was feeling from the spinal tap.

At ten, my aunt came into Area A, where I was sitting with my grandmother. I told her what had gone on the night before and that they still wouldn't admit her. My begging and pleading did not help. At this point, we'd waited four hours for an ambulance to take her home. Transportation arrived for my grandmother a little after noon, but it was an ambulette, not an ambulance. We might as well have taken her home in a cab if she was going to have to sit up on the way home. Tears streamed down my grandmother's face as we rolled her out into the sun; I'd never seen her in so much pain. The ambulette driver, a young black man who looked like he weighed 125 pounds soaking wet, eased her over every bump with such care it was as if she were a member of his own family. It was the first time I'd seen a professional treat her so gently. He brought her all the way up to the second floor of the walk-up on 152nd Street, sweat pouring from his forehead and arms. He wouldn't take the twenty dollars we offered him.

By Saturday night, my grandmother's wheezing had not improved, but her temperature was lower, so I went home. On Sunday morning, Mrs. Morgan called from my grandmother's house. Something had shown on the cerebro-spinal fluid culture, and the hospital had called asking if we could bring my grandmother in. I decided to go to the hospital on my own to see what this was all about. Maybe they would admit her after all! At the front desk, they told me that a doctor had recommended she be brought in for further evaluation. I called the physician and spoke to her. She told me that the cells on the CSF culture were not infectious and seemed to be epithelial. "From skin?" I asked incredulous. Yes, well, they thought it was just from skin on the needle, but just to make sure. . . . "And if I bring her in," I asked, "Will there be someone here to see her, or will she wait for twenty-one hours on a gurney in Area A and then be sent home again?" Well, the doctor admitted, "She will have to go through the usual emergency room procedure." I asked again if there was a way to get her admitted. Not without bringing her to the emergency room, I was told. But I had already done that, and they had released her after twenty-one hours of hell and a spinal tap! I called Dr. Evertze, and since my grandmother had an appointment with her on Monday morning at nine, we decided to wait and keep her home until then.

At eight-thirty that evening, Mrs. Morgan called again. I called for an ambulance from my house, and then went to my grandmother's. I called again at nine to make sure the ambulance was on its way. The police came and they waited with us. With Carol's stethoscope, I listened to my grandmother's chest, which was filled with fluid, and her heart, which was around sixty-five beats every minute. I kept thinking that the thermometer must be broken, because the mercury was all the way up to the top of the scale, 107 degrees. She was broken out with little red dots all over her body. Between nine and ten, I called Emergency Medical Services six times. When they arrived at 10:10 p.m., the emergency medical technicians came rushing in. They listened to her heart beat, took her blood pressure, and gave her oxygen. One EMT stood over my grandmother and shook his head. "It doesn't look good. Why didn't you call earlier?"

At CPMC they took my grandmother to Area A immediately and packed her in ice. The thermometer had not been broken; her fever was spiking at 107 degrees. Mrs. Morgan and I sat in the waiting room. Although this felt exhaustingly familiar, Sunday night was a different experience from Friday night. For one thing, my grandmother was in worse shape, so she was tended to quickly, and a new doctor was on duty—Dr. Luban. He came out to speak with us about forty minutes after we'd brought her in and took a short medical history. He let me in to see her. Watching Dr. Luban, I saw the little things that made him so different from the other physicians my grandmother had encountered that weekend: he looked tired, and at some points overwhelmed, like the others had; he had too much to do, as the others did, but he respected my grandmother. He draped a sheet over her when he could, after her temperature had fallen; he addressed her in a normal tone first, then gauged whether he'd have to raise his voice or not; he never called her "Sweetheart."

My grandmother was admitted to the Intensive Care Unit early Monday morning at 4:00 a.m. She was diagnosed with pneumonia in all lobes of her lungs that same day. By Tuesday, my mother had arrived from St. Croix and while we were visiting, some physicians and students were rounding. They mounted the chest x-rays they'd taken Friday night on a lightbox for viewing and I wanted to hear what they had to say. One of the doctors came over and threatened to have a security guard remove me from the hospital if I didn't move down the hallway, out of earshot. My mother and I did as we were told, as I'd done all weekend.

A couple of days later, I registered at the medical school and got a CPMC identification card. It was great: I could go visit my grandmother anytime. No one stopped me, and the guards were nicer to me. I felt as if I'd joined a magic club. A lot of family visited my grandmother that week she was in the hospital. They all told me how proud they were of me. Not only the first person in the family to become a doctor, but at Columbia! The hospital where everyone in the family had everything done from deliveries to gall bladder surgery! How wonderful! I just smiled and thanked them, but I was beginning to wonder whether this was really something I wanted to be a part of after all.

My grandmother died ten days after being admitted.

I'm still very angry about the way my grandmother and other patients I saw that weekend were treated at Columbia Presbyterian. But after five years at the College of Physicians and Surgeons, now I see this treatment in a much wider context. The manner in which people are treated when they need medical help says a great deal about the fabric of any society. I have come to understand the events surrounding my grandmother's illness and death as outgrowths of the way American medicine is organized at three levels: in our society generally, in neighborhoods and between individual doctors and patients.

The health-care delivery system in this country indicates that our society feels that the more needy one is, the less deserving of help one warrants. In the neighborhood around CPMC, there is not only a dearth of doctors, but a dearth of other medical facilities as well. There is no question that the Washington Heights community, and indeed, all of Harlem, are medically underserved. The absence of adequate health systems reflects societal priorities as well. When the New York City government tried to pull itself out of a financial hole, the first items to go were three hospitals in Harlem. CPMC, heir to the resulting overflow, is deeply affected as an institution by such prioritizing and so are the relationships within the hospital.

Anytime physicians are overworked, under-supplied and working with the bulk of the city's homeless, they will be less giving of their time, more harried and more unpleasant to their patients. Doctors in such straits tend to see patients when their health status is already much impaired. The economics of our society and lack of access to quality health care—especially in urban settings—leads to deficient health among the poor. Many physicians, failing to see the roots of substandard health among economically disenfranchised patients (or too busy to care about the roots of what he/she sees every day), perceive these inequalities as due to a lack of concern on the part of poor people.

The institution, in turn, sends out messages to its employees: it's OK to be abusive ("to folks who don't care enough to take care of themselves"). Guards do not kick patients' chairs in New York Hospital and tell them to sit up; visitors are not harangued at Beth Israel for trying to see their loved ones. In short, it seems that Columbia Presbyterian believes it is being drained by the community and conducts itself toward the community accordingly. There is no feeling that the hospital cannot exist without the community. Consequently, members of the community are treated differently from people who look and act as if they are from somewhere else. This dynamic colors patient-physician relationships all over the city. Nowhere is it more marked than in the city's emergency rooms.

On a smaller scale, the emergency room itself is the site of interface between two societies; one well-off, largely white, well-educated and fairly young; the other poor, largely black and Hispanic, less well-educated, and either very young or elderly. Race relations at Columbia Presbyterian operate against a backdrop of race relations in New York City and the social attitudes that these divisions of a split society bring to the institution. If this problem were acknowledged, change might be possible. For instance, CPMC medical students routinely make negative comments about the Washington Heights neighborhood in which the hospital is located. Since the students are, for the most part, white and upper-middle class, and the patients they will see for the first four years of their training are predominately black and Hispanic poor, a race-relations workshop to educate medical students about their racism should be a mandatory component of the first year curriculum. But no such workshop exists.

CPMC's position in the community has been adversarial for too long. The charitable contributions the hospital makes to community projects are helpful, but what CPMC really needs to do is to place itself in partnership with the community. Patients are well aware that they are a part of the teaching process, and that if they were private patients at another institution, they might be treated with greater respect during stays in the hospital and emergency room visits. Yet few students or staff view the opportunity to treat members of the community as an honor. Many physicians don't consider consent a real question for clinic and emergency patients, but a formality. For instance, Dr. Bass was shocked that I even considered saying "no" to my grandmother's lumbar puncture, when nothing in her history or physical exam indicated that it was necessary.

One of the physicians I spoke to on Sunday afternoon, when I tried to gain admittance to the hospital for my grandmother, asked if I was from the neighborhood. I told her "yes" and asked why she had asked. "We don't usually get such articulate people around here," she answered. What to conclude, but that this physician is filled with racist assumptions waiting to be confirmed? Or, more to the point, if she were fluent in Spanish, she might be surprised at how very articulate the patients "around here" are.

As a black woman who is now a physician, about to start training in the same institution that killed my grandmother, I find it difficult to reconcile the lessons I have learned from my observations. Do we, as black women (who are entering medicine in increasing numbers), turn away from monolithic medical institutions and attempt to found our own health-care delivery systems where our lives will be valued for the jewels they are—whether we are blind or seeing, ninety-one or thirty-five years old? (I recently found out that my grandmother, who was a Harlem businesswoman in the 1950s and 1960s, gave thousands of dollars to CPMC in my grandfather's name after his death in 1956). Do we attempt to educate the less-informed staff in an effort to make these institutions more responsive to our communities?

The only answers I've been able to formulate so far are personal: Respect my patients. Learn my craft so I can be as effective as I can possibly be. Be a black woman doctor who understands the roots of poor health in black, Hispanic, Native American and other communities of color. Take that knowledge to the emergency room in honor of my grandmother.

Menopause is a natural event spanning a period of a few months to several years that marks the end of menstruation and reproductive life. For many women, menopause also launches a new era of fertility filled with personal fulfillment, productivity and an increased zest for living.

In the following piece, a black woman shares her experiences of going through "the change" and offers words of support for sisters making the transition.

New Frontiers: Black Women and Menopause
Leora Myers

Menopause . . . a woman's passage into unfamiliar and mysterious terrain. In the past, many of our foremothers avoided even thinking about it, until they had their first hot flash and fashioned a home remedy or made a fast dash to a doctor for "immediate relief."

Today, as more baby-boomer women approach the BIG M, there appears to be a desire to know more about menopause and how to integrate it lovingly and healthily into a woman's life.

The physical changes that signal menopause begin with a drop in estrogen production. Estrogen is the dominant sex hormone that a female begins producing at puberty. Each month, estrogen levels rise as the uterus is prepared for ovulation and potential pregnancy, then fall when the egg is not fertilized and the menstrual period begins.

By around age forty, estrogen levels begin to decline markedly for most women, with menopause setting in between age forty-eight and fifty-two. Ovulation becomes sporadic but still may occur during this period. At the conclusion of menopause, menstrual bleeding stops entirely, signaling the end of fertility.

The lack of estrogen triggers menopausal symptoms such as hot flashes, vaginal dryness and soreness, mood swings and bone thinning or osteoporosis, which is caused by calcium loss. However, studies show that African-American women are less likely to suffer osteoporosis than white women.

Head to Toe Changes
My personal passage has been shocking, encouraging, depressing and comical . . . sometimes all at once. But one year after my first hot flash,

I know more about this stage in my life and find that I am filled with energy, vitality and hope about my future.

My flashes came after several months of irregular periods. My first clue that something major was happening was when I noticed that my hair looked like hell the day after I'd had it done. I've always had a beautiful and healthy head of hair that garnered me many compliments from friends. But something had changed. It no longer looked "good" when I shook it out the day after my hair appointment. When I mentioned it to my hairdresser she gave me a strange look (which I eventually came to know as the "you're probably going through the Change" look) and said: "Well, you may be going through some changes... that does happen."

My second clue was when I was teaching an exercise class and suddenly felt warm all over. When I said, "It sure is hot in here," one of my middle-aged female clients winked at me and gave me that look I'd come to recognize.

The real cooker was when I—who can sleep through a four-alarm fire—started waking up two and three times in the middle of the night drenched with sweat. My husband likes a cool bed, so during the colder months, when we sleep under an electric blanket, I turn it on only on my side. One night he rolled over and said, "Honey, turn off that damn blanket!" I immediately began to sob because the blanket wasn't on. I knew my body was going through a major change.

Frustration and Acceptance

At first I was defiant. "I am not going to go through this," I would say to myself. As a registered nurse and a professional fitness trainer, my head was filled with textbook knowledge about the challenges of menopause that I just put on the back burner, thinking: "I am in excellent shape. These imbalances and mood swings and physical changes I have been reading about will *never* happen to me." Of course my views were as futile and useless as those of a pre-teen girl hoping to stave off her first period. I had to get a grip.

Feeling hopeless and overwhelmed by a body I could no longer control, I sought spiritual guidance through my Buddhist practice and came to understand, as I was told: "Life is like the seasons and you are in the fall of your life. It is also like the night and day. It is very natural. We do not argue with the change in seasons or the change in the day, we accept it as what is natural at that time of the year or day. You can make this time of your life your friend or your enemy... it is your choice."

This was a turning point for me and I believe that every woman facing menopause can have such a moment as she approaches this stage of her life. It may be a person, an event or a particular insight. If you pay attention it will come to you and help you move forward into this incredible journey.

Taking Charge

There is plenty you can do to manage the symptoms of menopause. Remember that the process is individual and no two women will make the passage in the same way. While menopause is a natural event, not an "illness," you may want to consult a doctor about the process. As with any major transition in life, you may also find yourself saying, "I need to get away by myself just to sort things out." I believe this is a natural feeling that is rooted in our African culture where people often separate themselves from others or go into isolation during times of great change such as puberty, marriage and childbirth.

Hot flashes—sudden sensations of flushing and sweating—are one of the most common symptoms of the change. To reduce the intensity and frequency of hot flashes, try the following:

1. Wear loose, layered natural-fabric clothing that can be easily removed.

2. Limit consumption of alcohol, caffeine and spicy foods, which trigger hot flashes in some women.

3. Drink plenty of water and fresh juices.

4. Keep room temperature cool.

5. Exercise regularly—walking, jogging, cycling, dancing—which will improve your mood and sleep quality.

6. Practice stress management techniques such as deep breathing, massage, meditation, yoga.

7. Supplement your diet with vitamin E and herbs such as donquai, black cohosh, fennel, sasparilla and wild yam root.

8. Make the best of the situation (as sisters so often do) by carrying a decorative fan and starting a fashion trend.

As estrogen production declines, the vaginal membranes become thin and secrete less moisture, which can lead to soreness, itching, inflammation and painful intercourse. For relief try water-based lubricants such as K-Y Jelly or Astroglide. Replens, a moisturizer that adheres to vaginal cells, may also be helpful.

As with the onset of puberty, many women experience mood swings during menopause because of changes in hormone levels. You may also find yourself irritable and feeling like everyone is working your last nerve because of interrupted sleep. Regular exercise, meditation and proper diet can help you feel more balanced. You might consider joining a support group of sisters who are also going through the change.

Estrogen Replacement Therapy

One of the biggest controversies in medical treatment of menopause centers on the advisability of estrogen replacement therapy (ERT). Studies show that ERT can help relieve hot flashes, night sweats, insomnia and vaginal soreness. It can reduce the risk of osteoporosis, a factor in life-threatening hip fractures among older women. Research suggests that ERT reduces risk of heart disease, the leading killer of women over fifty. Women who receive hormone therapy also report less fatigue and depression.

But research shows that ERT may increase the risk of breast cancer, uterine cancer, gall bladder disease and fibroid tumors, a widespread health problem among black women. Discuss the advantages and disadvantages of hormone replacement therapy with your health-care provider. If you opt for it, take the smallest dosage possible.

A Smooth Transition

Every transition has a beginning and an ending. With the onset of our menstrual cycle women become able to "bear fruit." With menopause, we can now bear fruits of personal transformation. No longer restricted by the demands of motherhood or the concerns of our childbearing years we can blossom more fully and express the wisdom we've gained as we move into this new and joyous season.

For additional information about menopause here are some suggested readings:

The Pause by Lonnie Barbach (Dutton)

Menopause Naturally by Sadja Greenwood (Volcano Press)

The Menopause Self Help Book by Susan M. Lark (Celestial Arts)

The Silent Passage by Gail Sheehy (Random House)

Stemming from the slavery era, when slave masters treated light-skinned blacks (often their progeny) better than dark-skinned blacks, skin color conflicts have a long history in the African-American community. In addition to the prejudices we suffer at the hands of whites, intraracial color discrimination *has caused emotional pain and misunderstanding for black women all along the color spectrum. In the following discussion, two black women, self-identified as dark- and light-skinned, talk about the impact of "color consciousness" on their lives. Twenty-nine-year-old Tamara works as a paralegal. Trained as a lawyer, thirty-nine-year-old Michele is a food writer.*

The informal conversation took place over a kitchen table one sunny afternoon in Oakland, California and was moderated (loosely) by editor Evelyn C. White.

Color, Color, Color
Michele Anderson and Tamara Ingram

Evelyn: Let's begin by having you both talk a little bit about your background. Your family, where you grew up, schooling, etc.

Tamara: I was raised right here in Oakland. My father is a retired airplane mechanic who grew up in Mississippi. My mother is from Arkansas and is a tax auditor. They are divorced. Both of them arrived in California in the mid-1950s and got to know each other. Both my mom and dad come from a long line of very dark African people. But a lot of the people on my father's side purposefully married light people. I am the darkest one in my family.

Evelyn: You're saying that some of the people on your father's side set out to "whiten up the race?"

Tamara: That's exactly what they did. My father told me that his father always told them that they should marry somebody light to lighten up the family. My grandfather told my father not to ever marry a dark woman. But my father rebelled and married my mother who is dark and very pretty.

Michele: I grew up in Buffalo, New York. Both my parents are light-skinned, though my father is darker than my mother. My maternal grandmother looked white. She had long, straight, dark blonde hair and white skin. She attended Fisk University and was very active in civil rights efforts. She used to say that because she was so fair, white people didn't know she was black. So she got to overhear what they said about blacks and it made her mad. Even so, I do think my grandmother was a little colorstruck. Most of my relatives are very into the "pale" thing and are very class conscious. They really don't mix too closely with what they would classify as "commoners."

Evelyn: Meaning, darker-skinned black people?

Michele: Well, it's more based on class. But the way it goes down is that most of the upper or middle-class people are light-skinned and the darker-skinned people are not. So, it's all intertwined.

Evelyn: What kind of work do your parents do? Where did they meet?

Michele: My father is a retired lawyer. My mother is a retired school-teacher. They met in church. I'm one of four kids and I guess the palest of the crew. What I hear is that when I was a baby, my paternal grandmother, who was kind of dark, used to brag about the whites who stopped her on the street when she was out with me. She said they would say: "She's your granddaughter, but she looks white." My mother didn't like that, so she apparently put a stop to my grandmother taking me out.

Evelyn: Tamara, how did your paternal grandfather respond to your father's marriage and to your family?

Tamara: He never liked us. When I was a kid, he would say, "Get that dark thing out of here." When my parents divorced, my grandfather said to my father: "See, that's what happens when you marry a black girl. It's doomed to fail." He was so happy when my parents got divorced. My grandfather's views really affected my father. So, when I was about seven, my father looked at me one day and said: "Tammy, you're so black, you're so very, very dark."

Evelyn: How did that make you feel?

Tamara: It really hurt. You know, I was a child, innocent. And then my father makes this comment about my dark skin. I'd always known it, but I didn't think it was any big deal until my father pointed it out by saying, "You're really dark. You're the darkest one in this family." Then after that point, I realized I was really dark. Then the kids in the neighborhood started bothering me about being dark. I hated it. They used to call me "tar baby." They ridiculed me constantly. My family did, too. We would get in arguments and they could just shut me up by calling me "black."

Evelyn: Was there anyone in your family who would intervene?

Tamara: My mother. But only as a mother would. She'd tell us to stop arguing, never mentioning the color thing. All through my life, I've just had to take it. There was a little boy who lived next door and he was very nice. We became friends. He was darker than I was. We would watch television together and play. Then one day I realized that people just expected us to be friends because we were both dark. Then all of a sudden I wanted to push him away, even though he was my friend. I wanted to push him away because people had made me feel bad about my color. And I figured that if they hated me and called me ugly and black then they must hate my friend more. I thought that he must be even uglier because he was darker than I was and so I didn't want to be around him. That's when I stopped liking black kids altogether. They hated me and they made me hate my best friend. I remember everything about my childhood. It's like a diary. I was conscious of the whole thing because I kept telling myself: "There's got to be a way to get over this. One day this is going to stop." But it never did. As I grew older, it just got worse.

Evelyn: How did you deal with it?

Tamara: I took it in. Separated myself from people and rebelled. When someone would call me "Blackie," I wouldn't say much. Touché, more or less. Sometimes I'd cry. But I wouldn't let anybody see me cry. I'd walk away and go in my room and shut the door. My mom says I spent half my life with the door shut being anti-social. I just recently realized that I was anti-social because of the way I was humiliated about my skin color. All I ever heard was, "You're dark. You're cute but you're so dark." So I shut the door. I'd sit right up in my room and not talk to anybody. It's like I have a photographic memory of how I was ridiculed. I remember everything.

Evelyn: Michele, what was it like for you as a kid? Did you get taunted because of your light complexion?

Michele: Well, I was one of about three black children in my entire grade school. I didn't get teased by other black kids because there really weren't any to speak of. And I really didn't hang out with the kids in my neighborhood. I sort of stuck close to my white friends at school. I think I just sort of blended in. It must have been third or fourth grade when I remember one of my classmates said to me: "Nigger, nigger,

nigger" and that was the first time I felt any discrimination.

Then later, a girl came to school who was darker. I remember hearing someone comment that she was "loud." It struck me because I didn't think she was any louder than I was. I was a very talkative child. I think that the girl was perceived as being unruly and rowdy because she was dark. I feel shame about this now, but I remember thinking that maybe she would make things bad for all black people. There was so much emphasis on being a "good" black kid, mainly to be indistinguishable from the white ones.

Evelyn: You said you are the lightest in your family. What did your parents or siblings make of that?

Michele: Well, one of my brothers is about your color (medium brown). And one day he said to my sister that she was more Negro than he because she was darker.

Evelyn: What did he mean by that?

Michele: That he was closer to being a white person and therefore better. It's strange. Because on the one hand, light-skinned blacks resent it when people say we are trying to be or act white. Because for the most part, light-skinned blacks dislike whites just as much as anyone else. On the other hand, society, both black and white, gives us these messages that we are "better" than darker-skinned blacks. It's sort of like we're in limbo.

Tamara: I've never thought that light-skinned black people are trying to be white. I was never ridiculed by a light-skinned black person. I was mostly ridiculed by darker people.

Michele: Oh, that's just not done. Light-skinned black people try not to do that to dark-skinned people. At least not to their faces.

Evelyn: Well, what was the message you received from your light-skinned family about black people that look like me and Tamara.

Michele: I can't say there were any overt messages. I don't think anyone ever said out loud: "You shall not marry a dark-skinned person." I don't think there was any blanket ostracism of a person who married someone dark. In fact many of my light-skinned aunts thought they were dark in comparison to lighter folks in the family. So it's all very skewed. In fact, I don't think I'm that pale. Recently, a white woman said to me, "Well, things just look so good on you because you're 'dark-skinned.'" I said, "I guess."

Evelyn: I can't imagine there have been many times in your life when you have been called dark-skinned.

Michele: Only by whites.

Evelyn: How do you deal with the confusion about your race, your identity. How does it make you feel?

Michele: One of my friends said to me: "You're in the twilight zone of racial identity." That's how it feels, like I'm in the twilight zone. People dance around trying to place me. They ask if I'm Indian, Italian, anything but a sister.

Even to this day, every time I mention meeting somebody to my mother, she always asks, "Do they know that you're black?" I mean, how the hell should I know?

I do believe that my skin color has helped me professionally, especially in my former life as a lawyer because white people felt more comfortable with me. It has complicated my relationships with men.

Evelyn: Meaning?

Michele: Oh, a lot of black men get a certain gleam in their eye. I can tell that they are making certain assumptions about me. I feel that they think I'm attractive, some kind of "catch." It's like I'm some kind of fantasy for them because being light is the closest thing to being white. They react to my skin color before they even know anything about me. I resent it. It makes me feel like a piece of meat. I have not gone out with a lot of black men because I have found their attitudes about my skin color so appalling.

For instance, I went out with this dude recently. Mr. Fiction Writer, Would-be Lawyer, whatever. We met at a cafe, no sooner had we sat down than he puts his arm out and says, "Umm, I like that. It's not often I get to go out with a person around the same shade as I am." I thought, "Oh My God, this man is colorstruck." All he could talk about was color, color, color. But I should have known, because I'd seen that gleam in his eye when we first met. I was so mad. I was so offended. We are just obsessed with shade.

Tamara: I agree. By the time I reached high school, I'd just had it. I'd been so ridiculed that I started acting out and being totally rebellious. I was sick of being teased by black people; then I was in predominately white schools where I never heard anything positive about black people either. I essentially gave up on education. In high school, I dated Latin men. My first real boyfriend was Czechoslovakian. I felt much safer with white boyfriends. The black guys would just dog me. I'd be out with my friends and they'd say, "Hey baby, come here." And I'd look up and they'd say, "No, not you, the light one." I can't tell you how many times that has happened to me. I became so self-conscious that I tried to cover up my entire body. I tried to hide everything except my face. To this day, I still find myself walking with my head down and trying to cover up my body.

Evelyn: You mentioned to me that you used to pray to get lighter.

Tamara: Oh sure, I prayed not to be dark. I used to try to wash my black skin away. I told my aunt how much I hated being dark and she said, "Tamara, you're black now, but when you grow up, you're going to get lighter because your skin will stretch and the darkness will thin out."

Evelyn: You're kidding.

Tamara: I'm serious. I hoped and prayed for it to happen. I was eleven.

Michele: When I was about thirteen a black kid called me a "white bitch." I ignored it because somebody had told me that I would get darker as I grew older.

Evelyn: Well, there you have it. Lunacy on both sides. What about your relationships today, especially with other black women?

Michele: I think my relationships with other black women are good. I have black women friends. I think my friendships are solid because I don't wring my hands about my skin color. While I am upfront about my experiences, I don't do the "tragic mulatto" thing or whine about being light-skinned. I don't try to "outblack" people or compensate for being light. I think a lot of light-skinned blacks do that out of guilt. I refuse to feel guilty about the way I came out of the womb.

Tamara: Having this talk has been good for me. It feels good to be with other black women. In the past few years I have begun to like myself more. I am beginning to realize that I have choices about how I feel about myself. The most important thing is how I feel about me. I believe that I am beginning to heal.

It is possible for black women to have healthy bodies, minds and hearts. The process begins with self-love. In the following excerpt, from her Pulitzer Prize-winning novel Beloved, *Toni Morrison offers powerful words that can help bring black women to wholeness.*

We Flesh
Toni Morrison

"Here," she said, "in this here place, we flesh; flesh that weeps, laughs; flesh that dances on bare feet in grass. Love it. Love it hard. Yonder they do not love your flesh. They despise it. They don't love your eyes; they'd just as soon pick em out. No more do they love the skin on your back. Yonder they flay it. And O my people they do not love your hands. Those they only use, tie, bind, chop off and leave empty. Love your hands! Love them. Raise them up and kiss them. Touch others with them, pat them together, stroke them on your face 'cause they don't love that either. *You* got to love it, *you!* And no, they ain't in love with your mouth. Yonder, out there, they will see it broken and break it again. What you say out of it they will not heed. What you scream from it they do not hear. What you put into it to nourish your body they will snatch away and give you leavins instead. No, they don't love your mouth. *You* got to love it. This is flesh I'm talking about here. Flesh that needs to be loved. Feet that need to rest and to dance; backs that need support; shoulders that need arms, strong arms I'm telling you. And O my people, out yonder, hear me, they do not love your neck unnoosed and straight. So love your neck; put a hand on it, grace it, stroke it and hold it up. And all your inside parts that they'd just as soon slop for hogs, you got to love them. The dark, dark liver—love it, love it, and the beat and beating heart, love that too. More than eyes or feet. More than lungs that have yet to draw free air. More than your life-holding womb and your life-giving private parts, hear me now, love your heart. For this is the prize."

Resources

Here is a selected list of organizations that address black women's health issues. For more comprehensive information contact a culturally sensitive health care provider or agency.

Best of Health
*A Quarterly Newsletter for Black
  Women*
P.O. Box 40-1232
Brooklyn, New York 11240-1232

Black Women Physicians Project
3300 Henry Avenue
Philadelphia, Pennsylvania 19129
(215) 842-7124

Heart and Soul
*A Health Magazine for African-
  Americans*
33 East Minor Street
Emmaus, Pennsylvania 18098
(215) 967-8486

The Holistic Health Directory
342 Western Avenue
Brighton, MA 02135
(800) 782-7006

Institute on Black Chemical Abuse
2614 Nicollet Avenue S.
Minneapolis, Minnesota 55408
(612) 871-7878

Lupus Foundation of America, Inc.
1717 Massachusetts Avenue, NW
Washington, D.C. 20036
(202) 328-4550
(800) 558-0121

National Abortion Rights Action
  League (NARAL)
1101 14th Street, NW
Washington, D.C. 20005
(202) 371-0779

National Association for Sickle Cell
  Disease, Inc.
4221 Wilshire Blvd., Suite 360
Los Angeles, California 90010
(213) 936-7205

National Black Nurses Association,
  Inc.
1012 Tenth Street, NW
Washington, D.C. 20001
(202) 393-6870

National Black Women's Health
  Project
1237 Abernathy Boulevard
Atlanta, Georgia 30310
(800) 275-2947

National Dental Association
5506 Connecticut Avenue, NW
Suite 24-25
Washington, D.C. 20015
(202) 244-7555

National Medical Association
1012 Tenth Street, NW
Washington, D.C. 20001
(202) 347-1895

National Minority AIDS Council
300 I Street, NE, Suite 400
Washington, D.C. 20002
(202) 544-1076

National Women's Health Network
1325 G Street, N.W.
Washington, D.C. 20005
(202) 347-1140

Planned Parenthood
810 Seventh Avenue
New York, NY 10019
(212) 603-4600

Save Our Sisters
Minority Breast Cancer Screening
    Program
2131 South 17th Street
Wilmington, North Carolina 28403
(919) 343-0161, ext. 253

Women's Cancer Resource Center
3023 Shattuck Avenue
Berkeley, California 94705
(415) 548-9272

Additional Reading

Here is a selected list of books that offer guidance to black women. The books should be available at book stores and at your local library.

In the Company of My Sisters: Black Women and Self-Esteem by Julia A. Boyd, (New York: Dutton, 1993).

Women of Color: Integrating Ethnic and Gender Identities edited by Lillian Comas-Diaz and Beverly Greene, (New York: Guilford Press, 1994).

The Measure of Our Success: A Letter to My Children and Yours by Marian Wright Edelman (Boston: Beacon Press, 1992).

*Black Women in America: An Historical Encyclopedia edited by Darlene Clark Hine (Brooklyn: Carlson Publishing, 1993).

Sisters of the Yam: Black Women and Self-Recovery by bell hooks (Boston: South End Press, 1993).

Sister Outsider: Essays and Speeches by Audre Lorde (Freedom, CA: Crossing Press, 1984).

Soul To Soul: A Vegetarian Soul Food Cookbook by Mary Burgess McKinney (P.O. Box 11476, Colton, California 92324).

Race-ing Justice, En-Gendering Power: Essays on Anita Hill, Clarence Thomas and the Construction of Social Reality edited by Toni Morrison (New York: Pantheon, 1992).

A Hunger So Wide and So Deep: Eating Problems and Recovery in Women's Lives by Becky W. Thompson (Minneapolis: University of Minnesota Press, 1994).

Body and Soul: The Black Women's Guide to Good Health edited by Linda Villarosa (New York: Harcourt, 1994).

In Search of Our Mothers' Gardens by Alice Walker (New York: Harcourt, 1983).

Chain Chain Change: For Black Women Dealing with Physical and Emotional Abuse by Evelyn C. White (Seattle: Seal Press, 1985).

The Alchemy of Race and Rights by Patricia J. Williams (Cambridge: Harvard University Press, 1991).

Crossing the Boundary: Black Women Survive Incest by Melba Wilson (Seattle: Seal Press, 1994).

*This is an excellent two-volume reference work that costs about $200. Please urge libraries, academic institutions and professional organizations you are affiliated with to purchase a set. If the book is within your budget, buy it. It is a landmark work about black women that informs and inspires.

Contributors

Opal Palmer Adisa, Jamaican born, is a writer and story teller. Her published works are: *Tamarind and Mango Women,* 1992; *traveling women,* 1989; *Bake-Face and Other Guava Stories,* 1986; and *Pina, The Many-Eyed Fruit,* 1985. She lectures at the University of California at Berkeley and has three young children.

Denise Alexander, D.D.S., is a family dentist with a private practice in Berkeley, California and the mother of a son, Kadeem.

Michele Anderson is an editor/writer at *The San Francisco Chronicle.* Born in Buffalo, New York, she is a graduate of Yale University (B.A. English) and of the University of California at Berkeley School of Law (Boalt Hall).

Georgiana Arnold, M.S., is a Seattle-based health consultant. She views health education as a tool for healing and empowerment and is committed to helping people improve the quality of their lives.

Byllye Y. Avery is the founder of the National Black Women's Health Project in Atlanta, Georgia.

Sheila Battle, M.S.W., works as a medical social worker for the San Francisco Department of Public Health. She plans to begin doctoral studies in the near future.

Melissa Blount, M.D., is completing a pathology residency at Emory University. She holds degrees from Brown University and the University of California at San Francisco Medical School.

Lorraine Bonner, M.D., is a New York native who practices general medicine in Oakland, California. At present, she is remodeling her house, writing poetry and reflecting on everything.

Julia A. Boyd, M.Ed., is the author of *In The Company of My Sisters: Black Women and Self-Esteem* (Dutton, 1993). A practicing psychotherapist in Seattle, she has also written several articles on feminism and women of color.

Forrestine A. Bragg, lives in New York City where she is involved in literacy programs.

Andrea R. Canaan is a black lesbian southern feminist mother writer and political activist. She lives in San Francisco.

Betty W. Carrington, C.N.M., Ed.D., is a certified nurse midwife and is Director of Midwifery Service in the Department of Obstetrics and Gynecology at the Harlem Hospital Center in New York.

Lucille Clifton is the author of several award-winning collections of poetry and a two-time nominee for the Pulitzer Prize.

Angela Y. Davis has been teaching, writing and lecturing about African-American and women's social theories and practices for the past twenty years. She has also been active in numerous organizations concerned with social justice. She teaches in the History of Consciousness Program at the University of California at Santa Cruz.

Bridgett M. Davis, a Detroit native, is a journalist who has worked for numerous metropolitan newspapers. At present, she is an Assistant Professor at Baruch College of the City College of New York, where she teaches English and Journalism. She is writing her first novel.

Marian Wright Edelman is founder and president of the Children's Defense Fund in Washington, D.C. A leader in the Black Community Crusade For Children, Edelman holds degrees from Spelman College and Yale University Law School. She was a 1985 recipient of the prestigious MacArthur Fellowship.

Janis Coombs Epps lives in Atlanta, Georgia where she is the Associate Academic Dean of DeKalb College's Central Campus. She is the mother of a son and a daughter.

Lulu F. requests anonymity.

Vanessa Northington Gamble, M.D., Ph.D., is Associate Professor of the History of Medicine and Preventive Medicine at the University of Wisconsin-Madison. Her research includes health policy and the history of African Americans and American medicine. She still believes in dreams.

Joyce Gardner is the Maternal and Child Public Health Nutrition Consultant for the State of Washington Department of Health. Having breastfed her daughter Nia, she is a strong advocate of breastfeeding and healthy infant feeding practices. She is active in numerous organizations dedicated to improving the health status of women and children.

Jewelle L. Gomez is originally from Boston. She is the author of *The Gilda Stories*, a novel, and *Forty-Three Septembers*, a collection of essays.

Evelynn M. Hammonds, a longtime feminist activist, is an Assistant Professor of the History of Science in the Program in Science, Technology and Society at the Massachusetts Institute of Technology. She has published several articles on AIDS in the black community and is working on a collection of essays on race, gender and science.

Imani Harrington is a San Francisco Bay Area actress, dancer and writer. She works as a substance abuse and HIV counselor. Her first book of poetry is forthcoming.

Jessica B. Harris is a culinary historian who has written extensively on African-American foodways. Her publications include *Hot Stuff: A Cookbook in Praise of the Piquant, Iron Pots and Wooden Spoons: Africa's Gifts to New World Cooking, Sky Juice and Flying Fish: Traditional Caribbean Cooking* and *Tasting Brazil: Regional Reminiscences and Recipes*.

Rev. Linda H. Hollies is a pastor at First United Methodist Church in Arlington Heights, Illinois. She is also founder and director of Woman to Woman Ministries, Inc., a support and resource group for women of color. Her publications include *Inner Healing For Broken Vessels* and *Womanist Rumblings, Womanist Care: How to Tend The Souls of Women*.

Linda Janet Holmes has been writing about and advocating for midwife practices for nearly twenty years. At present, she is writing a book with a black, octogenarian midwife in Greene County, Alabama. While pursing doctoral studies at Columbia University, Linda lives with her daughter Ghana in East Orange, New Jersey and works at the N.J. Department of Health.

bell hooks is a teacher, author and speaker on the issues of personal empowerment and the politics of race, gender and class. Her publications include: *Ain't I A Woman, Black Looks: Race and Representation, Yearning: Race, Gender, and Cultural Politics* and *Talking Back: Thinking Feminist, Thinking Black*. She has taught at Oberlin College, Yale University and City College of New York.

Zora Neale Hurston authored several books including *Mules and Men, Tell My Horse, Jonah's Gourd Vine* and *Their Eyes Were Watching God*.

Tamara Ingram is a San Francisco Bay Area resident. She works in a law firm.

Francesca A. Jackson, D.C., practices chiropractic, homeopathy and other healing arts in Oakland, California. She is on the volunteer staff of the Charlotte Maxwell Complementary Clinic.

Vida Labrie Jones, Ph.D., did research on lupus for her doctorate in medical sociology at the University of California at Berkeley. She is involved in various efforts designed to educate the public about lupus.

Cheryl M. Killion, R.N., Ph.D., is on the faculty of the School of Nursing at the University of Michigan, Ann Arbor. At present, she is conducting research on the co-existence of pregnancy and homelessness; multigenerational house sharing among African-Americans; and childbearing folk beliefs of African-American women.

Mary Lou Lee lives in Flint, Michigan where she is active in numerous church and girl scout activities. She writes that at eighty-one she and her eighty-eight-year-old fiancé are "madly in love with each other and life."

Marsha R. Leslie is a journalist and writer who lives in Seattle with her teenage daughter, Michaela. She is the editor of an anthology on single mothers and works in program development at a public television station.

Andrea Lewis is a San Francisco-based editor and writer. She has worked on the editorial staffs of *Mother Jones* and *OUT/LOOK* magazines. She is currently of the staff of HarperCollins Publishers.

Gloria Lockett worked as a prostitute for eighteen years and is one of the nation's leading advocates for sex workers. She lives in the San Francisco Bay Area.

Patricia O. Loftman, M.S., C.N.M., is a certified nurse midwife and Director of the Midwifery Service in the Department of Obstetrics and Gynecology at the Harlem Hospital in New York.

Audre Lorde (Gamba Adisa) was an internationally acclaimed author of numerous books of poetry and prose. Her collections of poetry include *The Marvelous Arithmetics of Distance, Undersong, Our Dead Behind Us, The Black Unicorn* and *From A Land Where Other People Live*, which was nominated for a National Book Award. *The Cancer Journals* and *Zami: A New Spelling of My Name* are among her most influential prose works. She lectured widely on lesbian and gay rights, sexual, political, racial and economic oppression.

Elizabeth Lorde-Rollins, M.D., works as a resident in obstetrics and gynecology at Columbia Presbyterian Medical Center. After receiving her B.A. in psychology from Harvard in 1985 she taught third grade at Public School 46 in New York City for three years. She received her

M.D. from Columbia's School of Physicians and Surgeons in 1993. Her research interests include the use of acupuncture in obstetrics.

Janet L. Mitchell, M.D., M.P.H., is Chief of Perinatology (High Risk Obstetrics) in the Department of Obstetrics and Gynecology at the Harlem Hospital Center in New York. She is Assistant Professor of Obstetrics and Gynecology, College of Physicians and Surgeons and School of Public Health, Columbia University.

Toni Morrison, one of the world's most distinguished writers, received the Nobel Prize for Literature in 1993. Professor in the Council of Humanities at Princeton University, Morrison's novels include *The Bluest Eye, Sula, Song of Solomon, Tar Baby, Jazz,* and *Beloved,* which received the 1988 Pulitzer Prize. Her books of essays include *Playing in the Dark,* and her edited collection *Race-ing Justice, En-Gendering Power: Essays on Anita Hill, Clarence Thomas, and the Construction of Social Reality.*

Leora Myers, R.N., is an internationally recognized fitness specialist and trainer. She conducts fitness training workshops throughout the United States and Japan. Producer/host of a weekly cable television show in San Francisco, Myers's training programs are used in several corporate fitness centers including those of IBM, Levi Strauss, Lockheed and Apple Computers.

Pat Parker authored numerous collections of poetry and prose. Works include *Jonestown and Other Madness* (Firebrand, 1985), *Movement in Black* (Diana Press, 1978; Firebrand, 1990) and *Womanslaughter* (Diana Press, 1978).

Sean Reynolds, M.S.W., is a social worker with the Department of Social Work Services, Maternal and Infant Care, at San Francisco General Hospital. She is also a writer and photojournalist.

Beth Richie is on the faculty of the community health education program at Hunter College and a doctoral student in sociology at the City University of New York. She has been involved with the movement against domestic violence for more than a decade.

Kate Rushin grew up in Lawnside and Camden, New Jersey and attended Oberlin College and Brown University. She won the 1988 Grolier Poetry Prize and is the author of a book of poems, *The Black Back-Ups* (Firebrand, 1993).

Pamela Sherrod, a native Chicagoan, is a journalist, playwright and screenwriter who has authored several plays and screenplays. A features writer for the *Chicago Tribune*, she holds degrees from Michigan State University and DePaul University.

Judy D. Simmons has been an editor and writer for more than twenty years with *Essence, Black Enterprise, Emerge, Ms.,* and other national magazines. At present, she is a columnist and editor with the *Anniston Star* in Anniston, Alabama.

Barbara Smith is one of the leading activists in the feminist movement and editor/author of numerous writings. Her literary criticism, reviews and essays have appeared in many publications including *The New York Times*. She edited *Home Girls: A Black Feminist Anthology* and is a co-founder and publisher of Kitchen Table: Women of Color Press.

Beverly Smith has been a women's health activist and professional since 1975. She is currently the Prevention and Education Program Planner for the Boston AIDS Consortium.

Alice Walker is an internationally acclaimed author of numerous volumes of fiction, poetry, essays and short stories. In 1983 she won both the Pulitzer Prize and the American Book Award for her novel *The Color Purple*. Her most recent publications are *The Temple of My Familiar, Finding The Green Stone, Her Blue Body Everything We Know: Earthling Poems 1965 to 1990 Complete*, and *Possessing The Secret of Joy*. She is the co-producer of *Warrior Marks*, a film about female genital mutilation and author of a book about the film that bears the same title.

Faye Wattleton is the former president of Planned Parenthood. She appears frequently on national news shows. Her book about her experiences as a leader in the reproductive rights movement is forthcoming.

K. Malaika Williams is a Foreign Service Officer, currently serving as the commercial officer at the U.S. Embassy in Madagascar. She holds a degree from the University of California at Berkeley Graduate School of Journalism.

Acknowledgements

We gratefully acknowledge permission to reprint materials from the following sources:

Byllye Y. Avery, "Breathing Life into Ourselves: The Evolution of the National Black Women's Health Project." Originally appeared in *Sojourner* (1050 Commonwealth Avenue, Boston, MA 02215), Volume XIV, Number 5 (January, 1989). Reprinted by permission.

Melissa Blount, "Surpassing Obstacles: Black Women in Medicine." Originally appeared in the *Journal of the American Medical Association*. Volume XXXIX, Number 6 (November/December, 1984). Reprinted by permission of the author.

Julia A. Boyd, "Ethnic and Cultural Diversity in Feminist Therapy: Keys to Power." Originally appeared in different form in *Women and Therapy*, a journal published by Haworth Press. Reprinted by permission of the author.

Lucille Clifton, "New Bones" and "Roots." From *Good Woman: Poems and a Memoir* (Brockport, NY: BOA Editions, © 1987). Reprinted by permission of the publisher.

Angela Y. Davis, "Sick and Tired of Being Sick and Tired: The Politics of Black Women's Health." Originally appeared in *Women, Culture, and Politics* (New York, NY: Random House, © 1989). Reprinted by permission of the publisher.

Marian Wright Edelman, "The Black Family in America." Originally appeared in *Families in Peril: An Agenda for Social Change* (Cambridge, MA: Harvard University Press, © 1987 by the President and fellows of Harvard College). All rights reserved. Reprinted by permission of the publisher.

Janis Coombs Epps, "On Cancer and Conjuring." Originally appeared in *SAGE, A Scholarly Journal on Black Women*, Volume II, Number 2 (Fall, 1985). Reprinted by permission of the author.

Lulu F. as told to Rachel V., "Black, Female and Sober." Originally appeared in *A Woman Like You: Life Stories of Women Recovering from Alcoholism and Addiction* by Rachel V. (San Francisco, CA: Harper & Row, © 1985). Reprinted by permission.

Linda H. Hollies, "A Daughter Survives Incest: A Retrospective Analysis." Originally appeared in *SAGE, A Scholarly Journal on Black Women*, Volume IV, Number 2 (Fall, 1987). Reprinted by permission of the author.